Pediatric Physical Diagnosis

Balu H. Athreya, M.D.
Clinical Director
Children's Seashore House
Atlantic City, New Jersey
Chief, Pediatric Rheumatology Center
Children's Hospital of Philadelphia
Associate Professor of Pediatrics
School of Medicine, University of Pennsylvania
Philadelphia, Pennsylvania

Benjamin K. Silverman, M.D.
Pediatric Practitioner
Princeton, New Jersey
Clinical Associate
Children's Hospital of Philadelphia
Clinical Associate Professor of Pediatrics
School of Medicine, University of Pennsylvania
Philadelphia, Pennsylvania

With a chapter on *Examination of the Newborn* by:

Alan R. Spitzer, M.D.
Associate Physician
Children's Hospital of Philadelphia
Associate Professor of Pediatrics, Obstetrics, and Gynecology
School of Medicine, University of Pennsylvania
Philadelphia, Pennsylvania

ACC **APPLETON-CENTURY-CROFTS/Norwalk, Connecticut**

0-8385-7797-0

Notice: Our knowledge in clinical sciences is constantly changing. As new information becomes available, changes in treatment and in the use of drugs become necessary. The authors and the publisher of this volume have taken care to make certain that the doses of drugs and schedules of treatment are correct and compatible with the standards generally accepted at the time of publication. The reader is advised to consult carefully the instruction and information material included in the package insert of each drug or therapeutic agent before administration. This advice is especially important when using new or infrequently used drugs.

86 87 88 89 / 10 9 8 7 6 5 4 3 2

Prentice-Hall of Australia, Pty. Ltd., Sydney
Prentice-Hall Canada, Inc.
Prentice-Hall Hispanoamericana, S.A., Mexico
Prentice-Hall of India Private Limited, New Delhi
Prentice-Hall International (UK) Limited, London
Prentice-Hall of Japan, Inc., Tokyo
Prentice-Hall of Southeast Asia (Pte.) Ltd., Singapore
Whitehall Books Ltd., Wellington, New Zealand
Editora Prentice-Hall do Brasil Ltda., Rio de Janeiro

Library of Congress Cataloging-in-Publication Data

Athreya, Balu H.
Pediatric physical diagnosis.

Rev. ed. of: Clinical methods in pediatric diagnosis. c1980c.
Includes bibliographies and index.
1. Children—Medical examinations. I. Silverman, Benjamin K. II. Spitzer, Alan R. III. Athreya, Balu H. Clinical methods in pediatric diagnosis. IV. Title. [DNLM: 1. Diagnosis—in infancy & childhood. 2. Medical History Taking—in infancy & childhood. 3. Physical Examination—in infancy & childhood. WS 141 A871c]
RJ50.A839 1985 618.92'00754 85-15053
ISBN 0-8385-7797-0

Design: M. Chandler Martylewski

PRINTED IN THE UNITED STATES OF AMERICA

Contents

Preface

To the children all over the world for their
innocence, curiosity, humor,
and trust.

and

To the mothers of those children we know best
Ramaa
Beverly

This book provides a novel approach to recognition and description of physical findings. There are two components to this new approach. The first is the definition of normality for each organ system and its components. The second is the logical definition of abnormal physical findings based on the components of normality. This is different from the traditional description of physical findings on the basis of inspection, palpation, percussion, and auscultation.

The book is intended to encourage newcomers (medical students and house officers) and to refresh veterans in the skills of pediatric physical diagnosis. This revised new edition incorporates ideas received from the readers and reviewers of the first edition.

The ability of the human eye to recognize abnormality by "pattern recognition" is phenomenal. Both experienced and inexperienced clinicians often recognize abnormal physical findings by this method. But there are two problems when one relies primarily on pattern recognition. First, application of this method alone may fail us. Second, when you teach a newcomer, it is important to describe the normal features of the organ being studied so that the variation from normal is clearly appreciated. We give the descriptors for defining normality of the various systems and organs. The emphasis therefore is on the measurement of normality.

Good clinicians have been emphasizing a logical approach for many years. But it is hardly practiced today. For example, the logical descriptors for the characteristics of a swelling are: location, size, shape, consistency, color, temperature, and relationship to neighboring structures. We all know this but forget it quickly. This book emphasizes the logical approach to physical diagnosis.

Great clinicians such as Drs. S. T. Achar, S. M. Merchant, D. Buchanan, F. H. Wright, D. Cassels, and S. Tucker stimulated Dr. Athreya's interest. Dr. L. L. Coriell helped him think logically. Dr. H. S. Cecil showed him how to care for human beings. His brother, Professor N. H. Athreya, sowed the seed for this book.

Dr. Silverman is indebted to Dr. M. Baum who helped realize the dream of becoming a medical student; to Dr. A. J. Schaffer who induced excitement in pediatrics; to Dr. H. E. Harrison who integrated science, clinical acumen, and humility; to Dr. A. S. Nadas who molded a physician; to Dr. D. Cornfeld who artfully applied academia to clinical pediatrics; and to Dr. Athreya who perpetuated the love of learning.

Many house officers and medical students stimulated us with their enthusiasm. They helped us think critically. An additional note of thanks is due to Dr. S. Tucker for his review of the chapter on the central nervous system. We also thank Dr. Alan Spitzer for his excellent section on examination of the newborn.

Linda Timbers is known for her quiet efficiency. Her help in getting the manuscript typed so well and on time is greatly appreciated. Karen Ott is a fine medical illustrator and an artist. She has redrawn many of the line diagrams and has helped us improve the quality of the photographs.

The staff at Appleton-Century-Crofts has been extremely supportive of our project. Doreen Berne and Robin Millay have been of great help. The Van Nostrand Company was helpful in preparing the first edition.

Finally, the interest of the readers who shared their comments and suggestions and the comments of reviewers are greatly appreciated. We welcome ideas and suggestions on this new edition.

Balu H. Athreya, M.D.
Benjamin K. Silverman, M.D.

CLASSIC CLINICAL GUIDELINES

To see, to touch, to hear. —*Hippocrates*

To percuss. —*Auenbrugger/Skoda*

To auscultate. —*Laënnec*

To record. —*Louis*

To "observe, record, tabulate, communicate, use your five senses: see, then reason, compare and control." —*Osler*

INITIAL DIAGNOSIS A CLINICIAN'S LAMENT*

The patient's lying sick in bed.
The history we have not read
Nor laid a hand upon his head.
Whatever should we do?
Well, first we'll do a CBC
Hematocrit (HCT) and MCV
An LE prep—or maybe three—
And serum iron too.
And then we'll do his LFT,
A thymol flocc. and BSP,
A BUN, and IVP,
And urinalysis.
Electrolytes, blood volume too
(A little touch of Evans blue),
A pH and a CO_2
We really mustn't miss.
We ought to do a PBI,
It might be low—or even high.
And after all we've got to try
To do the most we can.
And if results don't quite agree
We'll blame the lab. (Forget the fee.)
We'll start again with fiendish glee.
And do them all again.
We'll culture urine, blood, and stool,
Measure the labile iron pool,
Use every diagnostic tool
And every function test.
An EKG, if we are wise,
Before and after exercise.
And if the patient up and dies
We'll have to leave the rest.
But if he lives, it might be fun
To give him some I^{131}
And maybe we could even run
A total body scan.
Then just to make us feel secure
I think we really should procure
Some chromosomes and make quite sure
He really is a MAN.

Lorna G. Macdougall, M.D.

*Reprinted with permission from Journal of Pediatrics 86:582, 1975. Copyright by The C. V. Mosby Company, St. Louis, MO.

SECTION I

Introduction to the Concept of Normality

CHAPTER 1

Objectively Describing Normality

The human organism thrives on contact and nurturing from the moment of birth. Particularly during an illness, human touch as in a gentle squeeze of the hand, a warm pat on the shoulder, and a little ruffling of the hair by a loved one or by a physician, has always played a great part in recovery. In the modern technological world, carried away by the precision with which we physicians can make a diagnosis, we may be forgetting to touch and to hold hands. Kindness and expressions of caring should remain the pilings on which the structure of medical care is supported.

During a major portion of the history of humankind, human infants got their nourishment directly from their mothers. This process is a natural one, facilitating not only nutrition but also human contact and nurturing. With advances in technology an artificial container for food, the feeding bottle, came between the mother and the infant. This is not all bad, particularly under certain circumstances. But when a child is left in a seat made of plastic to drink from a bottle made out of plastic held at an appropriate distance by two steel wires, civilization has gone too far and is out of touch with human needs.

A similar situation exists in the way a physician practices the profession. Gone are the days when physicians listened, felt the pulse and the abdomen, placed an ear against the chest of the patient, and held hands when things were not going well. Now, physicians can do much more than just hold hands—what with the equipment to localize precisely a lesion, medications to work precisely at the molecular level, and ultraprecise surgical techniques. The physician can now get a history through a computer, get a multichannelled recorder to give data on all the vital signs, listen to the heart through special devices, get an electrocardiogram, a laboratory report to look at most of the important biochemical markers, and an axial tomography scan or a nuclear magnetic resonance scan to look at the interior of the organs in precise details. There is now a machine or machines between the physician and the patient, very much like the baby in the mechanical seat with the bottle holder, one step removed from the mother. Dr. Lewis Thomas (1983) has beautifully pointed out how he would like to make sure that the physicians in training are not left to look after machines instead of taking care of people. Solid grounding in techniques of taking good history and performing a good physical examination will assure physicians and patients that physicians indeed will continue to take care of people. We must not forget how to hold hands.

A good history and physical examination lead to proper diagnosis in most situations. Time spent on these fundamentals helps bridge a relationship with patients and facilitates future communication. A thorough physical examination, in addition, is an essential part of reassurance therapy, particularly for patients with psychosomatic illness.

There are many books on physical diagnosis, though few on pediatric physical diagnosis. What is unique about this particular book is that we move away from the traditional subjective approach to an objective description of the findings of a history and physical examination. We describe an objective and more logical approach for observing and recording the findings of a good examination.

Traditionally, physical findings are acquired under four categories: inspection, palpation, percussion, and auscultation. These approaches are based on the faculties of the examiner (sight and hearing). They are examiner (physician)-oriented, and they are subjective. When the medical student is asked to inspect, a framework is not given within which to understand the inspection of that particular organ. For this reason, one physician's inspection is likely to be more or less complete and revealing than another's.

A more objective and logical way is to define the normal characteristics of the organ or physiologic function being scrutinized. For example, when describing the head, the traditional approach asks for a description of findings from inspection, palpation, percussion, and auscultation. In the approach described in this book, the first paragraph will describe normal dimensions or characteristics of the head that should be looked for. Normal characteristics of the head should include a description of its size, shape, continuity, and hair. These can again be logically divided into subheadings. For example, the size of the head can only be normal or abnormal; abnormality can be in relation to increased size or decreased size. The shape has to be even and symmetrical or uneven and asymmetrical. If it is uneven we wish to know whether the head is longer (from front to back) or broader (side to side) or conical. Continuity can be described as intact or as a loss of continuity: *projection* of the surface or a *depression* below the surface.

Once the normal characteristics of the organ to be looked at are defined, it does not matter what subjective modality the physician uses in a description of that normality. This description of the normal components of a part makes it easy to teach medical students. In addition, a constant reminder to oneself of these characteristics of an organ will make sure that one recognizes normality and, therefore, an abnormality, quickly. This is the approach we present in this book.

CHAPTER 2

Defining Normality: What Is Normal?

Before one can recognize abnormality, one has to know normality. We are not referring to normality in the philosophic sense. We are referring to the recognition of normal structure (anatomy) and function (physiology and biochemistry). Many of us intuitively know what normal is for a particular part of the body, but we cannot describe it. To understand and to teach, we must be able to communicate an explanation of normality.

The following real-life episode points out the importance of the above statements. A five-year-old child with seizures was taking phenobarbital for 2 years prior to being seen in our clinic. The house officer looked at the mouth, saw something like hypertrophic gum and wrote that the child had "dilantin hyperplasia." The child was not on dilantin. Here is an example of reverse logic: since the child was on anticonvulsant therapy there must be hyperplasia of the gum. The house officer, of course, did not know the characteristics of a normal gum and therefore did not know that the child could not have hyperplasia. The child was retarded and had bruxism; therefore, the teeth were ground to a smaller size. There was relatively more gum than teeth, but the gum was not red and it did not overhang the tooth, two of the characteristics of dilantin-induced hyperplasia.

Students and trainees seem to be more aware of physiologic normals than they are of normal anatomic characteristics. This may reflect in part the emphasis on the physiologic basis of disease in modern medicine. In pediatrics there is an additional problem: the variations depending on age. One has, therefore, to be aware of normal values for physical, behavioral, intellectual, emotional, physiologic, and biochemical characteristics at various ages.

The clinician interprets laboratory values on the basis of normal values. Unless the clinician knows that the normal value for blood urea nitrogen is 8 to 18 mgm% in the laboratory, recognition of an abnormal value is impossible. Similarly, one cannot recognize an abnormality of the ear or the eye or the gum unless one knows the characteristics of the normal structure of these parts of the body. For example, knowing that the ear makes an angle of 10 degrees or less with the scalp will help identify a protuberant ear. Knowing that all the metacarpophalangeal joints should be in an almost straight line when the hand is fisted should help identify a short fourth metacarpal, but this should be confirmed by actual measurement.

In an editorial (1983) Murray Feingold made the following comments: "It is no longer acceptable to describe *dysmorphic physical findings without using proper measurements.* Claims, such as low-set ears, wide-spaced eyes and long fingers, should not be made unless they are accompanied by accurate measurements. Incorrect clinical impressions, because of lack of measurements, have been responsible for persistent misinformation about specific syndromes. For example, many clinicians are still under the *false impression that children with Turner's syndrome have wide-spread nipples and an increased carrying angle.* Studies using proper measurements have shown that these observations are not correct."

"The method used to obtain clinical measurements varies. Direct measurements are more practical than measurements by radiologic examina-

TABLE 2-1. POSSIBLE ALTERATIONS IN ANATOMIC STRUCTURES

Descriptors	Size	Number	Shape	Position
	Normal	Normal	Normal	Right/Left Anterior/Posterior Superior/Inferior
Variables	Abnormal (large or small in relation to itself and in relation to other structure) Rate of growth	Fewer (fused, absent) More (split, extra)	Uniformity (defines entire organ) Concave Convex	In relation to other structure: Far off Elevated Depressed Moved in Moved out Rotated In relation to itself (pushed or twisted): Forward Backward Inward Outward Multiple (combinations)

tion. . . . The only measurements that should be used are those that have a significant number of normal controls."

These comments introduce the importance of knowing what is normal. They also emphasize the importance of observation and measurement. It is no use merely knowing the normals, one has to apply this knowledge again and again. A good clinician should be a little compulsive. A good clinician should be like the decorator who can recognize and cannot tolerate a slightly crooked picture on the wall.

Being a good clinician requires a sense of pattern recognition. Pattern recognition demands formation of mental images of normal features of various parts and organs of the body, so that if a pattern with minor variation appears it is quickly recognized.

One way to systematize our observations of normal structures and functions is to define the variable under the following headings:

1. Anatomic Variations
2. Physiologic Variations

Table 2-1 lists various characteristics that describe anatomic structures and their variations.

Color	Texture/ Consistency	Continuity	Alignment
Normal	Normal	Normal	Normal
Less of normal color More of normal color Abnormal color Black Green Dark Red Blue Yellow Cherry red Milky white Brown Pink	Soft Firm Hard	Abnormal (a) Extra growth (not normally present) including skin rash, swellings, and projections Location Size Shape Rate of growth Flat or elevated Margin-regular/irregular Surface-smooth/rough Consistency (as listed) Color (as listed) Temperature (hot, cold) Tenderness Pulsation Attachment to skin and to surrounding structures (b) Loss of continuity such as ulcers and fractures	Abnormal In relation to itself In relation to other structures

DESCRIBING ANATOMIC STRUCTURES

The following must be considered in describing an anatomic structure: size, number, shape, position in relation to itself, position in relation to other structures, color, texture, continuity, and alignment. Let us take the *eye* as an example and define the descriptors. One can then say whether the eye is small or large (size). The very rare cyclops is recognized by answering questions on number. Hypotelorism and hypertelorism are recognized as alterations in position in relation to the other eye. Proptosis and enophthalmos are recognized as alterations in position in relation to the eye itself (forward and backward) and any color change in and around the eye is recognized. Firmness of the eye is a feature of conditions associated with glaucoma. The item on continuity is not applicable, but the alignment of the eye on the face in relation to other structures defines conditions such as mongoloid slant and antimongoloid slant. Recognition of abnormality in the structural components of the eye according to the descriptors given above is more important than remembering words such as microphthalmia, macrophthalmia, cyclops, hypotelorism, hypertelorism, proptosis, exophthalmos, and phthisis bulbi. Instead of trying to remember Latin and Greek names, one can try to remember the anatomic basis of variation.

An anatomic description of normality gives a logical basis for describing abnormality. This can be taught easily. Such a base is applicable to all anatomic structures. For example, a normal finger can be described by:

- *Size:* Small or large in relation to the hand and to other fingers.
- *Number:* Extra fingers or fewer than five fingers? If fewer than five, is it because fingers are fused (as in Apert syndrome) or lost because of an accident?
- *Shape:* Does the finger look fusiform or tapering?
- *Position:* Is one finger placed more proximally or distally than others?
- *Color:* Are the fingers blue or red or pale or mottled?
- *Texture:* Is the finger stiff? Is the skin soft or coarse or peeled?
- *Continuity:* Is there any disruption of continuity (e.g., fracture of phalanx)? Is there a rash or a nodule? Is there any other swelling?
- *Alignment:* Is the finger straight or curved? Is it curved in a front-back direction (flexion contracture) or in a side-to-side direction (clinodactyly)? Are the fingers aligned normally in relation to the forearm and wrist (ulnar deviation-radial deviation-volar subluxation)?

An explanation is needed about continuity and alignment. As indicated in Table 2-1, extra growth as a descriptor is used under "continuity" to define the characteristics of rash, swellings, and other projections. Every extra growth has to be described under subheadings such as location, size, margin, shape, or surface. Continuity is also used when describing ulcers in the skin and mucous membrane because ulcers signify loss of surface continuity. Displaced fractures also are to be described under this heading. Alignment as a subheading is included mainly to describe deformity of extremities but can be applied to other organs, as shown earlier in describing the normal eye.

DESCRIBING PHYSIOLOGIC FUNCTIONS

Alteration in physiologic functions can be explained in a logical fashion using the characteristics listed in Table 2-2. For example, a function such as movement of an extremity may be present, lost, or only partially present. Complete loss of ability to move an extremity is called paralysis and a partial loss is called paresis. In the present system, instead of focusing on the meanings of words (*paralysis* and *paresis*), we focus on the logical possibilities and their precise descriptions.

TABLE 2-2. POSSIBLE ALTERATIONS IN PHYSIOLOGIC FUNCTIONS

Present				
Loss of				
Partial loss of				
Function present—painful				
Function present—difficult (all those symptoms due to difficulty in functions like dysphagia, dyspnea, etc.)				
Function present—abnormal (applicable to rate, volume, size, depth)				
Reduced	(slow)	(short)	(less)	(small)
Elevated	(fast)	(excess)	(large)	
Combination of slow and fast rhythm				
Irregular:	regularly irregular irregularly irregular			
Sounds:	normal sound absent sound abnormal sounds and murmur			
Voluntary movements:	contraction relaxation	smooth irregular		
Involuntary movements:	At rest—twitch tremor writhing fasciculation convulsions			
Abnormal sensations (specific types):	Pain—intensity, characteristics, aggravating factors, relieving factors, frequency, spread, etc. Dizziness Vertigo Parasthesias			

To explain this example further, a function may be present but painful or difficult. For example, passing of urine may be painful (as in dysuria) or difficult (as seen after surgery). Finally, function may be present but abnormal: A patient may have normal micturition but it occurs too often or too infrequently.

A function such as the rate of breathing or the heart rate may be less than normal or more than normal, just as volume of urine per day may be more than or less than normal. The depth of respiration may be shallow (decreased) or deep (increased). One may have a combination of these characteristics.

When describing functions with a rhythm (respiration, heart rate, etc.) one looks for regularity or irregularity. If irregular, one has to know whether it is regularly irregular or irregularly irregular.

When describing sounds heard with or without a stethoscope, one has to describe whether the sounds are present or absent; if present, whether they are normal or abnormal, and in what way the sounds are abnormal.

Voluntary and involuntary movements may then be described under various subheadings. Involuntary movements present spontaneously are described, not those elicited by special stimuli such as tendon reflexes. *This classification does not lend itself to describing elicited responses.*

The final heading in Table 2-2 describes abnormal sensations such as pain or paresthesias.

TABLE 2-3. EXAMPLES OF LOGICAL DESCRIPTION OF SYMPTOMS AND SIGNS BY DEFINING CHARACTERISTICS

Traditional Term	Structure/Function	Alteration(s)
Dyspnea	Respiration	Difficult
Hyperpnea	Respiration	Rate—fast Depth—increased
Tachypnea	Respiration	Rate—fast
Diarrhea	Bowel movement Bowel movement Bowel movement	Rate—increased Consistency—decreased Volume—increased
Polyuria	Urine	Volume—increased
Melena	Bowel movement	Color—black
Hematochezia	Bowel movement	Color—red (bloody)
Hypertelorism	Eyes	Position—far off (in relation to each other)
Proptosis	Eyes	Position—forward (in relation to itself)
Ulcer	Skin	Continuity—loss of
Jaundice	Skin	Color—yellow
Papule	Skin	Extra growth—elevated—smooth
Purpura	Skin	Extra growth—flat—red (blood)

As can be seen from the above examples, defining normality helps a clinician become more exact in diagnosing abnormality. Further examples of descriptions of abnormality defining the anatomic or physiologic characteristics and their variations are given in Table 2-3.

Using this categorization, normal bowel movements should be described under the following headings: frequency, consistency, and volume. Increased frequency and decreased consistency imply diarrheal disease. Large volume implies bulky stool; decreased frequency and increased consistency imply constipation.

"The clinician tries to be scientific in the use of inanimate objects, but not in the use of his own sensory organs and brain," said Feinstein (1967). In the proper use of the sensory organs and brain the clinician has to start defining symptoms and signs as well as possible, so that others will understand what is said. Signs and symptoms are words used to categorize alterations in structures or functions of the body; one therefore has to first define the attributes of normal structures and functions. One should be as precise with this as one is in describing results of laboratory investigations.

BIBLIOGRAPHY

Feingold M: Proper measurements in physical diagnosis. Am J Dis Child 137:828, 1983.

Feinstein AR: Clinical Judgment. Baltimore, Md., Williams & Wilkins, 1967, p. 29.

Thomas L: The Youngest Science. New York, Viking Press, 1983, p. 60.

SECTION II

Taking the History

CHAPTER 3

Techniques in History Taking

GENERAL CONCEPTS

History taking is an art and ideally should be learned from working with good clinicians in action. Some modern methods of taking medical history emphasize psychiatric concepts at the expense of clinical accuracy, particularly some of the newer methods of teaching history taking through simulation exercises and computers. Before going into the details of history taking, some *general remarks about concepts* that have been very useful will be given.

One of our professors once said: "Go after the symptom like a hound dog." That is what we should do. We should go after the scent, dashing out occasionally, only to get back on the trail. Failure to keep on track is responsible for many errors in diagnosis and unnecessary laboratory procedures. For example, during system review of a patient with a history of constipation if one finds that the hands get blue on exposure to cold, one has to dart off the track and ask leading questions to establish whether the patient may have Raynaud phenomenon. Before arranging for elaborate immunologic studies, however, the physician should complete the whole picture and see how each complaint fits.

Another very important point to remember is not to accept the diagnosis many parents bring with their children. During initial history taking it is common for a parent to say that the child has arthritis or urinary tract infection. It is an essential clinical habit to go back to the original symptoms and signs that led the parent to that conclusion. It is especially important to do this if the child has already been diagnosed by another physician. Keep an open mind and follow the scent, detective style.

Another important clinical habit is to learn to focus on only the crucial points when you are working in the emergency room or during an acute office visit. Go for all the details at the time of hospital admission or when you have an appointment with an hour or more at your disposal. Good clinicians learn to modify their pace with the prevailing circumstances, but they always sniff out the relevant details. During a visit for an acute problem in a busy office, history taking can be quite informal and proceed while the child is being observed and examined. As an example, a six year old presents with fever. Observe the child's alertness and sensorium and look for rashes and petechiae while you ask when the fever began and whether there are associated symptoms, such as pain, coughing, vomiting, diarrhea; gently palpate the abdomen, as you continue to question both patient and mother as to whether the child has had other illnesses recently; ask if anyone else in the family is sick as you watch the respirations and softly flex the neck; ask about specific pain sites—sore throat, earache, headache—as you soothingly run your hand across the child's face and tenderly palpate the cervical nodes. Establish confidence. Take a relevant history. Under busy office circumstances, make maximal use of your time by focusing your history taking and combining it with the preliminary steps of the physical examination.

When evaluating a child with chronic complaints, it is important to ask why the child was brought at this time. This has to be done gently and with a proper choice of words. History obtained with such questions may reveal precipitating factors, such as stress in the family or anxieties.

This leads to another important point in the personal growth and development of a clinician. When a parent calls in the middle of the night with what appears to be a simple complaint, it is not unreasonable for a physician to get upset, but it is not reasonable to express it in unhelpful ways. The physician should be able to control the anger and ask very relevant questions to find out what specific anxiety brought the family to the emergency room at that hour for a minor complaint. At a later stage in personal growth the physician has no anger at all for having been awakened in the middle of the night for a trivial complaint. This growth is very crucial because when the physician is angry, however well concealed, it will create an atmosphere of guilt and antagonism. But when there is no anger, the family will be able to share their real anxieties with greater ease.

It is also essential at the end of history taking to find out what the real concerns of the parents are. Very often you will find the parental concerns are far removed from the presenting complaint and from what the physician's concerns are. A good question to ask parents is, "What do you wish this is not?" Usually, this question provides them with an opening to express their anxieties.

TECHNIQUES OF INTERVIEWING

The most important means of *gathering data* is through obtaining a good history. A good history leads to a proper diagnosis. In formulating a management plan, one has to take into account the family's strength and weaknesses, their level of understanding, their support systems, their social situation, and their economic conditions. Information on all these areas has to be obtained during the interviews. Developing skills in talking with people and obtaining information is an essential part of a physician's work. Some have these capabilities as part of their nature. Others can learn by observing expert clinicians at work, by reading available literature on interviewing techniques, and by interviewing trained volunteers who act as the parents of sick children.

In human relations, the first contact is the most important contact. Getting the interview started in a positive way is therefore essential. The techniques vary depending on the setting and the time available. In an emergency room, obviously the focus should be on the most important and urgent problems requiring immediate care. By its nature, the atmosphere is tense and the distractions are many. When seeing a child for developmental problems or behavior problems, however, the atmosphere should be relaxed and there should be no time pressure.

It is important to talk to the parents and whoever is accompanying the child to obtain the necessary information. It is equally important to talk with the child directly, particularly an adolescent. One should remember to have periodic communication with the child even though the parents are talking. The physician should also be able to gently request the parent's permission to talk to the child separately, if indicated. In the initial stage it may be better not to approach the child too quickly, particularly a toddler or preschool child. When talking to children, one should be talking to them at a level appropriate to their stage of development.

In asking questions, it is important to use both open-ended questions and leading questions. To arrive at a medical diagnosis in organic disease, it is necessary for the physician to lead the way and ask specific questions. In developmental issues and in learning about the child's family and social situations and problems, it is important to ask open-ended questions and allow time for the family to respond. In other words, it is very important to be flexible in one's approach, depending on the urgency, the time, the place, and the problem. Remember to use a language that lay persons can understand and do not use words that can be misinterpreted.

It is not always *what* questions are asked that are important, but the *way* the questions are asked. If we would like to get an answer in order to set an appropriate plan, we must ask the question correctly.

Not only must we look at what answers are given but the way they are given. We should be alert to the body language of the parent but without overinterpreting it. If a parent does not look in our eyes directly, it may mean evasion. On the other hand, this is an appropriate behavior for certain cultures. We should be alert to remarks and clues and follow through with leading questions.

We often ask the right questions, but hurry in listening. Constant interruptions with phone calls and paging systems will leave the parents often wondering whether their history is being listened to or not. We can show the parents that we are listening by using various techniques: looking at their faces, if appropriate; asking questions that clarify the statements they make; and periodically summarizing what they said. This in turn will help them provide a better history.

In talking to the child, begin with easy subjects. Talk about the child's name and those of brothers and sisters, the family pets, and the attractive clothing being worn. It is good to find out where the child hurts and to avoid touching that area until the latter part of the physical examination. The child's speech, affect, and position during these talks will give us many clues to diagnosis. Ask the child to draw a picture of a person or anything else. Though one should be cautious about overinterpretation, children's drawings can give clues to their mental age and to the presence of problems in visual-motor integration. Also, when the child picks up a crayon or a pencil, we can determine the handedness and any abnormalities in the pattern of holding of the pencil suggestive of cerebral palsy or chorea. Handwriting itself may give clinical clues (the unsteadiness of chorea, reversing of letters, mirror-image writing).

Asking children about their wishes, if it were possible to get these wishes, will open our eyes to what is significant to them, though this may have no relation to their primary complaints. Asking gently about good and bad dreams, with reassurance that dreams do not come true, will help us determine the child's level of anxiety and fears. Another very interesting question I have found useful to ask is, "What does Mommy say to you often?"

DETERMINING THE CHIEF COMPLAINT

Inquiry into the reason for the current visit is associated with eliciting the chief complaint. Often when the question is asked regarding the chief complaint, a diagnosis is given. Accepting the diagnosis as given by the family may lead us into blind alleys. Our mind becomes closed and often we end up following the wrong track. It is necessary, therefore, to ask what are the actual symptoms and signs which led to that particular diagnostic categorization. This is particularly important when a child has come through a number of other physicians who might have made a diagnosis.

Make note of the persons giving the history, their ability to communicate properly, particularly if they are not able to speak the local language, and their mood, affect, and apparent reliability. Recognize that the stated reason for the visit may not be the same as the hidden reasons for the visit.

In addition to finding the chief complaint, one should find out its *duration.* In obtaining a complete history of the chief complaint, one should know the characteristics of the *onset.* A symptom that comes on very suddenly will be remembered clearly. The parent and the child may know exactly what they were doing and at what time of the day this symptom was noticed. On the other hand, symptoms which have been coming on gradually will be hard to define, and the parents may not know exactly when they started. Next, one should define the *intensity* of the symptoms. For example, if a child has pain one should find out how severe the pain is. Questions such as the behavior of the child during the onset of the pain, whether the pain interferes with activity, and whether it interferes with sleep will help to define the intensity. One should question the *periodicity* and *frequency* of these symptoms. Recurrent bouts of fever once a month have a different connotation from daily fevers experienced for 6 to 8 weeks. One should find out what factors *aggravate* the main symptom and what factors *relieve* the symptom. An abdominal pain made worse by squeezing the abdomen is likely to be inflammatory in nature, whereas an abdominal pain relieved by holding the abdomen is probably due to some spastic condition. One should note whether the illness has been getting worse or better in the *general trend.* One should also know about *other symptoms* which have been *added on* to this chief complaint. If so, the description of those symptoms in terms of the onset, the course, the chronology, and the intensity should be obtained. On other occasions, the child may have had a number of symptoms that were not of concern initially, but the appearance of a dramatic new symptom was what brought the child to medical attention. Details of these associated symptoms that brought the child to this visit should be obtained.

Find out where the child and the family were getting their medical care prior to this visit and what are the reasons for the change. A relocation, a need for specialty care, and cost are understandable reasons. A history of repeated dissatisfaction and changes of physicians should alert us to potential problems in relationships. Always quiz gently, but carefully and firmly. If aspects of the history seem incongruous, try for verification. Particularly with a family that has been "doctor-shopping," be aware of the possibility of the pediatric version of the "Münchhausen syndrome."

SPECIFIC ASPECTS OF HISTORY TAKING

In pediatric history taking, questions about related areas should be asked to obtain a complete history.

Pregnancy and Delivery

What para? What gravida? (these questions may relate to genetic and chromosome diseases and Rh incompatibility). Was this a wanted or an unwanted pregnancy? (psychologic problems are a possibility—this question has to be asked at the appropriate time and discretely). What was the mother's age at the time of the birth of this child? (age is significant if the mother was an adolescent or over 40 years of age). Did the mother have any illness during pregnancy? (possible congenital malformation and con-

TABLE 3-1. EXAMPLES OF DRUGS THAT, IF TAKEN BY THE MOTHER DURING PREGNANCY OR DELIVERY, MAY AFFECT THE FETUS OR NEWBORN

Drug	Effect on	Type of Problem Encountered
Adrenal cortical steroids	Fetus	Cleft palate
Ammonium chloride	Newborn	Acidosis
Cyclophosphamide	Fetus	Malformations
Immunosuppressives	Fetus	Abortion/Malformations
Morphine (or other narcotics)	Newborn	Withdrawal
Potassium iodide	Fetus	Goiter
Reserpine	Newborn	Drowsiness and nasal congestion
Tetracycline	Newborn	Effects on skeletal growth and on teeth
Vitamin K	Newborn	Hyperbilirubinemia
Dilantin	Fetus	Cleft palate, lip and other malformations
Alcohol	Fetus	Facial abnormalities Growth retardation
Thalidomide	Fetus	Phocomelia

genital infections must be considered). What drugs were taken during pregnancy? (Table 3-1 summarizes various diseases associated with maternal drug ingestion). Also ask about over-the-counter drugs and about drug abuse. Was there exposure to x-rays or injurious chemicals? Was there any emotional stress during pregnancy such as divorce, death, or change of location? Was the pregnancy full term, or premature, or overterm?

Was labor induced? If so, why? Was the delivery normal? Were forceps used? Was the baby delivered by C-section? Was the presentation normal? What was the total duration of labor and delivery (neonatal asphyxia, cerebral palsy)? Did the obstetrician report polyhydramnios (tracheo-esophageal fistula) or oligohydramnios (renal agenesis)?

Did the baby breathe spontaneously at birth? What was the Apgar score at birth? Was the cord around the neck? Was the baby meconium-stained? (suggesting asphyxia). Were the cord and placenta reported to be normal in appearance? (looking for evidence of infection, postmaturity, abnormality of placental vessels).

Neonatal History

How long did the baby stay in the nursery? (If a good neonatal history is not available, prolonged stay in the nursery should arouse suspicion of some problem.) Were there any infections? Did the baby have convulsions? How severe was the jaundice? Was bililite used or was the baby transfused? Were there any bleeding problems? Were there breathing problems?

Nutritional Record

Was the baby breast-fed or bottle-fed? If bottle-fed, what type of formula was used? How good an eater was the baby? When were solids introduced and in what sequence? How easy was it to introduce new food? Was there any food intolerance? What was the pattern of weight gain?

Past Medical History

Details of any prior illness, hospitalization, infectious diseases, surgery, accidents, allergies, and immunization should be determined.

Most families will not remember details of minor *illnesses.* One should, however, ask for details of past, more serious, illness, including the nature of the diagnosis, the age of the child at the time of the illness, the treatment given, and any complications that ensued. If the illness was considered serious, one should get details of the diagnosis, hospitalization, tests performed, treatment given, duration of illness, and complications. If possible, the records should be obtained and reviewed. Often the illness is considered serious, but the child might have been treated at home. The family's perception of the seriousness of the illness may not match the description. After a serious illness, the family may think that the illness is still present even if it has been cured. Also, after recovery from a serious illness the family may consider that particular child as always vulnerable.

If any *surgery* was performed one should know the diagnosis, nature of the procedure done, when it was performed, the hospital in which it was performed and the complications, if any.

A history of *accidents* such as an automobile accident, sports-related injuries, and ingestions of poisons should be sought for. A history of repeated accidents should alert the physician to problems, either in the child or in the family situation. A history of repeated ingestion of poison should suggest social and family problems. Injuries out of proportion to the accident may indicate a defect in the child such as osteogenesis imperfecta or a bleeding diathesis or child abuse.

A history of *allergies* to medicines, food, and environmental agents should be sought for with leading questions. This is one area where overdiagnosis and overinterpretations are common. The descriptions of symptoms considered indicative of allergy, time relationship to the allergen, experience with repeated exposures, response to treatment, and family history are important clues to establishing the accuracy of allergic history.

A history of *immunization* should include dates for primary immunization, completion of boosters, and the location where they were completed. It is important to review the past records or look at the immunization card the parent may carry.

If the patient is an *adolescent,* one should get details of sexual habits, contraceptive use, pregnancies (completed or not), and venereal diseases.

Developmental Milestones

One needs details of milestones of development, particularly if a child is brought for evaluation of developmental delay, behavioral problems, for adoption, for school problems, or for learning problems. The usual questions are designed to find out the date of the first smile, age at first vocalization, age when baby attained head control, age at which baby turned over, sat up unsupported, stood up and walked, and age at which the child attained full control over bladder and bowel for night and day (Tables 5-1 and 5-2, pp. 47–50).

Behavioral and Emotional History

It is hard to assess a child's behavior during a short office visit. Behavioral and emotional history, nevertheless, is of enormous importance in certain situations, such as failure to thrive, recurrent abdominal pain, learning problems, encopresis, and childhood psychosis. In addition, an understanding of a child's behavior and primary reaction pattern helps in counseling mothers during routine office visits.

Dr. H. S. Cecil suggests the following outline for organization of an emotional and behavioral history:

1. Child's assets and liabilities based on:
   a. Primary reaction pattern (see the next paragraph)
   b. Secondary reaction pattern (in older children)
   c. Level of sensory motor integration
   d. Physical status, physiologic function, and health condition
   e. Social responsiveness—in older children, history of relationship with siblings, peers, and adults; progress toward self-care and reaction to discipline
   f. Nature and degree of disordered functioning or developmental deviations
2. Family assets and liabilities based on:
   a. Past history of rearing this child. Start with history of pregnancy including details such as whether this was a wanted child, whether there were any disappointments, whether there was stress during pregnancy
   b. Current state of child-rearing behavior with this child
   c. Mother's sources of support
   d. Mother's life situation apart from child rearing
   e. Mother's experience in being reared

Many of these items are self-explanatory. Understanding of the primary reaction pattern (item 1a) of a child is, however, an important subject that all pediatricians should master and deserves further explanation.

Most mothers know instinctively that babies differ in their style and quality of response to environmental stimuli. There are intrinsic patterns of behavior for each child, and it is the interaction of these with the characteristics and behavior of the mother that determines child-rearing practices and outcome. Dr. Stella Chess (1959) organized these predictable patterns of behavior of children in nine categories. These categories are: (1) *Activity/Passivity:* Some children are by nature very active; some others are quiet and do not move around that much. One can ask the mother how active the baby is when she tries to bathe the baby or change a diaper and get an idea of behavior in this area; (2) *Regular/Irregular:* Some babies wake regularly every morning and ask for their food at about the same time. Others are very irregular. Questions to elicit information on sleep-wake cycles, hunger frequency, regularity in urination and bowel movement will give answers to understand this aspect of a child's behavior; (3) *Approach/Withdrawal* is shown by the *initial reaction* to a new stimulus. Does a child approach new people, new toys, and new food quickly or is it usually a negative or cautious approach the first time? (4) *Adaptive/Nonadaptive:* The ability of the child to relate to a new situation *after the initial contact* may be adaptive or not. Some children may be nervous the first time they see a new person or taste a new food. But they quickly relate to the situation or repeated contacts. Some others take a few days or weeks to adjust to a new stimulus even if it is presented many times in a predictable fashion. (5) *Low threshold/High threshold:* The threshold describes the intensity level of stimulation necessary to evoke a discernable response (auditory, visual, cutaneous sensory stimuli). One of the simplest ways of learning the threshold level of the baby is to find out how soon after wetting does the baby cry to be changed. Some babies will scream as soon as they wet the diaper. Others will stay in wet diapers for a long time without a whimper and get diaper rash if the mother is not sensitive to the subtle clues given by the child. It is easy to see how parental behavior can be affected by the child's threshold for stimuli. (6) *Intense/Mild:* The energy content of the response may vary in degree. Some babies are mild in their response to various stimuli. There are others who are intense and let you know without doubt. Questions on how intensely a baby responded to a new food, a wet diaper, or a new face will give clues to this aspect of behavior. (7) *Positive/Negative:* Some babies are smiling all the time and friendly. Others cry more often and are unfriendly. Everybody wants to carry the smiling baby, and that infant gets the socialization. The crying unfriendly baby is often left alone and often lacks socialization. A quiet, high-threshold, unfriendly baby is likely to be a neglected child, particularly if the mother is not a sensitive person. An active, low-threshold, intense baby is likely to be abused! The importance of taking a history of these aspects of behavior is obvious when evaluating children with emotional problems who fail to thrive, who have poor maternal–child bonding, and who are subject to child abuse. (8) *Attention Span/Persistence:* The attention span measures the difficulty with which an established line of functioning can be altered. For example, a child's attention span in listening to a story or music and the child's ability to stay with one activity for a long time give clues regarding the extent of the attention span. (9) *Distractability:*

The effectiveness of an environmental stimulus to interfere with the ongoing behavior of a child indicates the child's distractability. Questions on how easily one can alter the child's progress toward or demand for an object give clues to this area of personality.

Social and Personal History

Details of the child's social history include development, behavioral and emotional patterns, interpersonal relationships, habits, living arrangements, school performance, economic situations, strengths, and weaknesses. Details of child development have already been mentioned in the preceding section.

In obtaining a history of the child's *personality characteristics* some sample questions might include: "How does the child compare with other children the same age?" "What are some of the child's strengths?" "What are some weaknesses?" "What are some items that scare the child?—that raise anxiety?" "How does the child show anger, fear, and anxiety?" "What are the usual moods?" "How are they shown?" "What are favorite activities?" "How does this child relate to the family?—to strangers?" "How does the child behave in a new situation?" "Who is the child's favorite person in the family and why?" "How do the parents discipline this child and for what things?" "How does the child respond to these measures?"

In obtaining a history on *personal habits* one needs information on:

- *Feeding:* What is the usual eating pattern? Are there any problems with feeding? What kinds of problems? Are there any favorite likes and dislikes? What is the eating pattern of the family?
- *Sleeping:* Is the child a good sleeper? Does the child share a bedroom or bed with someone else? If so, with whom? When does the child go to bed? When does the child go to sleep? What does the child do in bed? What kind of TV shows are watched or what books read before sleep time? Is there any bed-wetting? Are there any bouts of night terror?
- *Toileting:* When did the child get bowel control? Bladder control? Does the child have accidents? If so, under what conditions?
- *Games and Play:* What are favorite toys and games? Does the child have friends? How does the child relate to them?
- *Living Arrangements:* Is this a nuclear family, single parent family, or an extended family? Who are the current household members? What are their ages? What is their health status, both physically and emotionally? Who are the primary care givers? Is a baby-sitter or grandparent involved in this patient's care?

What are the *sources of support* for the mother in physical, emotional, and financial areas? What is the family's religious affiliation? Religious affiliation is important to know, partly because of the emotional support religion plays in many lives. Also, the practices of certain religious sects may provide clues as to the etiology of disease and its management. For example, infants raised completely on breast-feeding without vitamin supplementation are susceptible to tetany, and those raised totally on an unsupplemented diet free of animal protein might have rickets. Other sects will not allow the use of blood transfusions.

The sources of economic support, the nature of the parents' job, the availability of medical insurance and any local or federal aids the family receives are of great importance, particularly in the management of chronic and catastrophic illness. One should therefore be aware of any agencies the families may be already connected with for counseling or supportive purposes. Details of the agency involvement, years of contact, reasons for referral, and the name of the primary contact person should be obtained.

The *school history* should include details of the name and address of the school, the grade level, the mode of transportation, any special emotional or physical needs at school, and any behavioral problems and learning difficulties. If appropriate, it is a good practice to call the school teacher, school nurse, or the gym teacher to get more details.

We should look for *strengths and weaknesses*. We are trained to look at defects and weaknesses to help diagnose and treat the abnormal. In the process we forget we cannot only support the weaknesses, but we can build on the strengths. We should therefore look for strengths in the patients (inner, innate strengths) and in their support network, such as a strong grandparent or neighbor who is very involved with the family.

Family History

Obtain a history of siblings. How many brothers and sisters does the child have? What are their ages? What sex? Are there or has there been any illness in the siblings? If so, what? Recently or earlier? Did any sibling die due to any unknown or undiagnosed diseases?

What are the ages of the parents? Is there any consanguinity between the parents? (important in taking a genetic history). Are these the natural parents? Depending on the time available, get details of the parents' occupations, time spent by the parents at home, and a health history of grandparents and of baby-sitters. In a detailed workup of an undiagnosed or puzzling illness, details of health of close relatives of the mother and father are also needed.

Genetic History

In certain situations a detailed genetic history is essential. A history of members of the maternal and paternal side of the family should include details about the spouses and the children of all the members. A pediatrician should be able to make a reasonable map of the family tree (Fig. 3-1). In certain situations where genetic counseling is indicated, a more detailed history and subtle questioning is desirable, based on a knowledge of patterns of inheritance of the suspected syndrome.

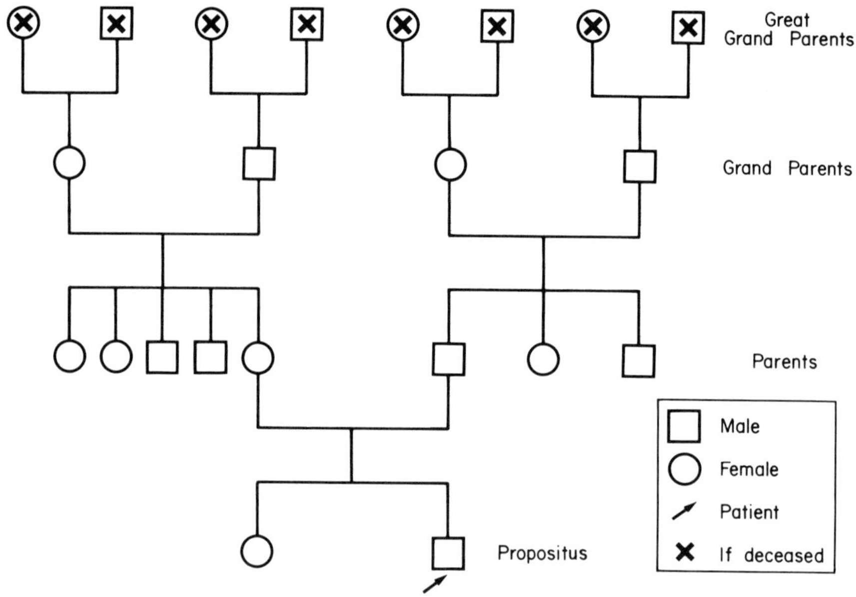

Figure 3-1. Genetic family history.

Dr. R. Juberg (1972) has suggested a three-step approach in obtaining a genetic history depending on the clinical situation. The first step is applicable to *all* pediatric patients. In routine history-taking, the following pieces of information on all first-degree relatives are to be obtained irrespective of the nature of the problem: given names, surnames, date of birth (or current age), age at death and cause of death, presence of any disease or defect. The second step is designed to survey the family history for the occurrence of diseases or defects, particularly when the child has a set of symptoms and the diagnosis is not certain. This applies to *most* situations but not to every one. There are five questions designed to elicit the necessary information: (1) Is there *any* relative with any identical or similar trait? (2) Is there *any* relative with a possibly related trait? (For example, when taking a history from parents of an infant with anencephalus, ask about other central nervous system malformations in the family.) (3) Is there *any* relative with a trait that is generally recognized to be genetically determined? (4) Is there *any* relative with an unusual disease or has any relative died of any unusual condition? (5) Is there any consanguinity in the pedigree?

The first two steps require very few minutes and are adequate for most clinical situations. However, if there are questions about the patterns of inheritance of a defect or questions on possibilities of recurrence, maximal family history and construction of a pedigree is required. This includes details on as many relatives for as many generations as possible. This third step is reserved for those working in the genetic clinics.

System Review

After getting the family and genetic history it is appropriate to obtain a history on certain overlooked items and also to make sure that no associated related or unrelated problems are coexistent. A few crucial questions about each system should be adequate, but the interviewer should be flexible enough to pursue leads brought out during this review. Some examples are:

- *General:* Weight loss, activity level, fever, appetite, poor weight gain, excess weight gain, delay in growth, delayed developmental milestones
- *Skin:* Rash, birthmarks, pigmentations, hair loss
- *Head and Neck:* Headache, any head injuries
- *Ears:* Past infections, hearing, drainage
- *Eyes:* Infections, injury, squint, visual problems, does the child wear glasses?
- *Nose:* Infections, bleeding, nasal block, mouth breathing, snoring
- *Mouth, Teeth, and Throat:* Ulcers, caries, thumb sucking, sore throat, hoarse voice
- *Neck:* Stiffness, pain, glands
- *Respiratory System:* Cough, wheeze, dyspnea, chest pain
- *Cardiovascular System:* Cough, dyspnea, cyanosis, pallor, squatting, tolerance for physical activity
- *Gastrointestinal:* Vomiting, abdominal pain, diarrhea, constipation, jaundice, exposure to parasites, pica, food intolerance
- *Urinary Tract:* Usual habits, color of urine, burning, frequency, discharge, excess volume, thirst, enuresis, edema of hands and feet
- *Genital Tract:* In prepubertal female ask about discharge, itching, pinworms. In pubertal and adolescent female get history of menstrual periods (onset, frequency, regularity, pain, etc.), date of the last period, sexual activity, contraceptive use, prior pregnancy, venereal diseases, history of vaginal discharge and itching.
  In male ask about history of sexual activity, discharge, pain or swelling of testes, nocturnal emissions, contraceptive use.
- *Endocrine:* Breast development, asymmetry, pain or discharge, change in growth pattern, masses in the neck, nervousness, sleep habits, bowel habits, cold intolerance, delay or accelerated development of secondary sexual characteristics, loss of hair, excess hair, acne.
- *Central Nervous System:* Headache, visual disturbances, seizures, ataxia, paresthesia, personality changes, mental deterioration, school failure, speech problems, weakness.

- *Blood:* Pallor, easy bruising, unusual bleeding, large nodes, bone pain
- *Musculoskeletal:* Pain in bone, joint, or muscle; swelling of bone, joint, or muscle; limping, stiffness, limitation of motion
- *Immunologic:* Recurrent infections, rash, failure to thrive
- *Travel:* Foreign travel
- *Pets:* At home
- *Psychologic:* Memory loss, behavioral change, sleep problems, eating problems, school failures, hallucinations, mood changes, temper outbursts, enuresis, encopresis
- *Any Current Medications:* When started? For what purpose? What dosage? Any side effects?

BIBLIOGRAPHY

Chess S, Thomas A, Birch H: Characteristics of the individual child's behavioral response to the environment. Am J Orthopsychiatry 29:791–802, 1959.

Chess S, Hassibi M: Normal and Abnormal Psychological Development in Pediatrics, 17th ed. Rudolph AM (ed). Norwalk, Conn., Appleton-Century-Crofts, 1982, pp 43–81.

Garrett A: Interviewing: Its Principles and Methods. New York, Family Service Associates, 1970.

Goodall J: Opening windows into a child's mind. Dev Med Child Neurol 18:173–181, 1976.

Juberg R: Making the family history relevant. JAMA 220:122–123, 1972.

Kleinman A, Eisenberg L, Good B: Culture, illness, and care. Ann Intern Med 88:251–258, 1978.

Korbin JE, Johnston M: Steps toward resolving cultural conflict in a pediatric hospital. Clin Pediatr 21:257–263, 1982.

Levine MD: Developmental dysfunction. In Levine MD, Carey WB, Crocker AC, Gross RT (eds): Developmental-Behavioral Pediatrics. Philadelphia, Saunders, 1983, pp 709–742.

Ludwig, S, Fleisher, G: Understanding the unique needs of children. In *Textbook of Pediatric Emergency Medicine.* Baltimore, Md., Williams & Wilkins, 1983, pp 25–32.

Maguire, P, Rutter D: Training medical students to communicate. In Bennett AE (ed): Communications between Doctors and Patients. Oxford, Nuffied Provincial Hospitals Trust, 1976, pp 47–74.

Simmons JE: Psychiatric Examination of Children. Philadelphia, Lea & Febiger, 1969.

CHAPTER 4

Three Basic Steps in Diagnosis

Diagnosis means "to know through." Derivatively, the word implies differentiation. In usage, however, the term *diagnosis* primarily denotes the initial impression based on the presenting symptoms and signs. The words that describe the process of establishing the specific cause of a symptom–sign complex are *differential diagnosis.*

The use of computers in medical diagnosis has increased the interest in differential diagnosis. The mental processes involved, however, in the initial diagnosis have not been scrutinized closely.

The three basic questions which a clinician has to ask when presented with a symptom, a sign, or a complex are:

- What is *it?*
- What is it *not?*
- How do you know?

Let us take two examples to explain mental processes: Assume that a patient comes with pain in the joints (arthralgia). The first question is: what is *it?* The obvious initial assumption is "arthritis." But to be sure of this, the physician has to *define* the word *arthritis*. Arthritis is defined as a nonbony swelling of the joint or as the presence of two of the following three findings: limitation of passive movement of that joint, tenderness or pain on motion, and heat. If only one condition is present, the patient does not have arthritis.

The first mental step assumes that the physician knows the definition of the condition he is naming. You can therefore, rewrite the first question as:

"What is *it?—Define.*"

The condition of a 12-year-old girl was diagnosed as acute rheumatic fever. She was put on bed rest for 2 years. The diagnosis was based on a history of joint pains, elevated sedimentation rate, and a high ASO titer. She had joint pain but not true arthritis. If the physician had used the criteria for arthritis (as described in the preceding paragraph), bed rest need not have occurred. If the physician's first impression is wrong, the entire problem will be mishandled.

The second question about our hypothetical patient, assuming the presence of arthritis, is "What is it *not?*" In other words, what are the conditions which may give symptoms easily confused with those of arthritis? Bone pain is one. Tendon pain is another. Periarticular pain is a third. In this step, we are excluding conditions that may mimic the symptoms of the condition that the clinician thinks the patient has. You may, therefore, rewrite the second question as:

"What is it *not?—Exclude.*"

The third step is, "How do you know that the initial impression is correct?" In this hypothetical case of arthritis, the ideal proof is to show that the synovial fluid from the affected joint has all the characteristics of an inflammatory fluid. Also, one would like to see an increase in the level of acute phase reactants in the serum of the patient. If one or both of these factors are positive, we are certain the patient has arthritis. We are now ready to proceed with the differential diagnosis of arthritis to establish the cause. In other words, the third step may be rewritten as:

"How do you know?—*Confirm.*"

Another example illustrating these points is that of a patient who has a history of yellow skin and highly colored urine. The initial question is, "What is it?" The answer obviously is "jaundice." We know that yellow skin and highly colored urine are caused by jaundice. The next question, of course, is "What is it not?" We have to exclude conditions (such as carotenemia) that produce discolored conjuctiva and occurrences (such as ingesting certain food items or drugs) that result in discolored urine. This is where laboratory support comes in to confirm or exclude our initial impression.

CHAPTER 5

History Taking by Systems

In this chapter some common symptoms and diagnostic labels under which children are likely to be seen by physicians are grouped according to the various systems of the body with which they are likely to be associated. For each symptom or diagnostic category, an appropriate definition is given. Wherever it is appropriate, the definition is followed by a list of conditions that may resemble that particular symptom or diagnostic category. Following this list of "exclusions" are questions that are usually asked to obtain details of that particular symptom or diagnostic label. These questions are to be asked in addition to the initial questions about the duration, onset, severity, periodicity, aggravating factors, and factors that relieve the symptom. Answers to these questions are important in arriving at a proper diagnosis. The significance of some of these questions is given within parentheses.

GENERAL

Crying

A good clinician can recognize certain problems just from the sound of the cry. Descriptions of the natural cry in newborns and infants are available in the book *The Infant Cry* by Wasz-Höckert et al. (1968). There is a 45 rpm recording of various types of crying of newborns which accompanies that book.

Important Questions to Ask. Is the child comforted by cuddling? Does the child cry on handling? (meningeal irritation, septic arthritis, fractures); Is it a shrieking cry? (CNS insult); Is it a mewing cry? (as in *cri-du-chat* syndrome); Is it a weak cry? (lipoid proteinosis, various debilitating conditions and neuromuscular conditions); Is it a cry without noise? (vocal cord paralysis, laryngitis, babies of diabetic mothers, babies born of mothers on "drugs," and respiratory distress syndrome); Is it a hoarse cry? (laryngitis, hypothyroid, congenital laryngeal stridor, epiglottitis, foreign body in larynx, vocal cord weakness, papilloma of larynx, congenital vascular ring).

Difficult to Feed

When a mother says that her infant is difficult to feed, the reason may be anything from simple maternal anxiety and lack of understanding on the part of the mother about developmental needs, to a major medical problem such as congenital heart disease or severe hypotonia.

Important Questions to Ask. What exactly is the problem? Is he a slow feeder? Or is he too fast so that he swallows air? Is he too sleepy to feed? Can he suck? (neuromuscular weakness); Does he have tongue thrust? (cerebral palsy); Can he move tongue from front to back? Is there nasal regurgitation? (palatal defects); Does he get tired easily so he has to rest frequently during feeding? (congenital heart or pulmonary disease); Are there choking spells during feeding? (tracheoesophageal fistula); Are there maternal anxieties? Does the quantity he eats fall below what the mother expects in quality or quantity? Are her expectations realistic?

Edema

Definition. Soft swelling of the various parts of the body due to accumulation of fluid.

Exclusion. Nonpitting, nonsoft swelling due to other causes (tumors, inflammation, tissue infiltration).

Important Questions to Ask. Where is it? Is it generalized edema or localized? Does it involve only one side? (venous or lymphatic obstruction); Does it involve only the feet? (exclude vascular causes); Is it only facial edema? (exclude superior vena cava obstruction); Is there abdominal distension? (ascites); It there scrotal edema? (nephrosis); Is there anemia? Dietary history? (nutritional); Is there dyspnea and cyanosis? (heart disease); Does the child have jaundice? (liver disease). Is it confined to one eye or one ear lobe? (insect bite, infection).

Fatigue

Parents often say the child tires easily. This has to be assessed carefully. We know of a boy whose main interest was music. His mother's interest was for him to go out and play. She interpreted her son's desire to stay home as caused by fatigue. She ignored the fact that he stayed home to play the guitar that he loved. (This is another important example to show why parents should be asked to elaborate on symptoms—particularly vague symptoms such as "fatigue," "weak," "tired.")

Fever

Definition. Elevation of the body temperature to above normal (98.4°F or 37°C orally or 99.8°F or 37.6°C rectally).

Exclusion. Adults can have fictitious fever; rare in children.

Important Questions to Ask. Was the onset sudden (infection) or gradual? (collagen disease); Does the temperature curve show high fever (infections) or low grade fever? (minor infections); Are there associated chills? (TB, infections); Are there convulsions with fever? (central nervous system infection); Does the temperature curve show remittent fever with fluctuations more than 1.5°F but not touching normal? (various infections); Is the fever intermittently touching normal for part of the day? (malaria, rheumatoid arthritis); Is it continuous fever with fluctuations less than 1.5°F? (as seen in typhoid); Does the child sweat when the fever subsides? (any high fever, TB, malaria); Has the fever been present for short duration (infection), or has it been present for weeks and months? (rheumatic disorders).

Growth Retardation

This may relate to height, weight, or both.

Definition. Any child who is below the third standard deviation for that age in height and weight.

According to Barbero and McKay (1983), "Failure to thrive" is used to describe "infants and children who, without superficially evident cause, fail to gain and often lose weight."

Know the sizes of the parents (constitutional).

Headache

This is a common enough symptom. Headache can be due to a psychologic cause (stress and anxiety) or it can be due to a brain tumor. Therefore it cannot be ignored.

Important Questions to Ask. Is it frontal (eye strain, regular headache, brain abscess), temporal (migraine), or occipital? (tension headache); Does it start in one place and spread? (more significant than if it stayed in one place); Is it so bad that it makes the patient vomit (migraine, brain tumor/abscess) or is it mild headache? (most viral illness); Does light bring it on (cerebral irritation) or cough make it worse? (increased intracranial pressure); Is it worse early in the morning (brain tumor/abscess) or is it at the end of the day? (visual problems/tension); Are there any associated symptoms such as diplopia, noise in ears, vertigo, paralysis? (these signify more urgent problems); Is there pain in other parts of the body?

Remember that small babies with headaches cannot express pain and may only be irritable. Also, it is interesting to watch and notice frowning and tightening of the muscles of the *eyebrows and forehead* with headache, whereas *muscles of the lower face* are involved in the grimacing of children with pain around the abdomen.

Jaundice (icterus)

Definition. A syndrome characterized by hyperbilirubinemia and deposition of bile pigment in the skin and mucous membrane with resulting yellow appearance of patient. This can be a symptom or sign or both.

Exclusion. Carotenemia or lycopenemia (sclera not colored in these two conditions). Also exclude other causes of colored urine—such as concentrated urine, hematuria, hemoglobinuria.

Important Questions to Ask. Present at birth? (infectious and hemolytic problem); Age of onset? (acquired conditions, hemolytic, infections, and obstructions); Color of stool? (jaundice with clay-colored stool suggests biliary obstruction); Color of urine? Itching? (itching with jaundice suggests obstructive cause for jaundice); Abdominal pain? (calculi); Hemoglobinopathy in family? Any drug ingestion recently?

Obesity

Definition. There are differences of opinion in defining obesity. Three different criteria have been used based on triceps skin-fold thickness, weight for age, and weight for height. Values over the 95th percentile or 2 standard deviations over the mean for each of these criteria are considered abnormal. One of the commonly used clinical definitions considers a person whose weight is more than 10 percent above the median for that person's age and height as obese.

Important Questions to Ask. Family history, dietary history, emotional and behavioral history. Dietary history should be in detail including early feeding history. Sample menu for one 24-hour period includes volume consumed. Is there dry skin and intolerance to cold? (hypothyroidism).

Pain

Pain is a very common symptom. Ascertaining *location* of pain is very important and may be very difficult in the infant. Usually pain in one area indicates some pathology immediately underneath. In some situations, pain is perceived away from the anatomic location where it originates. Certain locations of referred pain are very typical, e.g., retrosternal pain of pericarditis; shoulder-tip pain of gall stone disease; abdominal pain in lower lobe pneumonia; knee pain in hip disease.

It may be located strictly in one area, as in pancreatitis and peptic ulcer, or diffusely, as in appendicitis and colitis. The *spread* of pain from one area to other areas may be characteristic and significant but not so common or useful in diagnosing illness in children.

Important Questions to Ask. It is important to find out *what brings the pain* on or aggravates it. For example, pain of pulp space infection or tenosynovitis gets worse on dangling the limb to the side; pleural pain gets worse on coughing; the pain of increased intracranial pressure gets worse on coughing. *Relief of pain* is another important clinical clue. The pain and stiffness of juvenile rheumatoid arthritis is relieved by walking and moving. Colicky pain in the abdomen is relieved by holding the abdomen, whereas pain due to intraabdominal inflammatory process will be aggravated by this maneuver. Dramatic relief of joint pain with aspirin is characteristically seen in acute rheumatic fever. The *severity* of pain can be of help also. In rheumatoid arthritis, the joint pain is not severe. In acute rheumatic fever and septic arthritis the pain is very severe. Pain due to sympathetic dystrophy is the worst. Pain that keeps children awake at night is probably due to infectious processes (exclude emotional causes). But pain that wakes a child from sleep is most commonly due to teething or otitis. Septic arthritis, osteomyelitis, or osteoid osteoma will also cause nighttime pain. Severe attacks of colicky intermittent pain are common in intussusception. Details on the *characteristics* of pain are hard to obtain from children. Dull aching pain of the joints is the usual picture in most rheumatic disorders. In reflex sympathetic dystrophy it is severe burning pain. Throbbing pain is usual with acute abscesses. The pain of oxygen want is literally like someone tightening the chest with an iron chain. *Timing* is another important factor. Morning headache is of more serious significance than evening headache. Pain in the abdomen after food is different from pain when the stomach is empty (gastric ulcer).

Pica

Definition. Altered appetite. History of child swallowing dirt, crayons, chalk, and any inedible thing.

Exclusion. Mental retardation.

Important Questions to Ask. Age at onset of pica? What items are consumed? Any anemia? Worms? Evidences of lead toxicity? Explore family set-up for emotional disorder.

Polydipsia

Definition. Excessive thirst and water drinking. This is a symptom with serious implications (diabetes). Most of the time it is a common behavior of children (6 to 10 years) to sip water many times a day even though the volume of water consumed is not high. On many occasions it is a parental concern rather than real. The volume consumed (not the frequency) and the history of polyuria are significant.

Exclusion. Psychogenic polydipsia (children with psychogenic polydipsia will drink any water, including water from a toilet bowl, whereas children with polydipsia due to diabetes mellitus or insipidus will never do this).

Recurrent Infections

This is a common complaint. Consider the frequency with which all children get various respiratory and gastrointestinal infections. It is important to know when to consider this a significant or serious problem.

It is known that young children, on the average, get three to six episodes of upper respiratory infection per year. Obviously this is a good guideline to remember.

Recurrent infection *at the same site* (other than upper respiratory infection) usually points to a local anatomic defect; recurrent infection with *the same organism* (pneumococcus, monilia) may suggest problems of immune deficiency.

Swelling

At any site, swelling may be of serious importance. Swellings in most places are due to trauma or congenital malformations or infection or malignancy.

Important Questions to Ask. Was the onset acute or chronic? (infection versus congenital). Was it present from birth? Is it growing or regressing?

Is it fluctuating in size? (infectious); Are there any color changes? Does the swelling feel warm? (infectious); Was there any injury to the site? Is it painful? Has similar swelling occurred in other places? (Also see edema).

Vomiting

Definition. Forcible expulsion of gastric contents.

Exclusion. Simple regurgitation in smaller babies.

Important Questions to Ask. Age of child? (certain conditions are characteristic of the newborn, such as congenital malformations); What was the age of onset? What is the frequency? Is there associated diarrhea? Is there loss of weight? (indicates severity); What is the urine output? (indicates level of dehydration); What are the antecedent symptoms? (pain in the abdomen indicating intestinal problems, and headache indicating meningeal or cerebral irritations); Does fluid come through the nose during vomiting? (if it does, it is indicative of definite and severe vomiting, not regurgitation); Is it projectile in nature? (pyloric stenosis or central nervous system disease); What is the relationship to feeding? (if it occurs soon after feeding, particularly in small infants, it may be because of faulty feeding techniques or acute gastrointestinal infections; if it occurs ½ to 1 hour later it is often caused by obstruction). Is undigested food or bile or blood seen in the vomitus? Is there history of treatment with any drugs such as digoxin or aspirin? Is there history of accidental drug ingestion? Does the child regurgitate food into the mouth and chew on it? (rumination).

CHEST (CARDIOPULMONARY)

Abnormal Noisy Respiration

Definition. *Stridor* is a harsh, high-pitched sound heard during or at the end of inspiration. It is commonly heard in association with conditions characterized by narrowing of the upper air passages (laryngotracheobronchitis, foreign bodies, epiglottis, diphtheria, vocal cord paralysis). "Snoring" is a form of stridor which occurs during sleep.

Grunt is a noise produced at the beginning of expiration.

Rattle is a rapid succession of short, sharp sounds usually heard in moribund and dying patients, due to air going in and out through pooled saliva in the throat.

Wheeze is a noisy musical sound (heard in asthma) and may be heard even without a stethoscope.

Cough

Definition. Paroxysmal expiratory movements.

Important Questions to Ask. What is the duration? (acute or chronic); How severe is the cough? Is it dry (pleurisy) or productive? (pneumonia, TB); What is the nature of the sputum? (purulent as in lung abscess and cystic fibrosis, frothy as in heart disease); Is there copious sputum? (lung abscess); What is the color? (blood tinged in mitral stenosis, greenish in cystic fibrosis); Is there frank blood in the sputum? (hemoptysis); Does the sputum have a very bad smell? (lung abscess); Is there associated fever? Is the cough worse in certain positions? (postnasal drip gets worse on lying down); Is there pain in the chest (pleurisy); What is the character of the cough? (hoarse cough as in laryngotracheobronchitis, whoop as in pertussis, aphonic cough as in vocal cord paralysis). Is the cough present all day but only while awake? (habit); Is it worse when asleep or at awakening? (postnasal drip).

Cyanosis

Definition. Bluish discoloration of skin and mucous membrane.

In central cyanosis, cyanosis is generalized (including tongue) and the extremities are warm; in peripheral cyanosis, tongue is not blue and extremities are cold.

Exclusion. Methemoglobinemia (when the patient is blue without dyspnea); cherry-colored lips of carbon monoxide poisoning.

Dyspnea

Definition. Difficulty in breathing or labored breathing. In infants, dyspnea is characteristically evidenced by inability to suck continuously and by grunting respiration.

Important Questions to Ask. Is there difficulty in feeding? Does the child get tired easily during feeding? Is there fever? Is there cough? (infectious pulmonary problems); What is the nature of sputum? (frothy in heart problems; purulent in pulmonary infections; pink in mitral stenosis); Is there pain in the chest? (pleural); Does the patient have orthopnea? (heart); Is there cyanosis? Does the child have generalized edema? What is the urine output? (heart failure); Does the patient have dyspnea at rest or only on exertion? (to indicate severity).

Hemoptysis

Definition. Blood in the sputum.

Exclusion. Swallowed blood from epistaxis. Hematemesis (frothy material with bright red blood is seen in hemoptysis; the blood is darker and non-frothy in hematemesis).

Important Questions to Ask. History of cough? History of tuberculosis in the family? History of rheumatic fever? Any bleeding diathesis? Bad odor in the breath? Foreign body ingestion?

GASTROINTESTINAL (GI)

Blood in Stools

Definition. Hematochezia is fresh blood in stool. Melena is altered blood in stool.

Exclusion. Dark stool due to ingestion of iron compounds or colored drinks such as grape juice or Hawaiian Punch.

Important Questions to Ask. When did it start? How often? Amount of blood? Is it frank blood (indicating bleeding from lower end, near rectum), or is it dark? (bleeding from higher up); Is there only blood or is there blood with mucus? (amebiasis, ulcerative colitis); Does the child have pain in the abdomen before passing blood? (intussusception, Meckel's diverticulum, anaphylactoid purpura); Is there a history of constipation (fissure) and severe pain during defecation? (fissure); Does the child have tenesmus? (ulcerative colitis, amebiasis).

Bulky Stool

Important Questions to Ask. Is it really bulky for the age and the size of the child? What is the frequency? Is it foul smelling? (cystic fibrosis); Does it float? (malabsorption syndrome); Is it greasy? (cystic fibrosis); What is the color? (pale in liver disease); What is the food intake? (in starvation the stool may look fat and bulky; in malabsorption syndromes, there is voracious appetite); What is the weight pattern? Is there prolapse of rectum? (cystic fibrosis); Does the child complain periodically of pain in the abdomen? (surgical malabsorption); (in some difficult cases of malabsorption syndrome, don't forget surgical lesions of the gut such as malrotation).

Constipation

Definition. Constipation is infrequent or difficult evacuation of the feces. Though the complaint of constipation by the parents is very common, true constipation is rare in normal children. If you consider normal bowel movement with its three variables, namely frequency, consistency, and volume (see page 13) and consider each variable within a range of normality, it is easy to see why these can be unduly misinterpreted. Add to these variables the usual maternal concerns with the functions of the bowel and you have all the ingredients for overinterpretation of this symptom. Before accepting the mother's diagnosis of constipation, one should ask enough questions to find out if this is indeed constipation. The pain of fissures can lead to holding of the stool, with resultant constipation, which in turn can aggravate the fissure and pain.

Important Questions to Ask. How many stools per day or per week? Consistency? Is blood present? If so, is it around the stool or mixed with the stool? Is it present from birth? (Hirschsprung); Did it start around 10 to 18 months? (during toilet-training pressures); Did it start around certain changes in family life? (new baby); What is the dietary history? (too much nonbulk food); Any periodic diarrhea or encopresis? (leaking); Any vomiting? Any loss of weight? In addition to the above questions, good family and emotional histories are needed.

Diarrhea

Definition. Using the same criteria as in constipation, diarrhea is characterized by increased frequency and decreased consistency. Increased volume of bowel movements may or may not be part of this picture.

Important Questions to Ask. Is it acute (infectious) or chronic (functional, parasites, malabsorption)? What is the frequency? Are the stools large and watery (severe diarrhea as in cholera), or is it small volume? What is the color? (green indicates rapid peristalsis; pea soup color in typhoid; rice water color in cholera); Is there vomiting? Is there pain in the abdomen? Is there blood and mucus? (indicates dysentery); Any history of ingestion of unusual food? (toxin); What is the urine output? (to estimate severity); Is there weight loss? (in young children, this is a very important question). Is the child well in every other way—afebrile, good spirits, active, alert? (functional).

Dysentery

Definition. Blood and mucus in the stool.

Important Questions to Ask. Same as for diarrhea.

Dysphagia

Definition. Painful swallowing. In practical use, dysphagia means difficulty in swallowing.

Important Questions to Ask. Duration of the disease (from birth (congenital) or acquired later)? Any history of lye ingestion? Does the food seem to stop in the upper portion (palatal paralysis) or lower portion (scleroderma)? Is there nasal regurgitation (palatopharyngeal paralysis)? Is there trouble with solids (strictures) or with liquids (muscle weakness)?

Hematemesis

Definition. Blood in the vomitus.

Exclusion. Swallowed blood in the vomitus (e.g., blood from epistaxis which was swallowed); colored drinks ingested recently (very common).

Important Questions to Ask. Earlier history of "stomach upsets"? History of bleeding diathesis? History of drug ingestion (aspirin)? Liver disease? What is the color of the blood? Is there bleeding elsewhere?

SKIN

Rash

Described in detail in Chapter 7D, page 167.

MUSCULOSKELETAL

Arthritis

Definition. Swelling of a joint or the presence of two of the following three: pain or tenderness on motion, limitation of range of passive movement, and heat.

Exclusion. Bone pain, periarticular pain, tenosynovitis.

Important Questions to Ask. Is there a history of trauma? Is there fever? (septic arthritis); Does it involve a single joint (septic) or many joints? (juvenile rheumatoid arthritis); Is it migratory? (acute rheumatic fever); Is it nonmigratory? What is the duration? (short duration in trauma and septic arthritis; long duration in rheumatic disorders); Are there any gastrointestinal symptoms? (ulcerative colitis, salmonellosis with reactive arthritis); Are there any low-back symptoms? (ankylosing spondylitis); Have there been any eye problems? (uveitis of juvenile rheumatoid arthritis and ankylosing spondylitis); Is there a bleeding diathesis in the family? (hemophilia) or hemoglobinopathy (sickle cell); Are there any oral lesions? (systemic lupus, mucocutaneous lymph node syndrome); Is there any rash? If so, what kind? (erythema marginatum of acute rheumatic fever, macular evanescent rash of juvenile rheumatoid arthritis, butterfly rash of systemic lupus erythematosus).

CENTRAL NERVOUS SYSTEM

Ataxia

Definition. Failure of muscle coordination. In practice, however, *ataxia* is used to indicate unsteady gait. Classified also as motor ataxia because of muscle incoordination, sensory ataxia caused by loss of proprioception, truncal ataxia due to weakness of muscles of the trunk.

Athetosis

Definition. Slow, writhing movements of the distal portions of the extremities.

Chorea

Definition. Purposeless, *nonrepetitive* involuntary movements of the extremities and face, which interrupt a normal activity.

Exclusion. Tics, which are purposeless, *repetitive* movements.

Coma

Definition. Loss of consciousness from which the child cannot be aroused.

Exclusion. Hysteria—not a major differential diagnostic problem in pediatric age group.

(*Important Questions to Ask* and the proper recording of the level of consciousness will be discussed in Chapter 7F, page 209).

Convulsions

Definition. Convulsions are violent, involuntary movements or a series of movements of the voluntary muscles with or without loss of consciousness.

Exclusion. Hysterical movements (no patterns; occurs only during the day when being seen; patient falls gently without getting hurt). Tetany (spasm with typical posturing of hands and feet).

(*Important Questions to Ask* will be discussed in Chapter 7F, page 208 as part of the discussion of seizures.)

Seizure is defined as a sudden attack or recurrence of a disease and this is the term preferred by neurologists to describe the general category of epilepsy and convulsions.

Delirium

Definition. A mental disturbance marked by delusions, hallucinations, cerebral excitement, physical restlessness, and incoherence. Particularly related to head injury, toxic infectious states (particularly typhoid fever), drug toxicity (atropine group), cerebral vasculitis (SLE).

Diplopia

Definition. Double vision.

Important Questions to Ask. Is there associated headache and vomiting? (increased intracranial pressure); Does the child have squint? Is there history of head injury? Does the child have buzzing in the ears? (labyrinthine involvement); Is the hearing normal? (eighth nerve involvement); Does the child have weakness of any part of the body? Is diplopia present all day (as in tumors and multiple sclerosis) or at the end of the day? (eye strain, myasthenia); Is diplopia present only during the movement of the eye in certain directions? (indicating lateral rectus paralysis, for example).

Tremors

Definition. Fine rhythmic involuntary movements with movements of agonists and antagonists of equal amplitudes. *Static tremor* is present at rest as in Parkinsonism. *Postural tremor* is observed when a limb is kept in a particular position for a long time. This is present in old age as exaggerated physiologic tremor. Tremor of thyrotoxicosis, cerebellar tumor, and asterixis or liver failure also belong to this group. *Intention tremor* is brought about by active movement toward an object and is seen in diseases of superior cerebellar peduncle. There may be a *functional tremor* associated with anxiety or tension.

Vertigo

Definition. A sensation as if the surrounding objects are going round and round (objective vertigo) or the patient himself is revolving (subjective).

Exclusion. Dizziness, which is a "funny" feeling within one's head—a sensation of unsteadiness.

Important Questions to Ask. Is it present at rest (tumors) or on movement? (labyrinthine); Is it on looking to one side? (labyrinthine); Is it associated with diplopia and vomiting? (more serious); Is it acute (infection-toxin) or chronic?; Is there past or recent history of head injury or meningitis? Did the child have recent respiratory or ear infection? (labyrinthitis); Are these recurrent attacks? (Meniere).

(It is hard for children to know that they have vertigo. Frequent falling to one side, unexplained crying episodes, or suddenly closing the eyes as if in terror may be the only evidences of vertigo.)

DEVELOPMENTAL

Delayed Development

Definition. Any child who fails to complete a developmental step (e.g., sit, stand) that is completed by 90 percent of children of the same age may be considered "slow" and delayed in development. Though there are limitations to the use of the Intelligence Quotient (IQ) as a criterion for the diagnosis of mental retardation, this diagnosis has to be considered in any child who performs at a level 2 standard deviations below the mean for that age in standard psychometric testing.

Exclusion. (Though any of the following may lead to delayed development):

- *Environmental deprivation.* History of poor socioeconomic conditions at home, broken home, inadequate parent–child interactions. Demonstrations of definite improvement of the child in a neutral and nurturing environment after a short period are suggestive of environmental deprivation or psychologic abuse rather than primary mental deficiency.
- *Cerebral palsy.* In an infant, developmental delay is in essence delay in motor development such as head control, turning over, walking, and talking. Though cerebral palsy and mental retardation can coexist, one has to differentiate these conditions.
- *Sensory defects.* It is obvious how a developmental delay or deficit in vision or hearing can lead to delay in language and communication development.
- *Primary personality disorder* (e.g., autism). Failure to relate to the environment appropriately and failure in development of interpersonal relationships are points in favor of this diagnosis.
- *Metabolic diseases.* Family history, other findings such as failure to thrive, diarrhea, and jaundice are clues to consider with reference to metabolic disease as a cause of developmental delay in the differential diagnosis.
- *Syndrome.* Presence of other physical stigmata should suggest the presence of a chromosomal abnormality or a nonchromosomal syndrome.
- *Isolated areas of delayed development.* This is *not* mental retardation. A child may be normal in every area except one, for example, confusion with right and left. If this is not part of a global delay, it is not mental retardation.
- *Variation in maturation.* There is no way of defining "normal" development. But one should be able to compare any particular child to the rate of development of an "average" child of the same age. As a child's development deviates farther away from the average, the child is less likely to be normal. (Normal milestones of development are given in Tables 5-1 and 5-2 and can be followed in the Denver Developmental Reference Chart in Figure 8-1, pp. 261–263.)

Important Questions to Ask. Prematurity? Illness during pregnancy? Family history? Parental age at birth of patient? Multiple pregnancy? Toxemia? Antepartum hemorrhage? Details of delivery—how prolonged, use of

TABLE 5-1. EMERGING PATTERNS OF BEHAVIOR DURING THE FIRST YEAR OF LIFE

	Neonatal Period (First 4 Weeks)
Prone:	Lies in flexed attitude; turns head from side to side; head sags on ventral suspension
Supine:	Generally flexed and a little stiff
Visual:	May fixate face or light in line of vision; "doll's eye" movement of eyes on turning of the body
Reflex:	More response; active stepping and placing reflexes; grasp reflex active
Social:	Visual preference for human face
	At 4 Weeks
Prone:	Legs more extended; holds chin up; turns head; head lifted momentarily to plane of body on ventral suspension
Supine:	Tonic neck posture predominates; supple and relaxed; head lags on pull to sitting position
Visual:	Watches person; follows moving object a few degrees
Social:	Body movements in cadence with voice of other in social contact; beginning to smile
	At 8 Weeks
Prone:	Raises head to slightly farther; head sustained in plane of body on ventral suspension
Supine:	Tonic neck posture predominates; head lags on pull to sitting position
Visual:	Follows moving object 180°
Social:	Smiles on social contact; listens to voice and coos
	At 12 Weeks
Prone:	Lifts head and chest, arms extended; head above plane of body on ventral suspension
Supine:	Tonic neck posture predominates; reaches toward and misses objects; waves at toy
Sitting:	Head lag partially compensates on pull to sitting position; early head control with bobbing motion; back rounded
Reflex:	Typical Moro response has not persisted; makes defense movements or selective withdrawal reactions
Social:	Sustained social contact; listens to music; says "aah, ngah"
	At 16 Weeks
Prone:	Lifts head and chest, head in approximately vertical axis; legs extended
Supine:	Symmetrical posture predominates, hands in midline; reaches and grabs objects and brings them to mouth
Sitting:	No head lag on pull to sitting position; head steady, held forward; enjoys sitting with full truncal support

(continued)

TABLE 5-1. *(Continued)*

	At 16 Weeks
Standing:	When held erect, pushes with feet
Adaptive:	Sees pellet, but makes no move to it
Social:	Laughs out loud; may show displeasure if social contact is broken; excited at sight of food
	At 28 Weeks
Prone:	Rolls over; may pivot
Supine:	Lifts head; rolls over; squirming movements
Sitting:	Sits briefly, with support of pelvis; leans forward on hands; back rounded
Standing:	May support most of weight; bounces actively
Adaptive:	Reaches out for and grasps large object; transfers objects from hand to hand; grasp uses radial palm; rakes at pellet
Language:	Polysyllabic vowel sounds formed
Social:	Prefers mother; babbles; enjoys mirror, responds to changes in emotional content of social contact
	At 40 Weeks
Sitting:	Sits up alone and indefinitely without support, back straight
Standing:	Pulls to standing position
Motor:	Creeps or crawls
Adaptive:	Grasps objects with thumb and forefinger; pokes at things with forefinger; picks up pellet with assisted pincer movement; uncovers hidden toy; attempts to retrieve dropped object; releases object grasped by other person
Language:	Repetitive consonant sounds (mama, dada)
Social:	Responds to sound of name; plays peek-a-boo or pat-a-cake; waves bye-bye
	At 52 Weeks (1 Year)
Motor:	Walks with one hand held; "cruises" or walks holding on to furniture
Adaptive:	Picks up pellet with unassisted pincer movement of forefinger and thumb; releases object to other person on request or gesture
Language:	Two "words" besides mama, dada
Social:	Plays simple ball game; makes postural adjustments to dressing

(From Vaughan VC III: Assessment of Growth and Development. In Behrman RE, Vaughan VC III (eds): Textbook of Pediatrics. 12th ed. Philadelphia, Saunders, 1983, p. 36. With permission from the publishers.)

TABLE 5-2. EMERGING PATTERNS OF BEHAVIOR FROM 1 TO 5 YEARS OF AGE

	15 Months
Motor:	Walks alone; crawls up stairs
Adaptive:	Makes tower of 2 cubes; makes a line with crayon; inserts pellet in bottle
Language:	Jargon: follows simple commands; may name a familiar object (ball)
Social:	Indicates some desires or needs by pointing; hugs parents
	18 Months
Motor:	Runs stiffly; sits on small chair; walks up stairs with one hand held; explores drawers and wastebaskets
Adaptive:	Piles 3 cubes; imitates scribbling; imitates vertical stroke; dumps pellet from bottle
Language:	10 words (average); names pictures; identifies one or more parts of body
Social:	Feeds self; seeks help when in trouble; may complain when wet or soiled; kisses parent with pucker
	24 Months
Motor:	Runs well; walks up and down stairs, one step at a time; opens doors; climbs on furniture
Adaptive:	Tower of 6 cubes; circular scribbling; imitates horizontal stroke; folds paper once imitatively
Language:	Puts 3 words together (pronoun, verb, object)
Social:	Handles spoon well; often tells immediate experiences; helps to undress; listens to stories with pictures
	30 Months
Motor:	Jumps
Adaptive:	Tower of 8 cubes; makes vertical and horizontal strokes, but generally will not join them to make a cross: imitates circular stroke, forming closed figure
Language:	Refers to self by pronoun "I," knows full name
Social:	Helps put things away; pretends in play
	36 Months
Motor:	Goes up stairs alternating feet; rides tricycle; stands momentarily on one foot
Adaptive:	Tower of 9 cubes; imitates construction of "bridge" of 3 cubes; copies a circle; imitates a cross
Language:	Knows age and sex; counts 3 objects correctly; repeats 3 numbers or a sentence of 6 syllables
Social:	Plays simple games (in "parallel" with other children); helps in dressing (unbuttons clothing and puts on shoes); washes hands
	48 Months
Motor:	Hops on one foot; throws ball overhand; uses scissors to cut out pictures; climbs well

(*continued*)

TABLE 5-2. (*Continued*)

	48 Months
Adaptive:	Copies bridge from model; imitates construction of "gate" of 5 cubes; copies cross and square; draws a man with 2 to 4 parts besides head; names longer of 2 lines
Language:	Counts 4 pennies accurately; tells a story
Social:	Plays with several children with beginning of social interaction and role playing; goes to toilet alone
	60 Months
Motor:	Skips
Adaptive:	Draws triangle from copy; names heavier of 2 weights
Language:	Names 4 colors; repeats sentence of 10 syllables; counts 10 pennies correctly
Social:	Dresses and undresses; asks questions about meaning of words; domestic role playing

(From Vaughan VC III: Assessment of Growth and Development. In Behrman RE, Vaughan VC III (eds): Textbook of Pediatrics. 12th ed. Philadelphia, Saunders, 1983, p. 37. With permission from the publishers.)

anesthesia, forceps, presentation? Neonatal problems? Neonatal infections? Emotional deprivation? Socioeconomic conditions? When did the child first smile? When did the child turn over? What was the age when the child could hold the head steady? When did the child sit? Take the first step with help? When did the child walk without help? When did the child talk the first meaningful word? Talk in sentences? How old was the child when dry at night? When was the child toilet trained?

Enuresis

Definition. Involuntary discharge of urine occurring during sleep at night.

Exclusion. Polyuria from any cause (we know of a child with sickle cell disease and hyposthenuria who was sent to a psychiatrist for bedwetting).

Important Questions to Ask. Is it during the day (more serious) or at night only? Did the child ever have bladder control and then lose it? Or did the child never obtain bladder control? (needs more investigation); What is the urine volume? (diabetic insipidus); Has there been any recent stress in the family? Is the child a very sound sleeper?

Hyperactivity

Definition. There are varying levels of activity of children. Some are more active than others; boys in general are more active than girls. Also, the irritability quotient of the parents determines the complaint about hyperactivity—one mother may complain about the normal curiosity of a 2-year-old boy and another father may find it cute to find his son punching every child on the street. Hyperactivity may imply an attention deficit disorder (ADD), but most hyperactive children are not to be classified as having ADD (see page 264 for more discussion).

Learning Disability

Definition. Children who have no neurologic disorder or mental retardation but still have problems in learning. They may also have various degrees of developmental delay and behavioral disabilities. This is a heterogeneous group consisting of many descriptive terms such as "hyperactivity," "dyslexia," and "minimal cerebral dysfunction." The latest addition to this list is "attention deficit disorder." There are controversies about the usefulness and need for these terms. A textbook by Levine, Carey, Crocker, and Gross describes these problems under the heading "developmental variations and dysfunctions in the school child."

Exclusion. Mental retardation; visual problems; cerebral palsy; neurologic disorders; hearing difficulties; behavioral problems; psychiatric illness; and environmental and social deprivation.

BIBLIOGRAPHY

Barbero GJ, McKay RJ: Failure to thrive. In Behrman RE, and Vaughan VC III (eds): Textbook of Pediatrics, 12th ed. Philadelphia, Saunders, 1983, pp 253–254.

Eviatar L, Eviatar A: Vertigo in children: Differential diagnosis and treatment. Pediatrics 59:833–838, 1977.

Hall M: Principles of Diagnosis, 2nd ed. New York, D. Appleton, 1835.

Knobloch H, Pasamanick B. Developmental Diagnosis, 3rd ed. Hagerstown, Md. Harper & Row, 1974, p. 153.

Levine MD: Developmental Dysfunction. In Levine MD, Carey WB, Crocker AC, Gross RT (eds): Developmental-Behavioral Pediatrics. Philadelphia, Saunders 1983, pp. 709–742.

Packman S: Diagnostic Evaluation of the Child with Mental Retardation. In Rudolph AM (ed): Pediatrics. 17th ed. Norwalk, Conn., Appleton-Century-Crofts, 1982, pp 399–402.

Taft LT; Mental Retardation. In Behrman RE, Vaughan VC III (eds): Textbook of Pediatrics. 12th ed. Philadelphia, Saunders, 1983, pp 123–129.

Wasz-Höckert O, Lind J, Vuorenkoski V, et al.: The Infant Cry: A Spectrographic and Auditory Analysis. Clinics in Developmental Medicine no. 29. London, Heinemann Med. Bks., 1968.

SECTION III

Physical Examination

CHAPTER 6
General Physical Examination

GENERAL COMMENTS

A 1976 editorial in the *Journal of the American Medical Association* was entitled: "Are Medical Schools Neglecting Clinical Skills?" The focus until recently has been on the technical aspects of care and on numbers. But fortunately, the clinical skills, human relation skills, and artistic skills that characterized physicians from an earlier era are once again getting the emphasis they deserve.

We believe that *all physicians* have to know how to examine *all systems* correctly. We may need a specialist to interpret unusual signs and symptoms, but every physician should be able to elicit common physical findings. To learn the correct approach is the first step, but without repeated application one tends to forget. The most important point in physical diagnosis, therefore, is not merely the knowledge but its application.

It is obvious that a cooperative patient is essential for a good physical examination. In the pediatric age group one does not always get a cooperative patient. Even the best of us will face a tough customer occasionally. Children in certain age groups do not like to be handled by strangers. However, there are certain useful approaches.

During the initial contact with the young child and the family, leave the child alone—do not even look straight at him—until you have had a nice relaxing talk with the parents. During this time let the child play around or sit on a chair or sit on a parent's lap until you are ready. The fact that the parents are talking to you freely relaxes the child.

On the contrary, with adolescents it is better to deal directly. Often you may have to gently remind the parents to let the boy or the girl tell their own story. This approach may be applicable to even younger children.

Any sudden movements may frighten the young ones. Beginning the physical examination without any instruments helps allay the child's anxieties. Allow the child to play with the stethoscope or flashlight or reflex hammer during your examination of the skin, abdomen, or the limbs. You may have to examine whatever part is available first and you cannot insist on going from head to foot in an orderly fashion. You have to examine them in whatever position they are in and cannot insist—at least initially—on having them lie down. You will have to examine the most painful parts last and look into the throat and the ears at the end of the examination. Allow them to cling to their parent or sit on a lap for as much of the examination as possible.

With all these tricks you may still miss many points in the first examination. In nonacute problems you may have to see a child more than once before you get a satisfactory, thorough picture. Time may be of the essence, however. The art of discovering the key findings in the initial examination of a difficult child is one of the hallmarks of a skilled clinician.

Each physician develops personal tricks to elicit and increase the cooperation of children during the examination. Here is a partial list:

1. Let the child play with the examining instruments.
2. Explain the procedures—particularly the painful ones.
3. Tell firmly what is expected; do not ask "Can you please open your mouth?" (That question always leaves the option to say "no!")
4. Have a colorful examining room with cartoon characters or toys.
5. Come *down* to their level—even if they are on the floor—both mentally and physically.
6. Never say "It won't hurt" if, in fact, the procedure will hurt. Deceiving the child will only lessen confidence in you.
7. With young children, allow as much parent contact as possible.
8. Another interesting approach to help relax the children and make them share some of their hidden fears and anxieties is the Winnicott squiggle game. In this game, the physician draws a squiggle and asks the child to complete it, to make a picture. Next, the child is asked to draw a squiggle and the physician completes a picture out of it. Even if no impressions can be made out of these pictures, certainly they will improve the physician–child communication and the child's cooperation during the physical exam.

This entire book is based on the systematic approach to symptoms and signs. We hasten, however, to state a favorite general rule in clinical practice. One has to be compulsive about getting all details on certain occasions when there is time: but being irrelevantly compulsive irrespective of the need, time, and place is *NOT* good clinical medicine. Knowing when to go for details and when not to, comes with practice and wisdom.

SOURCES OF ERROR

Before discussing the details of the physical examination, let us consider sources of errors in physical diagnosis. Errors may be due to faulty techniques in examination or in interpretation. Weiner and Nathanson (1976) observed 145 medical interns and residents and classified errors as follows: errors in techniques of examining various parts of the body, errors from omission (failure to examine certain areas), errors owing to failure to recognize signs, and errors because of incomplete and poor recording of physical examination. Comprising the first area, thus, are errors in the *technique* of physical examination. It is obvious that these errors can be corrected only by the combined efforts of the clinical teachers in emphasizing proper techniques and of the physician–students who should apply these rules methodically.

Weiner and Nathanson also included *interpretation* in their list of errors. This is the second and more sophisticated source. Experience is essential for the proper interpretation of physical findings, but, even after one gets experience, the following common pitfalls must be avoided:

1. All clinical findings must be interpreted within the context of the whole patient. It is easy, but erroneous, to accept those findings which confirm our suspicion and ignore those findings which seem contrary to our clinical judgment.
2. The specific interpretation and application of a clinical finding depends on the probability of the patient having a particular disease (given the rest of the clinical picture) and the probability of occurrence of that particular physical finding in that disease. For example, the presence of jaundice in a 3-year-old child in India has a higher specificity for hepatitis than for congenital hemolytic anemia. The reverse may be true in Mediterranean countries.

When a physician makes an initial working diagnosis based on symptoms and signs, the physician has developed a hypothesis or an unproved theory, which explains certain facts. This hypothesis—this working diagnosis needs confirmation. In this respect, the clinician is a scientist trying to prove a hypothesis. The clinician is liable to make the same mistakes that scientists are warned against, but the consequences of the action of the clinician can be more serious. Beveridge (1957) describes some of these pitfalls: (1) clinging to ideas which have been proved useless or untrue; (2) inability to subordinate ideas to facts; (3) inability to submit hypotheses to most careful scrutiny; and (4) inability to recognize that false hypotheses interfere with progress.

Ingle (1976) has listed fallacies in reasoning under the following headings: (1) fallacies that concern associated or correlated events, e.g., *post hoc, ergo propter hoc* [after this, therefore, because of this]; (2) fallacies of generalization, e.g., judging an individual on the basis of the general characteristics of the group; (3) fallacies of oversimplification, e.g., assuming that our "hypothesis must be true because there is no proof that it is not true"; and (4) fallacies that beg the question, e.g., the fallacy of hiding behind untestable hypotheses. Good clinicians have to guard against all these fallacies in the interpretation of physical findings.

SUBJECTIVE OBSERVATIONS

The first step in physical examination is to get the confidence and cooperation of the child. There is no known way to teach this important step. One has to love children and children should know and sense it. That is the only way to allow children to relax with you and make the examination easier.

During the physical examination, it is good for a beginner to start at the head and go down to the foot or vice versa but in an orderly manner. However, this may not be possible always, particularly with infants and toddlers. Therefore, one has to modify the approach and be able to collect all the information available in any sequence. As a famous comedian used to say, "What you see is what you get" with difficult children.

It is annoying to find a doctor whose pace never varies. A good clinician should be able to aim for the major problem very quickly in an emergency room setting but be able to take time in a thorough and routine examination when an hour or more is available.

The first step is to quickly ascertain whether the child is well, mildly ill, or severely ill. Simple observations made while you are talking to the parents will tell you many things. For example, a child lying comfortably on the back, with that special luster in the eye, cannot be sick. A child sleeping comfortably curled up in bed, or with legs tucked underneath the abdomen, cannot be seriously ill. On the other hand, children who are restless or cranky even when held by their parents, those who are limp, those with a shrieking cry, those with a grunting respiration or a grunting rather than lusty cry, and those who cannot lie flat on the back are seriously ill.

Dr. Irwin Redlener's (1972) mnemonics called "SCRAPE A" gives a list of seven items to help determine how sick a child is. Presence of any of the items in the following list should indicate that the problem is probably serious and requires immediate attention. (1) *S*kin: purpuric rash, jaundice, cyanosis, pallor; (2) *C*ry: shrieking cry, grunting cry, hoarse cry; (3) *R*espiration: grunts, retractions of intercostal spaces, gasping, nasal flaring; (4 & 5) *A*ctivity and *P*osition: some have been listed above; some will be described on page 59; (6) *E*ye: sunken eye, lusterless eye, sudden onset of squint, nystagmus, abnormal pupils, cataract; (7) *A*bdomen: distended or tender abdomen, concave abdomen.

The general nutritional status of the child is easily noted, even before the organized physical examination is started. One has to observe whether the child is overweight, lean or marasmic, or dehydrated.

Intellectual Functioning

If a child is not very ill, a quick assessment of the intellectual functioning is in order. Little extra time is needed to accomplish this. Table 6-1 lists some of the normal intellectual activities of children between 6 and 11 years of age. During the course of conversations with the child, you can easily include questions to elicit answers for items given in this table.

TABLE 6-1. SIMPLE TESTS OF MENTAL PROFICIENCY

Age	Numerical Skill	Other Concepts
6	Counts forward to 30 Repeats 4 digits	Tells right from left Tells AM from PM Draws a man with head, neck, hands, and clothing Defines objects in terms of how they are used
7	Counts by 2s and 5s Repeats 5 digits forward; 3 backwards	Copies a diamond Recognizes parts left out of a drawing
8	Makes change from a quarter Counts backward from 20	Knows days of the week Has an idea about distant places Can give similarity and difference between simple objects
9	Can do simple multiplication and division	Knows correct date Can arrange weights in order of heaviness
10	Uses fractions Knows numbers over 100 Repeats 6 digits forward	
11		Defines abstract terms such as honesty, fair play, deceit Can give the moral of fables

(From Blake FG, Wright FH, Waechter EH: Nursing Care of Children, 8th ed. Philadelphia, Lippincott, 1970, p. 442. Reproduced with kind permission from the publisher and the authors.)

Position/Posture

The position taken by the patient gives valuable clues to diagnosis. Irritability and dyspnea, worsening on lying flat, may indicate congestive heart failure. Asthmatic children sit on the edge of the bed with legs dangling, leaning forward with hunched shoulders, and hands supporting the body weight and placed slightly behind the midline. They may have a barrel chest and active accessory muscles of respiration. If children have colicky pain in the abdomen, they are restless and roll about, holding their hands over the abdomen; but if there is peritoneal irritation, they lie still and do not want their abdomen touched. The decerebrate posture is characterized by extended neck, extended shoulders and elbows, pronated forearm, with lower limbs in extension (Fig. 6-1). Decorticate posture is flexion at elbow and at wrist, with thumb adducted into the palm, with lower limbs extended (Fig. 6-2). Patients with spinal cord injury and amyotonia congenita have flail limbs and they lie in a "pithed frog" position. A child who wants to lie still in one position with eyes shut may have vertigo. Infants with sensory deprivation syndrome assume a posture characterized by "tonic immobility" of arms with elbows flexed, upper arm abducted and rotated outward, and the hands pronated (Fig. 6-3).

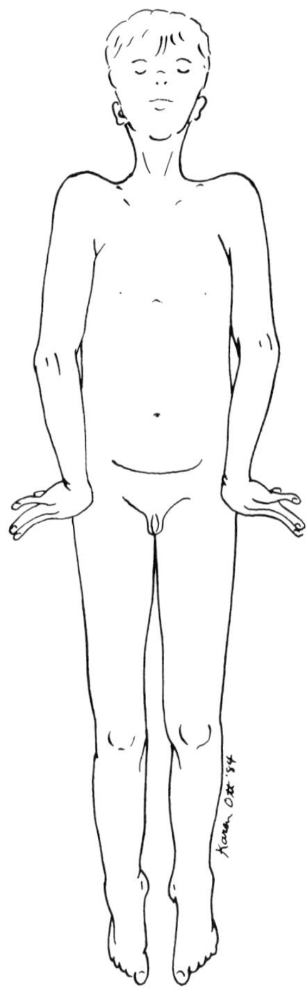

Figure 6-1. Decerebrate posture. Note extension of the neck, *extension at the elbows,* pronation of the forearm and extension of the lower limbs.

Cry

Many diagnostic impressions can be made by listening to the cry alone. The irritable cry of sick newborns is easily recognized with experience. Normal fussiness becomes less if a baby is picked up and handled. In contrast, the irritability and cry of cerebral irritation get worse with handling. In painful conditions of the skeletal system and joints, the child cries on handling. The cry is shrill, shrieking, and high pitched in diseases of the central nervous system. It is very weak in neuromuscular paralysis. It is voiceless in vocal cord paralysis and in the presence of tracheostomy. It is like that of a cat in *cri-du-chat* syndrome. It is hoarse in laryngotracheobronchitis and recurrent laryngeal paralysis.

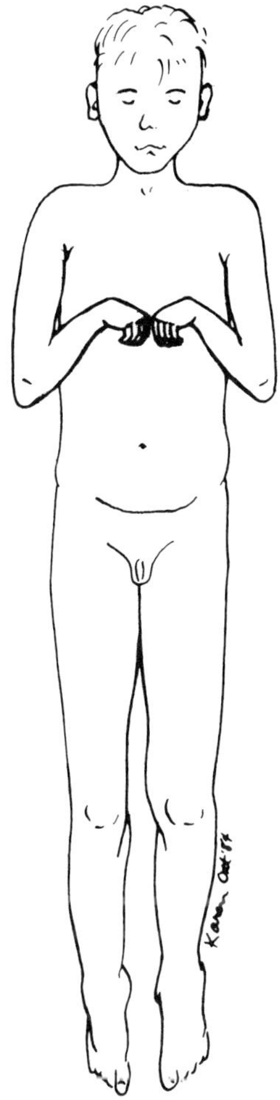

Figure 6-2. Decorticate posture. Note *flexion of the elbows* and the wrists, and extension of the lower limbs.

Alertness

Another thing to observe is the degree of alertness in children. A febrile child who is alert and responsive is less of a concern than one who is extremely lethargic or irritable. A blind child is extrasensitive to noise and jumps easily when there is sudden noise. On the other hand, a child who is extra-alert visually may be deaf.

A blind child has the following features: (1) a vacant distant look; (2) fine oscillations of the eyeball; (3) unusual alertness to sound. Children with autism make no eye contact. A child who has been placed in multiple foster homes is often in a dreamy state, though awake.

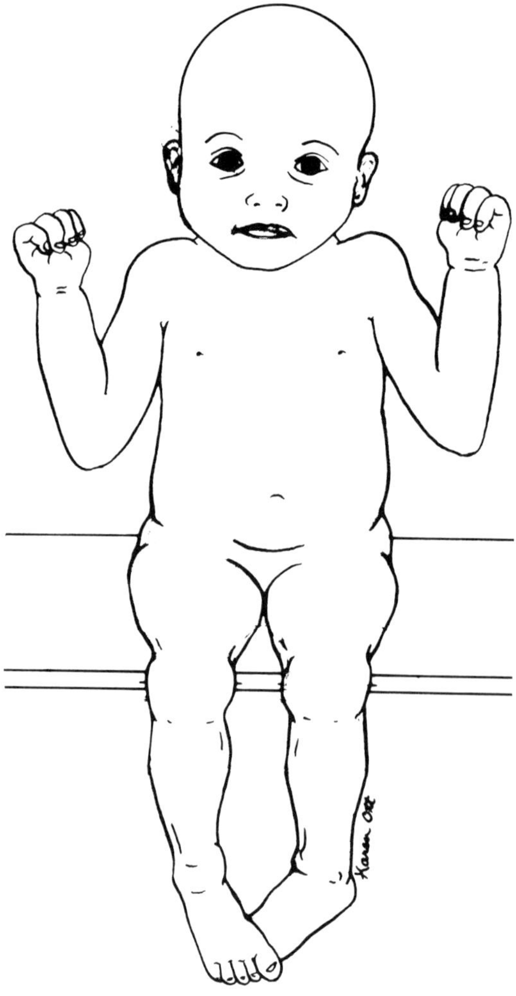

Figure 6-3. Infant with sensory deprivation syndrome. Note the posture characterized by flexion at the elbow, abduction and external rotation at the shoulder, and pronation at the wrist.

Odor

During this early observation period, be alert to recognize characteristic odors in the patient that may aid in the diagnosis. For example, smell of acetone in the breath of diabetes mellitus, fruitish smell of diphtheria, or smell of ingested toxin (kerosene) are well known. Other smells of diagnostic significance are given in Table 6-2, In addition, experienced clinicians can smell the characteristic odor of *Escherichia coli* diarrhea and the stool of cystic fibrosis.

Gait

As the child walks in, many impressions can be received on the basis of gait alone. Looking at the worn-out portions of the shoe gives many clues to

TABLE 6-2. CONDITIONS CHARACTERIZED BY CHARACTERISTIC ODOR OF THE PATIENT (BREATH, SKIN, OR URINE)

Disease	Odor
Diabetes Mellitus	Acetone
Diphtheria	Fruity
Maple Syrup Urine Disease	Caramellike (maple)
Phenylketonuria	Musky ("mousy")
Oasthouse Urine Disease	Dried malt (brewery)
Hypermethioninemia	Rancid butter

diagnosis. A shoe worn out in front without any marks on the heels indicates a tight heel cord (as seen in cerebral palsy) or a foot drop. In foot drop, the box of the shoe will also show marks of scraping on the floor. Children with arthritis and pain at the metatarsophalangeal joints learn to put weight on the outside so that the shoe is worn off on the outer side.

Abnormal gait has been classified traditionally as painful limp, paralytic limp, steppage gait, etc. The new knowledge developed by physiatrists, biomechanical engineers, and prosthetists in analyzing gait has not been adequately used by clinicians.

Gait cycle consists of the activity that occurs between heel strike of one limb and subsequent heel strike on the same side (Fig. 6-4). Heel strike is that moment when the heel touches the floor. During one gait cycle, each lower limb goes through two phases:

1. Stance phase, beginning from the moment the heel touches the floor (heel strike) and ending when the toe leaves the floor (toe off).
2. Swing phase, beginning with toe off until the heel strikes the floor.

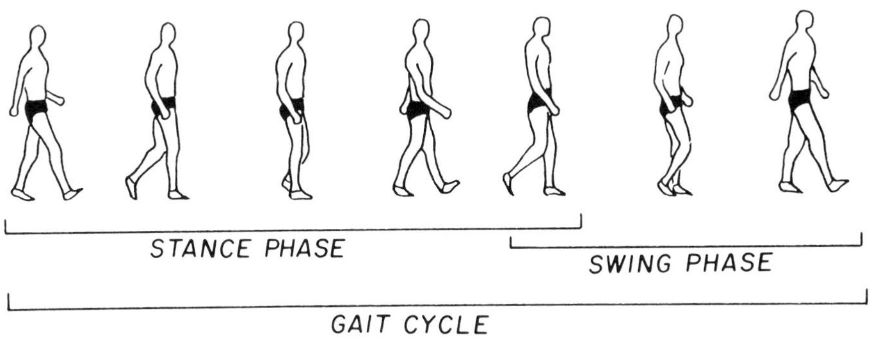

Figure 6-4. Normal gait cycle.

Whenever it is indicated, have the child walk about 12 to 24 steps and observe each limb in the stance phase and in the swing phase. It is also important to look at the ankle, knee, hip, and spine during the stance and the swing phase. If one does this systematically, one can observe many important clues.

Some abnormalities that can be detected during the *stance phase* include:

1. Lateral trunk bending during stance phase toward the side bearing weight suggests gluteus medius weakness on that side. The cause of this can be diseases of the hip, such as dislocation, or diseases of the muscles, such as dermatomyositis or muscular dystrophy.
2. Posterior trunk bending suggests gluteus maximus paralysis.
3. Excess lordosis suggests hip flexion contracture.
4. Hyperextended knee suggests weakness of quadriceps.
5. Slapping contact of the foot with the floor, where the toe touches the floor before the heel does, indicates anterior tibial weakness.
6. Excessive lateral foot contact suggests evertor weakness (peroneus) or pain on medial side of the foot.
7. Excessive medial foot contact suggests weakness of invertors of the foot or tightness of the evertors (peroneus) or knock-knee.

Some abnormalities that are observed during the *swing phase* are:

1. Lateral bending, away from the side which is in swing phase, denotes weak gluteus medius on the side which is bearing weight.
2. Hip hiking (lifting the hip vertically) suggests that the lower limb is longer on the side with hip hiking or shorter on the opposite side. Hip hiking may also indicate hip flexor spasticity or hamstring weakness.
3. Circumduction gait is seen in hemiparesis due to weakness of hamstring or flexors.
4. Anterior trunk bending suggests weakness of quadriceps.
5. Bobbing up and down with too much vertical movement of the hip above and below an imaginary line going through the umbilicus is seen in hip flexor weakness and hamstring weakness. This is different from hip hiking where the vertical movement is only upwards above the umbilical line from clearing the floor but no bobbing down.
6. Dangling flail foot suggests anterior tibial weakness which may be isolated, as in peripheral nerve disease, or part of a generalized weakness of muscles of the leg, as in polio or myelomeningocele.
7. Insufficient push off. This is characterized by the entire foot leaving the floor simultaneously instead of the heel first—and then foot and finally toes. This is seen in gastrocnemius weakness and painful foot syndromes.

When the length of step and period of time spent on one side are different from that on the other, look for pain anywhere in the limb, or fear of falling, or cerebellar dysfunction.

Face and Facial Expressions

Facial expressions are valuable guides to the child's emotions and aid in diagnosis. Facial expression is a composite of movements of various muscles of the face, the opening of the eyelids, and of the color and size of the pupils. The appearance of anxious, angry, and happy faces is obvious. In addition, it is known that when a child is in pain, muscles of the upper part of the face are wrinkled in painful conditions of head and neck, whereas the lower part of the face is also wrinkled when the pain is in the chest or abdomen. Spasm of the muscles of the jaw and of the face in tetanus gives rise to a facial expression characterized by clenched teeth, tightly pursed lips, and the drawing up of perioral muscles (risus sardonicus). The prominent eyes of hyperthyroid, the wide eyes with prominent forehead of Cruzon disease, the whistling face in Freeman-Sheldon syndrome, and the chubby cheeks of cushingoid facies are typical examples of how facial appearance can help in making a diagnosis.

Flattening of the face on one side, with wide palpebral fissure, enophthalmos, and ptosis are seen in Horner syndrome. Blue face, petechiae, and subconjunctival hemorrhage indicate thoracic outlet obstruction due to whatever cause, for example, cord around the neck, or whooping cough. Flame-shaped nevus on one side of the face is seen in Sturge-Weber syndrome; heliotrope (amethyst-violet) discoloration of eyelids is seen in dermatomyositis; an expressionless, flat, masklike face is seen in overdose of the phenothiazine groups of drugs.

The *cheek* is pink in normal and healthy children. Pale cheek is often an indication of fear or anemia or aortic regurgitation. In systemic lupus, one may see the butterfly rash (Fig. 6-5) characterized by discoloration, dryness, scaling, and follicular plugging, almost resembling acne, on either side of the bridge of the nose.

Other well-known facies described in the literature include: the elfin facies, masklike facies, and old-man's facies. These terms are used to give the description of a composite image of the face. If one has to give the details of abnormalities of the face, one has to take each component and give a description. For example, the appearance of "mongolian" facies in Down's syndrome is determined by the set, the slant, and the epicanthal folds of the eyes. Bilateral parotid swelling gives a "chipmunk appearance" to the child's face, as seen in mumps and Sjögren syndrome. (The best way to look for parotid swelling is to look from behind the patient to observe that the lower lobe of the ear is elevated laterally, away from the face.)

There are many symptoms in which there are combinations of abnormalities of forehead, eyebrows, eyes, nasal bridge, nose, philtrum, the lips, jaws, and the ears. In 1879, Galton had thought of an idea of creating

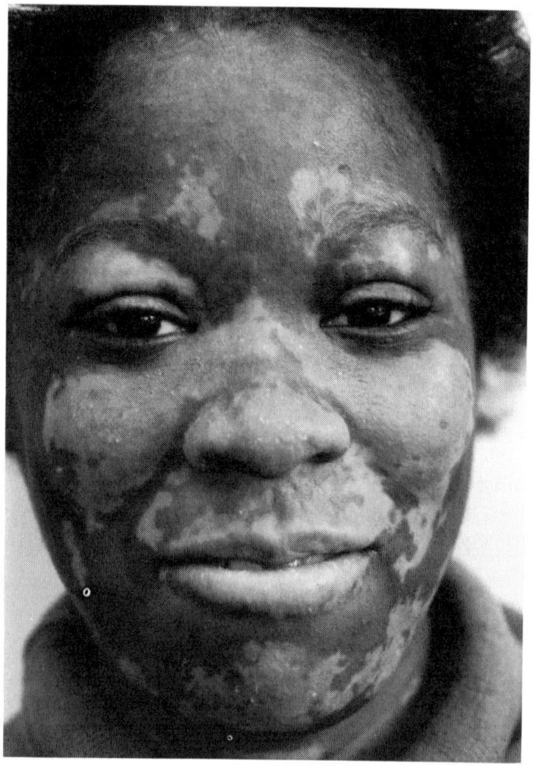

Figure 6-5. Rash in a girl with systemic lupus erythematosus. Discoid lesions causing depigmentation and atrophy. All of face involved, including the "butterfly" area of distribution.

composite photographs of normal individuals by superimposing many photographs. More recently, Leiber has reintroduced the idea. Until such composites are easily available one has to rely on some descriptive terms, ability to recognize normal and abnormal patterns, and some old-time clinical experience to make these diagnoses.

Hypertelorism and hypotelorism are part of what is described as "facies." Though a glance may give us an impression of hypertelorism, it can be often wrong, since the presence of a broad nasal bridge may simulate such an impression. It is hard to measure interpupillary distance, particularly in infants. Therefore, special graphs have been constructed based on measurement of distance between inner canthi and between outer canthi. Percentile values for various ages can be obtained on these graphs and have to be used for accuracy in cases where clinical observation alone is not adequate (Figs. 6-6, 6-7, 6-8).

The position of the *ears* and axial rotation of ears are features contributing to the total composite called "facies." Though relatively large ears and absent ears are easy to recognize, measurements are available to define low-set ears, small ears, and protuberant ears. Using a measuring instru-

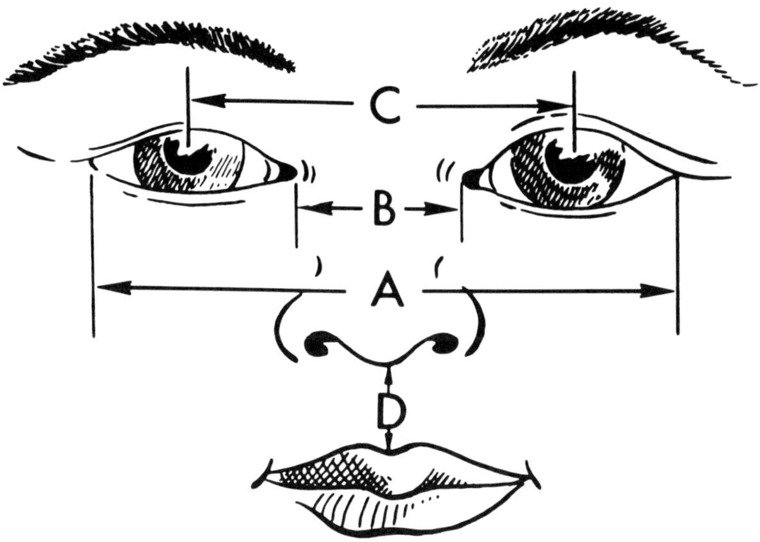

Figure 6-6. Measurements of the face. (A) Outer canthal distance. (B) Inner canthal distance. (C) Interpupillary distance. (D) Height of philtrum. *(From Feingold M, Bossert WH: Normal values for selected physical parameters. An aid to syndrome delineation. Bergsma D (ed). White Plains, N.Y.: The National Foundation, BD:OAS X(13):1–16, 1974.)*

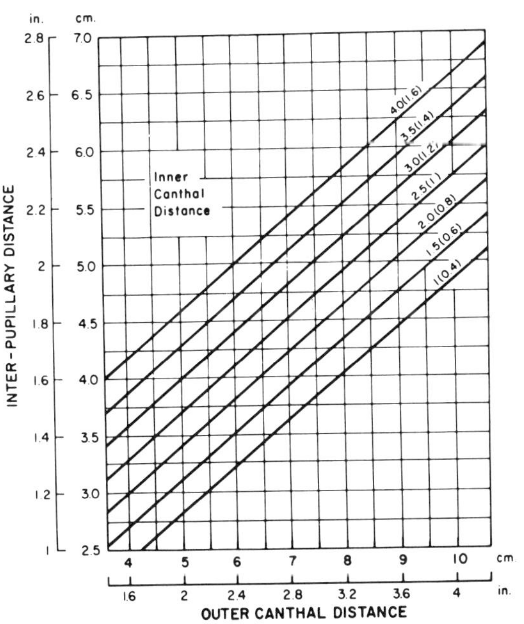

Figure 6-7. Relationship between outer canthal distance, interpupillary distance, and inner canthal distance. *(From Feingold M, Bossert WH: Normal values for selected physical parameters: An aid to syndrome delineation. Bergsma D. (ed). White Plains, N.Y.: The National Foundation, BD:OAS X(13):1–16, 1974.)*

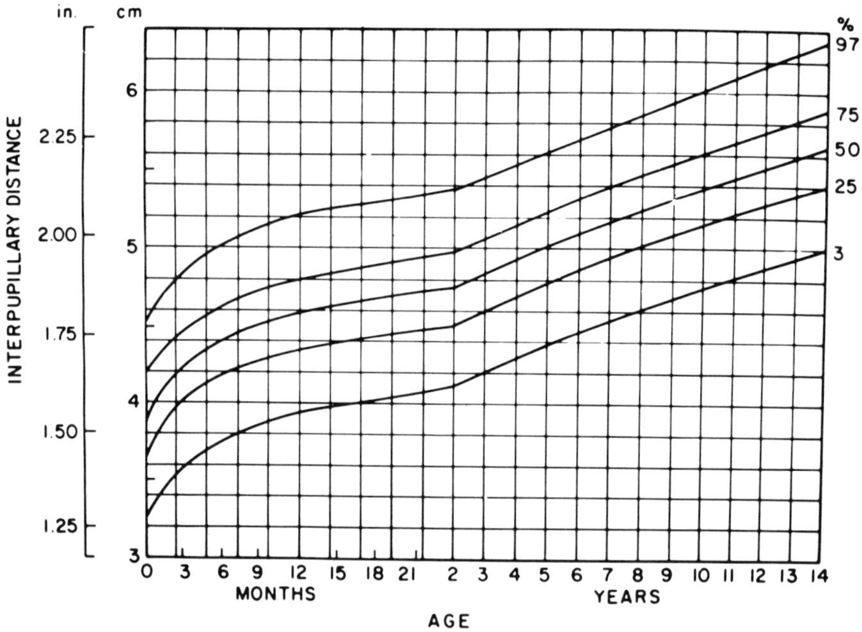

Figure 6-8. Normal values for interpupillary distance at various ages. *(From Feingold M, Bossert WH: Normal values for selected physical parameters: An aid to syndrome delineation. Bergsma D (ed). White Plains, N.Y.: The National Foundation, BD:OAS X(13):1–16, 1974.)*

ment that goes through *medial* canthi and measuring the total length of the ear, the percentage of the ear above the horizontal line connecting medial canthi can be calculated. Lateral canthus is not used as a reference point because this may vary in children with mongolian and antimongoloid slants of the eyes. Nomograms have been constructed using this calculation. Whenever ears appear to be low-set, these nomograms should be used for accuracy, but one can get a clinical impression by observing the helix of the ears in relation to a horizontal line passing through the medial canthi. At least 20 percent of the total height of the ear should be above this line in normal children. It is good to remember that ears may *appear* to be low-set (when they are *not*) whenever the neck is short or the cranial vault is high or the mandibular ramus is short or the auricles are rotated.

There are no available definitions of a prominent ear. When the ear sticks out more than usual, it is called "prominent ear" and may be seen in syndromes associated with Trisomy-13 and Trisomy-8. Occasionally one sees loss of supporting structures, such as absence of the superior crus and the antihelix, resulting in a "lop ear." This may also be interpreted as prominent ear. Normally the ear makes an angle of about 10° with the mastoid. There are also nomograms for total ear length at various ages (Fig. 6-9).

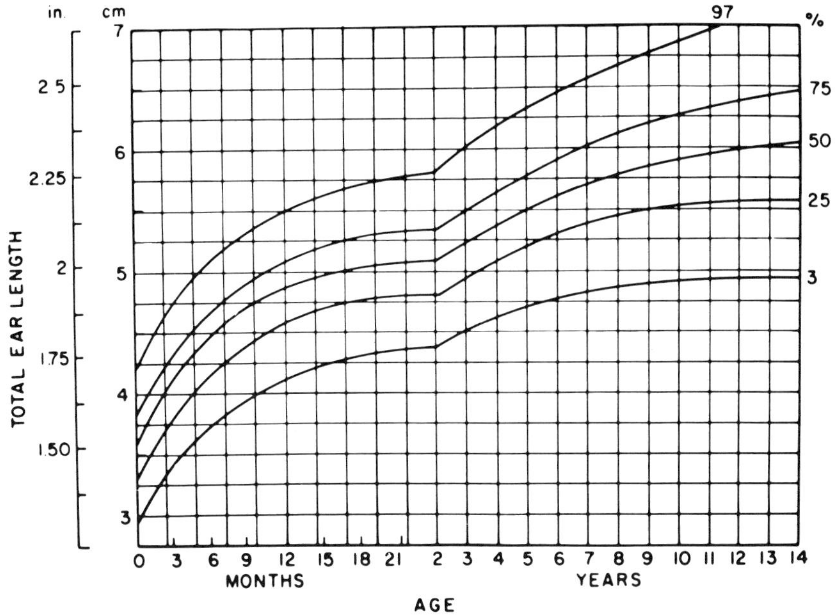

Figure 6-9. Ear length: normal values at various ages. *(From Feingold M, Bossert WH. Normal values for selected physical parameters: An aid to syndrome delineation. Bergsma D (ed). White Plains, N.Y. The National Foundation BD:OAS X(13):1–16, 1974.)* Total ear length is the distance between the most inferior and superior portions of the ear. Also refer to Figure 7A-6, page 109.

The shape of the *nose* gives clues to a number of syndromes. For example, the nose is unusually small or short in Apert syndrome and Trisomy-18 syndrome, and rather prominent in trichorhinophalangeal syndrome. The characteristics of the nose are determined by the length of the nasal bridge, height at the root of the nose, height of the septum, and the angle the septum makes to the coroneal plane of the face. For example, the root of the nose may be sunken (flat nasal bridge), as in achondroplasia or Down's syndrome, or broad, as in Trisomy-8 syndrome. The length may be long as a familial characteristic, in which case the septum makes a downward angle (as in Pfeiffer syndrome). In addition, the alae nasi may be well-formed or broad and flat bilaterally (as a familial or racial characteristic) or flat on one side (cleft palate).

The nasolabial distance (philtrum) is another part of the "facies" for which normal values for age are available.

There are certain other features of the facies that may suggest an abnormality to keen observers. For example, a vertical line drawn from the medial border of the pupil downward should touch the angles of the mouth. If the angle of the mouth lies lateral to this line the mouth is probably large (macrostomia) and if it lies medial the mouth is probably

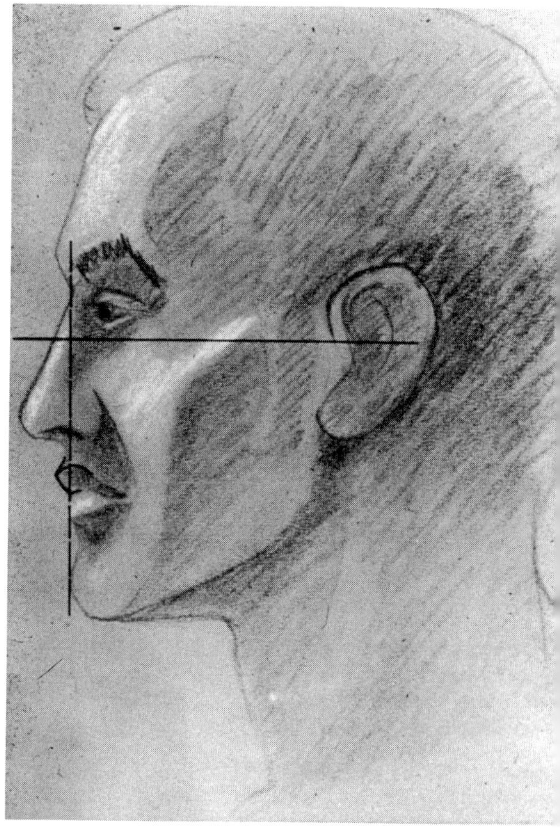

Figure 6-10. Idealized face in profile. Note the vertical line touching the lips and the chin. Also, note that the longitudinal axis of the ear is parallel to that of the bridge of the nose. (Courtesy of Dr. L. Whittaker.)

small (microstomia). A partially opened mouth in a child with nasal voice suggests adenoidal hypertrophy. When viewed in profile, a line drawn vertically from the glabella downward should touch the upper and lower lips and the chin. In cleft lip, the upper lip is behind the line. In micrognathia the chin is too far behind the line (Fig. 6-10).

Skin

The details of skin examination will be dealt with later in Chapter 7D. This section deals with observations that can be made during general evaluation of the patient. At this stage of the examination, one is interested to know whether the skin is pale, yellow, or cyanotic. It is good practice to look for eruptions early in the course of the examination. If an infectious disease is suspected, one can take precautions quickly before other children in the clinic or office get exposed.

At this time, look also for edema of the dependent parts—particularly over the anterior aspect of the leg and feet. Unilateral edema is seen in obstruction to venous flow. Bilateral edema denotes generalized disease such as heart failure, kidney disease, or hypoproteinemia. In a bedridden patient, the dependent part is the sacrum, not the legs. Edema of the scrotum signifies severe edema, as in nephrosis. The impressions made by socks and clothes on the body are good indicators of edema. Facial edema without edema elsewhere should indicate angioneurotic edema or thoracic outlet/superior vena cava obstruction. Presternal edema is seen in mumps.

If the neck and chin appear swollen, feel for crepitus, which signifies subcutaneous emphysema. Occasionally, if crepitus is not palpable, one can place the diaphragm of the stethoscope on the skin and press gently, eliciting a crackling noise.

Hand

During this period of general observation, the hand should be observed for clinical clues such as pallor and jaundice, which are noted on the palmar creases, and cyanosis, which is noted at the fingertips. Clubbing can be observed during this initial observation period. There have been many clinical descriptions of clubbing. The best clinical method is to look at the fingers from the side in profile (Fig. 6-11). The vertical height at the proximal edge of the nail (base) should be equal to or just less than the height at the distal interphalangeal joint in normal children. In true clubbing, the height at the base of the nail is taller than at the distal interphalangeal joint.

Another new sign described by a South African physician (Dr. L. Schamroth) on himself is elicited by apposing the dorsal surfaces of the terminal phalanges of corresponding fingers (Fig. 6-12). Normally, there is a diamond-shaped space at the base of the nail bed. In clubbing, the diamond-shaped space is lost.

Beaked nail also will appear clubbed, but the height at the proximal edge of the nail will not be taller than the height at the distal interphalangeal joint. In hyperparathyroidism, though the finger is described as clubbed, it is a rounded, spatulous finger—not a clubbed finger.

Tremor of the hands, flexion deformities, and unequal grip strength can be easily observed at this stage. Hand dominance can also be determined during this early stage by offering things and seeing which hand comes out first. If a child can write, give the child a paper and pencil and see how the paper and the pencil are held. Figure 6-13 shows the typical writing postures of left-handed individuals. Inverted position of left-handed writers is associated with an ipsilateral language hemisphere, and noninverted position denotes language control by the contralateral hemisphere.

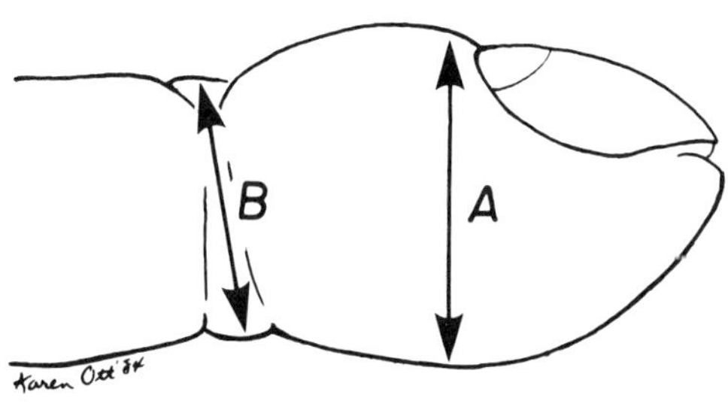

Figure 6-11. Clubbing of the finger. (A) Height at the base of the nail. (B) Height at the distal interphalangeal joint.

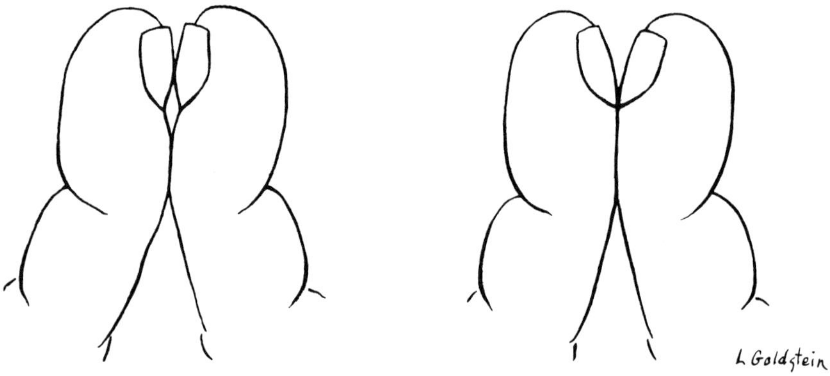

Figure 6-12. Schamroth sign for clubbing of fingers. The diamond-shaped space at the base of the nail bed, seen in normal fingers (*left*), is lost in the presence of clubbing (*right*).

Hip

Barlow's modification of Ortolani's maneuver is used to identify dislocated and dislocatable hips. This test should be done on all newborns and on all infants routinely.

How to Test for Congenital Dislocation of the Hip. Place the infant in the supine position on the examining table. Take a grip over the flexed hip with the thumb over the femoral triangle and the long middle finger over the greater trochanter (Fig. 6-14). Abduct the flexed thigh to midabduction position. (This may be difficult to do and unilateral limitation of abduction should suggest congenital dislocation of the hip.) When the thigh reaches the position of midabduction, press over the greater trochanter in a for-

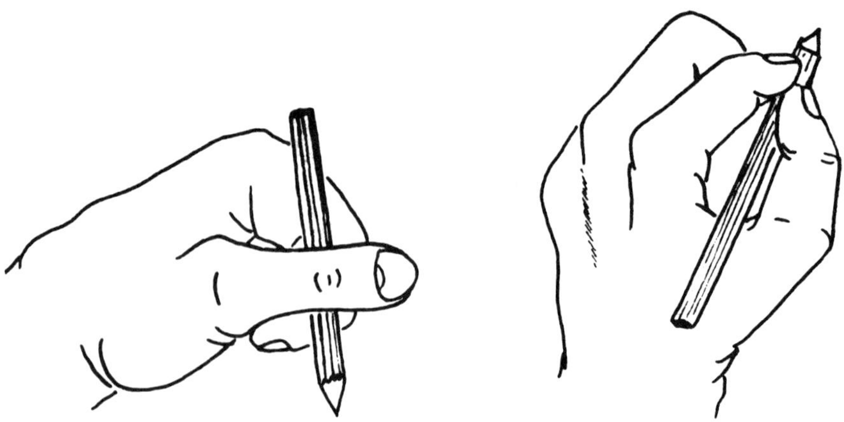

Figure 6-13. Writing postures of left-handed individuals.

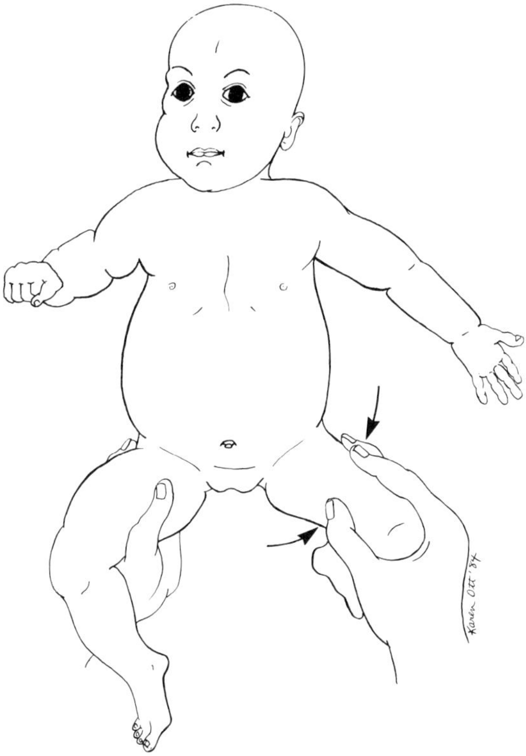

Figure 6-14. Examination of the hip for congenital dislocation. (See text for details.)

ward direction with the middle finger. If the femoral head moved anteriorly with this maneuver, it was out of place (dislocated) before pressure was applied.

If this portion of the test is negative, press gently with the thumb over the medial aspect of the thigh. If the femoral head moves out of the acetabulum with this pressure and returns back when the pressure is released, the hip is probably unstable. During this procedure, whenever the femoral head moves into or moves out of the acetabulum, or when the flexed hip is abducted and internally rotated, there may be a sudden "jerky" movement which can be felt by the examiner. This is called Ortolani's sign. This is different from the "click" that may be present even in normal hips of newborn infants.

In untreated congenital dislocation of the hip, there are many other physical findings: (1) The gluteal and thigh folds are asymmetric; (2) There is leg length discrepancy, with shortening of the affected limb; (3) There is limitation of abduction of the affected hip; (4) With the child supine, if the knee joints and the hips are flexed and the feet are held flat on the table, the knee on the affected side is at a lower level. This is called Allis sign (Fig. 6-15).

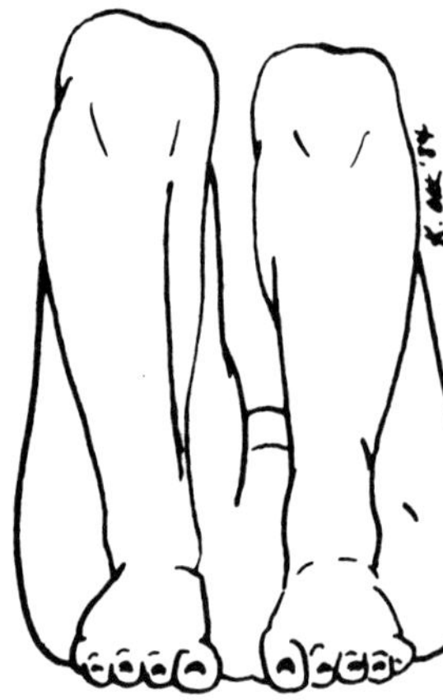

Figure 6-15. Allis sign. Note the lower level of the knee on the affected side.

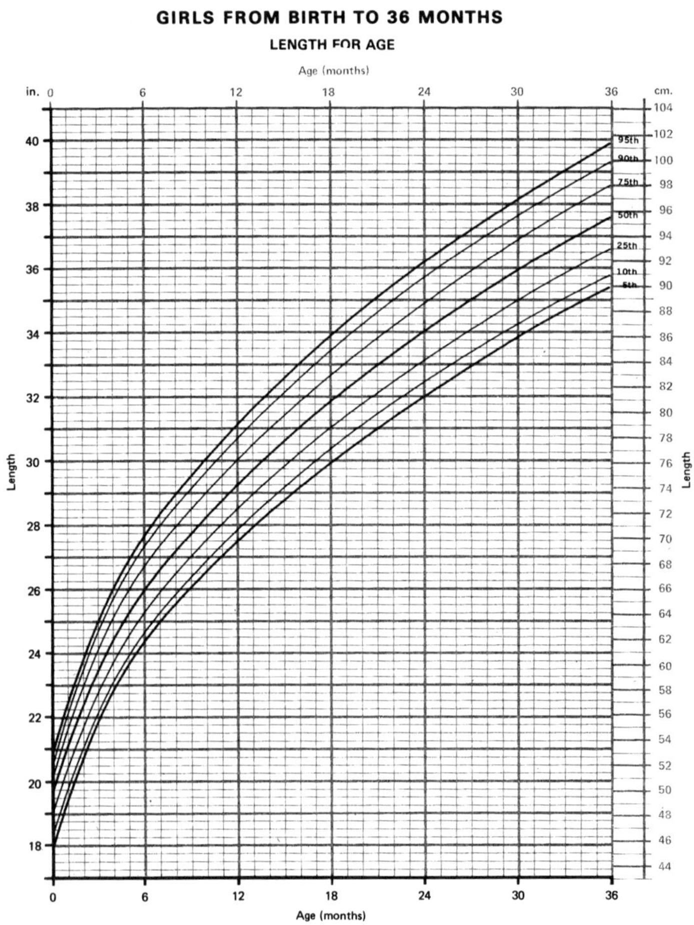

Figure 6-16. Girl's length in percentiles by age: from birth to 36 months.

MEASUREABLE OBSERVATIONS

Height

Height should be measured in infants and children below 3 years of age in a lying position (length) and in older children in a standing position (stature). The most important point to remember is the proper stance and position of the child: feet together, back straight, (occiput, back, and heels touching the measuring rod), eyes looking straight ahead so that a line joining the external auditory meatus to the lower border of the eye socket is parallel to the floor. When measuring height in the supine position, the feet are held against a fixed footpiece at 0 mark and a movable headpiece is brought to touch gently against the vertex. For measurement of standing height, the headpiece is brought to touch the vertex after asking the child to pull in the abdomen, stand as straight as possible, and stretch the neck.

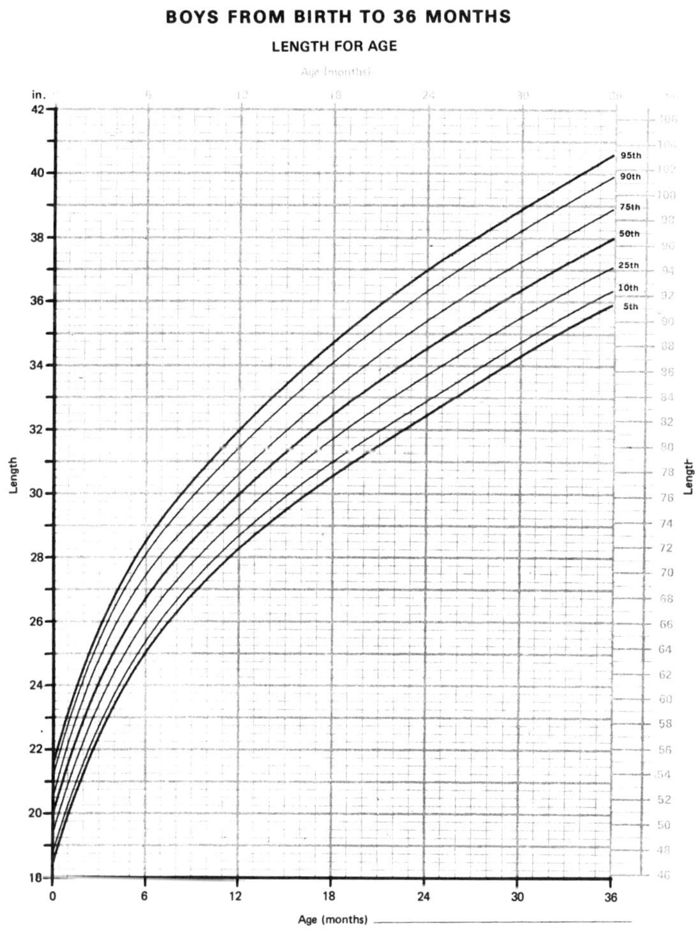

Figure 6-17. Boy's length in percentiles by age: from birth to 36 months.

The readings are recorded to the nearest 1 cm. Normal values for height in American children are given in Figures 6-16 to 6-19.

Weight

Weight is preferably taken on the same scale at the same time of the day (before breakfast) with minimal clothing. Weight should be taken to the nearest 10 gm in infants and to the nearest 100 gm in older children. The scale should be checked for accuracy by using standard weight every 3 to 6 months. When accurate follow-up is essential, as in heart failure or in estimating dehydration, attention should be paid to all details. For routine evaluation, one need not be this compulsive.

Normal values for weight in American children are given in Figures 6-20 to 6-23. A growth chart, for home use and for primary care centers,

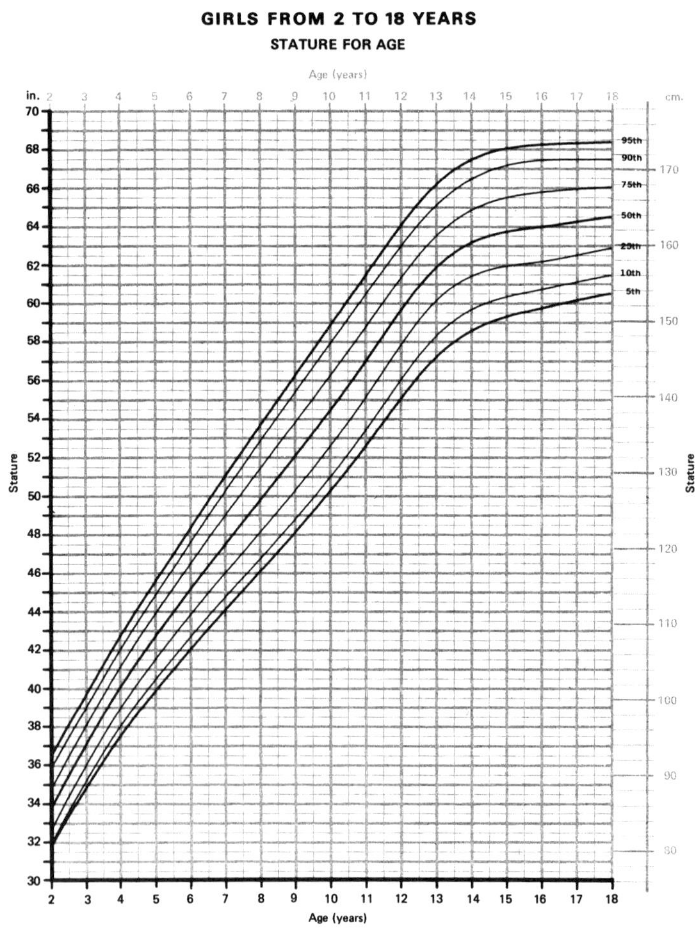

Figure 6-18. Girl's stature in percentiles by age: age 2 to 18 years.

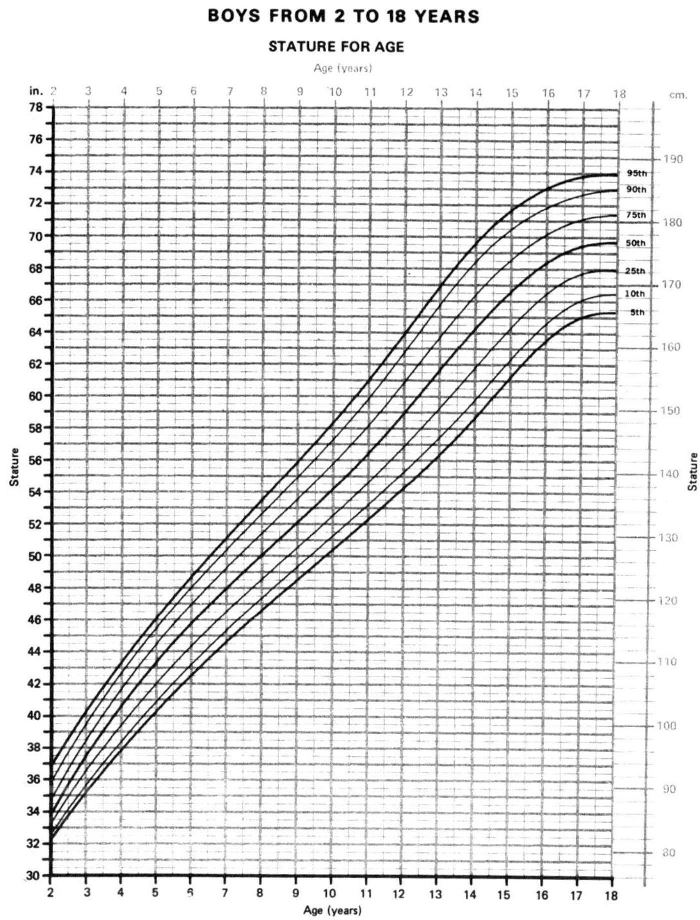

Figure 6-19. Boy's stature in percentiles by age: age 2 to 18 years.

which can be modified to the needs of the country, has been developed by the World Health Organization ("A Growth Chart for International Use in Maternal and Child Health Care." World Health Organization, Geneva 1978).

Head Circumference

Head circumference is measured at the maximum point of occipital protuberance posteriorly and at a point 1 inch above the glabella anteriorly.*

*It is important to note that data on head circumference published in earlier texts are based on measurements with the tape passing over the glabella anteriorly and maximum point of occipital protuberance posteriorly.

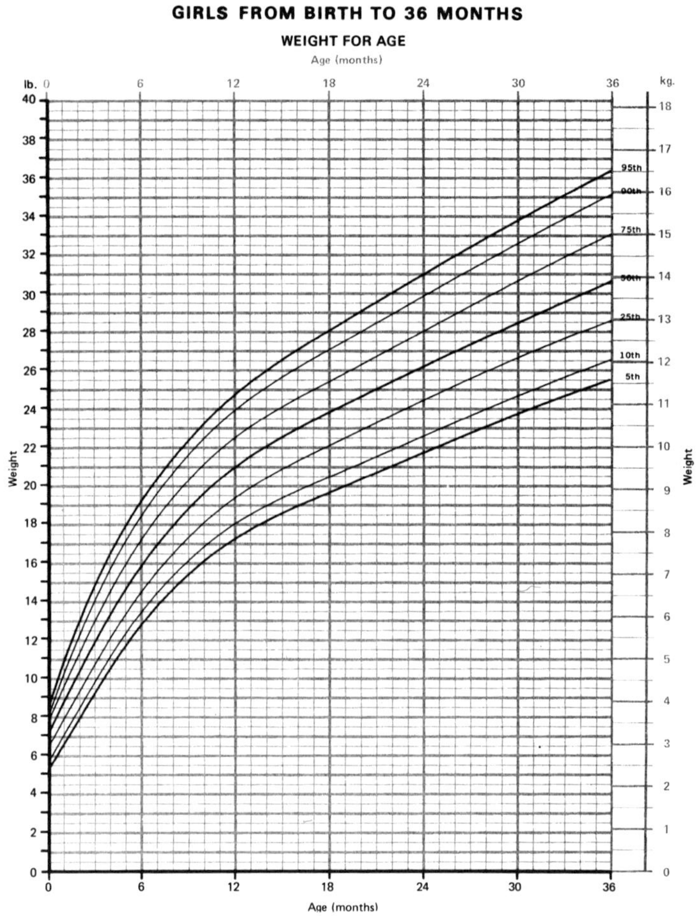

Figure 6-20. Girl's weight in percentiles by age: from birth to 36 months.

Cloth tape is safer to use in uncooperative children but stretches easily. The cloth tape, therefore, should be periodically verified for accuracy by comparing with a steel tape. Normal values for head circumference in boys and girls in the United States are given in Figures 6-24 and 6-25.

Chest Circumference

Chest circumference is measured at the level of the substernal notch in midinspiration. Normally at birth, head circumference is larger than chest circumference and remains so until 6 months of age. Later, chest circumference is larger than that of the head, except in the presence of malnutrition. However, in the presence of malnutrition, head circumference and chest circumference do not become equal until the first birthday. (The

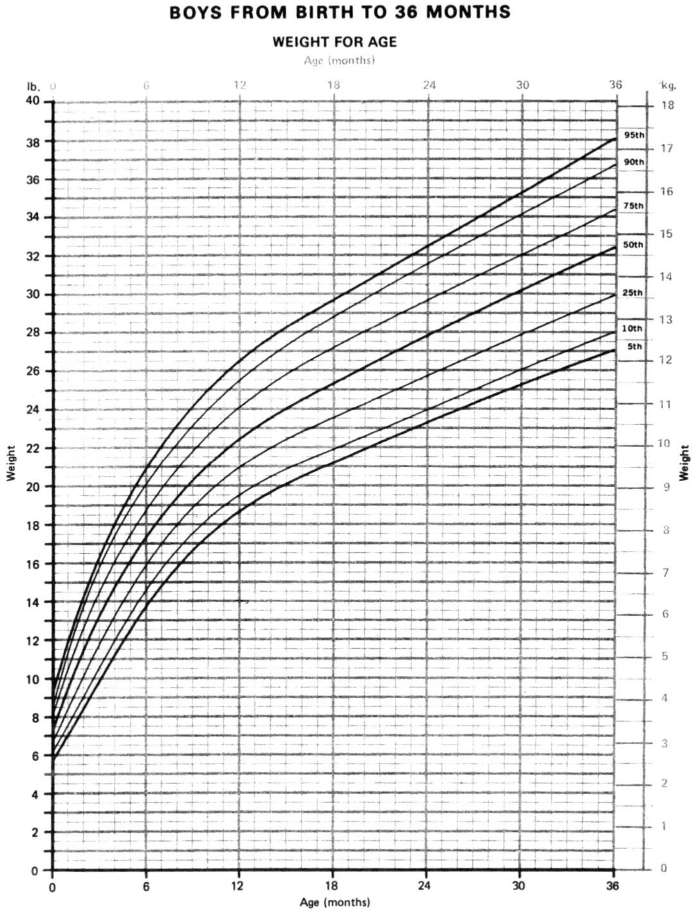

Figure 6-21. Boy's weight in percentiles by age: from birth to 36 months.

method for measuring chest expansion will be described in the section on examination of the chest, page 126.)

Other Measurements

1. *Arm span* is measured from the tip of the middle finger of one hand to that of the other hand with both shoulders abducted to 90° and palms supinated. Normally arm span equals total height. (Arm span significantly less than total height indicates various kinds of dysplasia affecting long bones.)
2. *Sitting height* versus standing height: Sitting height is measured as described under the section on height (page 75), except the child

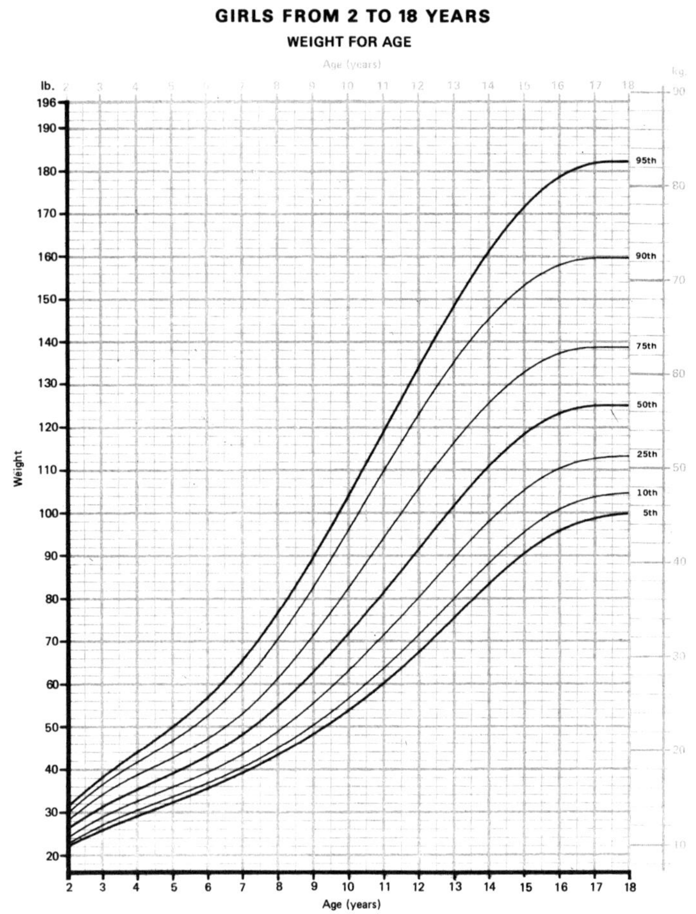

Figure 6-22. Girl's weight in percentiles by age: age 2 to 18 years.

is sitting close to the scale. Normally in a newborn, sitting height is approximately 70 percent of the total length. By age 3, it is only 57 percent of total height and at puberty it is 52 percent of total height.

3. *Skin-fold thickness* is a superior method for assessment of obesity, compared to weight for height or weight for age. There are three varieties of calipers available for skin-fold measurement (Lange, USA; Harpenden, England; and a plastic model). The inexpensive plastic model will be adequate to identify children with obesity in an ambulatory care setting. Measurements of skin-fold thickness over the posterior aspect of the upper arm and over the subscapular area give indications of varying distribution of fat in the limbs and in the trunk.

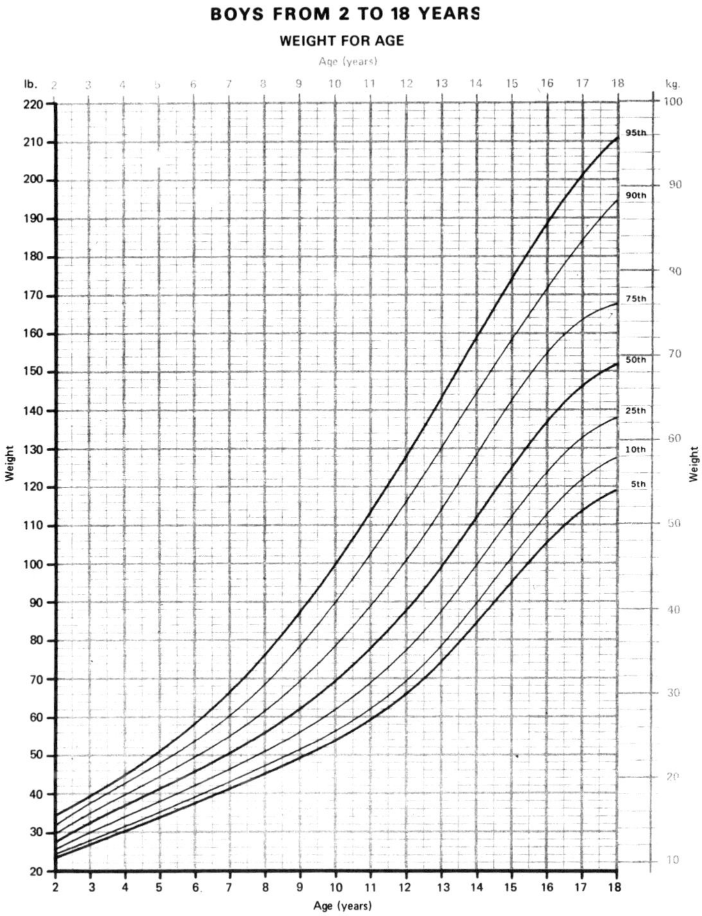

Figure 6-23. Boy's weight in percentiles by age: age 2 to 18 years

The accepted area for measurement is over the left triceps. With the elbow in 90° flexion, a horizontal mark is made at a point midway between the tip of the acromion process and the tip of the olecranon process. With the arm now hanging at the side of the body, a vertical line is placed to cross the horizontal line indicating the midpoint. A piece of skin just 1 cm proximal to the marked cross is pinched between the left thumb and index finger, and the caliper is used to measure the thickness of fat. Normal values for skin-fold thickness are given in Table 6-3.

4. *Muscle Bulk* is estimated by measurement of mid-upper arm circumference and is very useful in following children with malnutrition on treatment, combined with measurement of skin-fold thickness (which measures fat). Mid-upper arm circumference may help

determine the proportion of fat to muscle. The area to be measured is marked as described in the section on skin-fold thickness. With the arm hanging by the side, a steel tape is passed around the circumference of the arm (the tape should not be held tight enough to produce an indentation) and the measurement noted in centimeters.

Temperature

In 1868, Carl Reinhold August Wunderlich established firmly that body temperature is constant in healthy persons, and variation in temperature is evidence of a disease process. Before this time, fever itself was considered a disease. Dr. Wunderlich established the following norms: Temperatures below 36.6° (97.7°F) are considered subnormal; temperatures between 36.6° (97.7°F) to 37.4° (99.4°F) are considered normal; temperatures between 37.5° to 38°C (99.5° to 100.4°F) are considered subfebrile. Fever is considered to be present if the temperature is over 38°C (100.4°F); it is considered high fever if the temperature is over 39.5°C (103.1°F), and hyperpyrexia if the temperature is over 42°C (107.6°F). These values still hold today.

Three different thermometers are available for routine use in children: oral, rectal, and electronic. The oral thermometer has a long mercury section and a blue tip for identification. The bulb of the rectal thermometer is round, and there is a red identification on the tip. Electronic thermometers give a digital read-out of temperature. In very active and frightened children, trying to put a glass instrument into the rectum can be a traumatic experience and can be dangerous. There are reports of broken thermometers with rectal perforation. One therefore has to be cautious in the use of rectal thermometers. Generally, oral temperature cannot be taken in children who are young and cannot understand instructions. Therefore, most of the time, axillary temperatures are safest and equally efficient. If axillary temperature is to be taken, remember to hold the thermometer long enough (2 minutes at least in proper position) and to know that axillary temperature is at least 0.5°C lower than the oral temperature.

There are three classical patterns of fever: (1) continuous fever when daily fluctuations do not exceed 1°C (1.5°F); (2) remittent fever when daily fluctuations exceed 2°C but never touch normal; (3) intermittent fever when the temperature touches normal for several hours in a day. The intermittent fever is called quotidian if it occurs daily (as in juvenile rheumatoid arthritis—JRA), tertian if it occurs every other day (malaria), and quartan when it occurs every third day (malaria).

Daily rise of temperature in the evening is seen in tuberculosis and JRA. In JRA, the temperature returns to normal and actually goes subnormal the next morning. Double rise of temperature is also seen in JRA and typhoid fever, but in typhoid it does not reach normal at its low point.

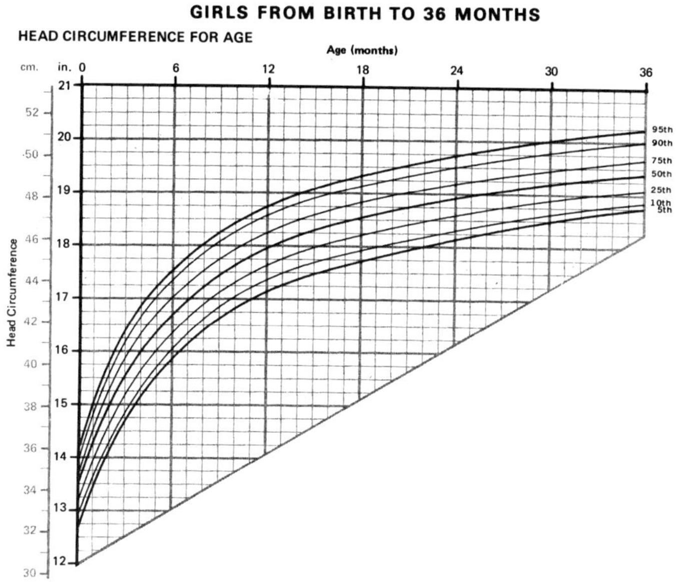

Figure 6-24. Girl's head circumference in percentiles: from birth to 36 months.

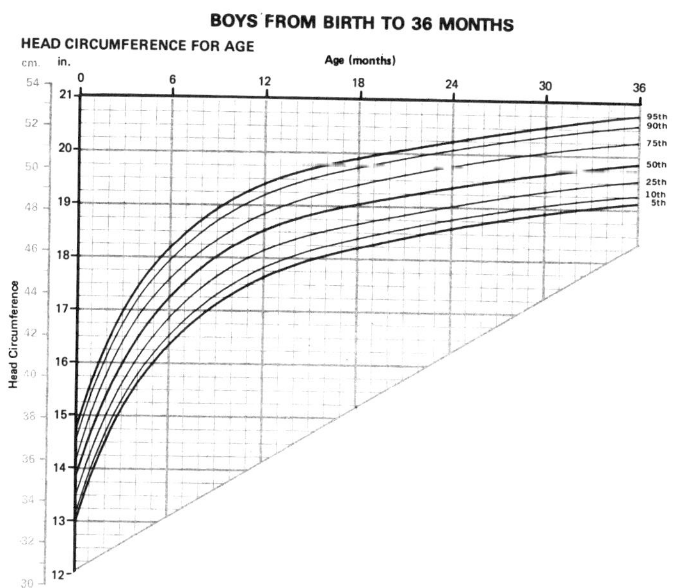

Figure 6-25. Boy's head circumference in percentiles: from birth to 36 months.

TABLE 6-3. TRICEPS FATFOLD PERCENTILES FOR WHITES AND BLACKS

Midpoint Age (yrs)	No.	Percentile Values 5	15	50	85	95	No.	Percentile Values 5	15	50	85	95
				White Males						*White Females*		
1	138	5	7	9	13	15	175	6	7	9	12	15
2	173	5	7	10	13	14	166	6	7	10	13	15
3	209	6	7	9	12	14	163	6	7	10	12	14
4	206	5	6	9	12	14	215	5	7	10	12	14
5	259	5	6	8	12	16	231	6	7	10	13	16
6	263	5	6	8	11	15	255	6	7	10	12	15
7	310	5	6	8	11	14	272	6	7	10	13	17
8	301	5	6	8	12	17	266	6	7	10	15	19
9	285	5	6	9	14	19	282	6	7	11	17	24
10	313	5	6	10	16	22	275	6	8	12	19	24
11	292	6	7	10	17	25	267	7	8	12	20	29
12	293	5	7	11	19	26	267	6	9	13	20	25
13	265	5	6	10	18	25	227	7	9	14	23	30
14	206	5	6	10	17	22	183	8	10	15	22	28
15	179	4	6	9	19	26	197	8	11	16	24	30
16	163	4	5	9	20	27	186	8	10	15	23	27
17	141	4	5	8	14	20	141	9	12	16	26	31
				Black Males						*Black Females*		
1	161	5	6	9	13	15	147	6	7	9	12	15
2	175	6	7	9	13	16	212	5	6	9	13	15
3	217	6	7	9	12	15	188	5	6	9	12	15
4	261	5	6	8	12	14	219	5	6	8	12	13
5	247	4	5	7	11	13	264	5	6	8	11	14
6	265	4	5	7	10	13	271	4	5	8	12	14
7	266	4	5	7	10	13	304	5	6	8	13	15
8	250	3	4	7	10	15	270	5	6	8	13	17
9	290	3	4	7	12	18	283	5	6	9	15	22
10	252	4	5	7	12	17	276	4	6	10	15	21
11	239	4	5	8	15	20	279	5	6	11	18	28
12	266	4	5	8	14	21	272	6	7	11	19	24
13	226	4	5	8	16	26	266	5	7	11	21	27
14	233	3	4	7	15	24	236	6	8	14	24	31
15	190	4	4	7	15	23	206	7	9	14	22	28
16	163	4	4	7	14	19	203	6	9	14	22	27
17	112	3	5	8	13	16	146	7	8	15	23	31

(Modified with permission from Garn S, Clark DC: Trends in fatness and the origins of obesity. Pediatrics 57:444, 1976. Copyright American Academy of Pediatrics, 1976.)

Fever with chills is seen in all infectious processes but one particularly likes to remember urinary tract infections, tuberculosis, and malaria.

Pulse

Sir John Floyer invented a watch with a second hand and published his article on "Physician's Pulse Watch" in 1707. Though it is a basic step in physical examination, some of the mysticism in taking the pulse and the psychologic advantages to the patient by the touch of the physician are lost with all the newer developments in electronic measurement.

The data to be collected while taking the pulse are: (1) rate; (2) rhythm; (3) volume; (4) tension. Normal pulse rates for various ages are given in Table 6-4.

The rhythm is either regular or irregular. If it is regular, it does not necessarily mean everything is fine with the heart. Actually, it is a good practice to always listen to the heart when counting the pulse to appreciate some missed beats. One can have an arrhythmia in which every other beat is not carried to the periphery as a pulse, so that the pulse rate is 50 percent of the heart rate. Thus, a regular rhythm may be perceived peripherally, even though a serious arrhythmia exists.

Sinus arrythmia is characterized by a rapid pulse during inspiration and a slower pulse during expiration. This is normal. A regularly irregular pulse may be observed when there are extra systoles at fixed intervals (every fifth beat or tenth beat). Irregularly irregular pulse is seen most often in auricular fibrillation.

Volume of the pulse is appreciated by the lift of the fingers as the pulse wave passes through. It is a composite of the force with which the fingers are lifted and the duration for which the force is maintained. Large volume pulse is seen in fever, thyrotoxicosis, anemia, patent ductus, and aortic regurgitation. Small volume pulse is seen in shock and aortic stenosis.

One can estimate tension by noting the intensity of pressure required

TABLE 6-4. NORMAL PULSE RATE

Age	Pulse Rate/Minute (Range)
Newborn	70–170
Up to 1 year	80–160
2 years	80–130
4 years	80–120
6 years	75–115
8 to 10 years	70–110
Adolescent years	65–110
18 years and over	55–95

to obliterate the pulse, but it is an unnecessary procedure to do. Measurement of blood pressure is more exact and will be dealt with later.

Certain types of pulse are diagnostically important:

1. *Sinus arrhythmia:* Pulse rate which gets fast with inspiration and slow with expiration is normal.
2. *Collapsing pulse* is best felt with the arm raised above the head and the pulse felt by the examiner's palmar aspect of the proximal interphalangeal joints. This type of pulse is felt in patent ductus and aortic regurgitation. Another method of feeling for collapsing pulse is to feel the superficial palmar arch as it crosses the metacarpal heads. Forceful pulsation of this arch is uncommon in infants below 2 years of age and if present, in the absence of fever and anemia, indicates patent ductus.
3. *Pulsus paradoxus* is said to be present when the pulse volume gets lower and even disappears at the end of inspiration. The presence of pulsus paradoxus is best confirmed by listening to the Korotkoff sounds, while measuring blood pressure during inspiration and expiration. A difference of over 10 mm between systolic pressure obtained during inspiration and systolic pressure obtained during expiration indicates the presence of pulsus paradoxus. If pulsus paradoxus is present, the differential diagnosis should include pericardial effusion and severe airway obstruction, as in bronchial asthma.

   After feeling the radial artery, one should also feel the pulse in the temporal arteries, femoral arteries, and dorsalis pedis during this examination.

How to Feel for the Femoral Pulse. The femoral pulse is felt at a point midway between the symphysis pubis and anterior superior iliac spine along the inguinal ligament. One should feel the radial artery while feeling the femoral artery. Strong arm pulses together with a delay between the pulse in the upper and lower limbs or a higher volume of the pulse in the upper limbs should indicate coarctation of the aorta.

Another simple method for suspecting coarctation of the aorta is to have the child lie prone, flex the knee joints, and place the palms of the patient's hands close to the feet. In the presence of coarctation of aorta, the pale color of the feet will contrast markedly with the normal colored palms.

Blood Pressure

With increasing knowledge of blood pressure control in adults, proper recording, follow-up investigation, and control of hypertension in children takes on increasing importance. However, this is an often neglected portion of the physical examination of children.

There are different types of instruments to measure blood pressure. Accurate systolic measurements can be obtained using Doppler instruments. Mercury or aneroid variety of sphygmomanometers are the commonly used instruments in clinical practice. A sphygmomanometer with a mercury column is the most accepted instrument.

To obtain a proper blood pressure recording in older children, blood pressure cuffs of the following sizes are available: 3 cm, 5 cm, 8 cm, 12 cm, and 18 cm. The 18-cm cuff is for recording pressures in the lower limb and for obese adolescents. The American Heart Association recommends that for adults, the inflatable bag of the cuff be 20 percent wider than the diameter of the limb on which it is used. This rule should be applied to children also. A narrower cuff will give spuriously high blood pressure and a broader cuff will give a lower blood pressure.

Other points to observe in taking blood pressure (BP) are:

1. Mercury type manometers are superior to the aneroid variety.
2. If an aneroid manometer is used, it should be checked for accuracy against a properly functioning mercury manometer.
3. The mercury manometer should be checked for leaking and zero line.
4. The patient preferably should be relaxed and lying down—not tense, crying, and agitated. Therefore, it is often hard to get reliable BP on infants and frightened children.
5. The mercury column should be vertical and the blood pressure reading read at the observer's eye level to avoid parallax error.
6. The cuff should be wrapped snugly around the limb with enough space at the antecubital fossa or popliteal fossa for the stethoscope.
7. Before auscultating for the blood pressure, it is a good habit to first estimate systolic blood pressure by palpation. This relaxes the child. One also gets an idea of how high one has to inflate the bag.
8. Systolic pressure in the lower limb is normally 10 to 40 mm higher than in the upper limb, but the diastolic pressure is the same.
9. In the presence of dyspnea and arrhythmia, the readings at which the sounds disappear should be recorded for both the stronger sound and the weaker sound.

For recording blood pressure, inflate the cuff rapidly for about 10 to 20 mm Hg above the point at which the pulse in the radial artery disappears. Place the stethoscope over the brachial artery. Slowly release the pressure (2 to 4 mm Hg per heart beat), while listening until the first sound (Korotkoff sound) is heard. This point, at which the first sound is heard, is the systolic pressure. Now continue to slowly release the pressure. As the pressure is lowered, the sound suddenly becomes faint or muffled and finally ceases. Diastolic pressure is best measured at the point of complete disappearance of the sound. Normal values are given in Figures 6-26 and 6-27. The techniques of measurement of blood pressure in the newborn are discussed in Chapter 9 (page 293).

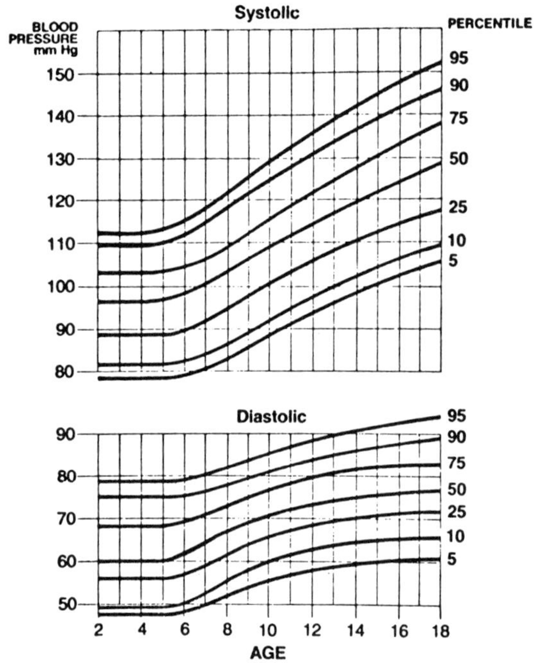

Figure 6-26. Percentiles of blood pressure measurement in boys (right arm, seated). *(Reproduced with permission from Pediatrics 59(5) (Suppl 2):803, 1977. Copyright American Academy of Pediatrics, 1977.)*

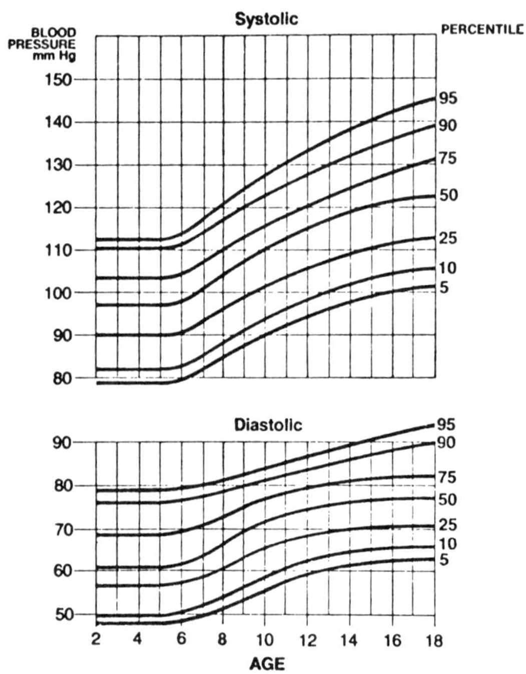

Figure 6-27. Percentiles of blood pressure measurement in girls (right arm, seated). *(Reproduced with permission from Pediatrics 59(5) (Suppl 2):803, 1977. Copyright American Academy of Pediatrics 1977.)*

TABLE 6-5. NORMAL RESPIRATORY RATE IN CHILDREN

Age	Respirations/Minute
Newborn	30–50
1 to 6 months	20–30
6 months to 2 years	20–30
Adolescent	12–20

Respiration

Count the respiration for a full minute when the child has been at rest for a few minutes or while sleeping. Normal rates are given in Table 6-5.

The other characteristics of respiration to be noted are: *rhythm, depth, positions of discomfort,* and *adventitious sounds.*

Alternate periods of deep and shallow respiration with recurring periods of apnea occur in left ventricular failure and in cerebral edema. This is called Cheyne-Stokes respiration. Biot breathing is characterized by periods of apnea alternating with four or five breaths of normal depth. This type of breathing is seen in association with intracranial pressure. Respiratory rhythm in the neonate is discussed in Chapter 9.

Rapid, deep respiration is seen in metabolic acidosis (salicylate overdose, diabetes). This is also called Kussmaul breathing. Shallow respiration is seen in narcotic overdosage and shock.

Orthopnea is indicative of pulmonary edema. An asthmatic child likes to sit up at the edge of the bed and lean forward with the palms on either side. The child with pleurisy or a fractured rib splints the side of involvement. This child feels more comfortable lying on the involved side. In the presence of massive effusion, the discomfort is increased if the child is made to lie on the opposite (uninvolved) side.

Adventitious sounds audible even without a stethoscope are due to pathology in the upper airway. (The only exception is the wheezing sound of an asthmatic.) The sniffling sounds of nasal obstruction, snoring noise of soft palate weakness, the rattling sound of mucus in the trachea, and the crowing inspiratory stridor of laryngeal obstruction are examples of this. Two interesting points to note are: (1) all noises due to upper airway problems are inspiratory noises, and (2) children with upper airway obstruction cannot appose the alae nasi to the midline cartilage by deep inspiration.

BIBLIOGRAPHY

Berger LR: The Winnicott squiggle game: A vehicle for communicating with the school-age child. *Pediatrics* 66:921–924, 1980.

Beveridge WIB: The Art of Scientific Investigation, 3rd ed. London, Heinemann, 1957, pp 48–52.

Blake F, Wright FH, Waechter EH: Nursing Care of Children, 8th ed. Philadelphia, Lippincott, 1970, p 442.

Clendening, L: Source Book of Medical History. New York, Dover, 1942, p 575.

Engel GL: Are medical schools neglecting clinical skills? An editorial. JAMA 236:861–863, 1976.

Garn S, Clark DC: Trends in fatness and the origin of obesity. Report of the Ad Hoc Committee to Review the Ten-State Nutrition Survey. Pediatrics 57:443–456, 1976.

Hall M: Principles of Diagnosis, 2nd ed. New York, D. Appleton, 1835, p 54.

Ingle DJ: Is It Really So? A Guide to Clear Thinking, 1st ed. Philadelphia, Westminster Press, 1976, pp 90–129.

Johnson CF: Diagnosing obscure syndromes: From professor to television to computer scan. Clin Pediatr 15:188–196, 1976.

Jung E, Mason Kauffman JJ, Narens D, Kaufman GE: Skin fold measurements in children: A comparison of Lange and McGaw calipers. Clin Pediatr 23:25–28, 1984.

Kreiger I, Sargent D: A postural sign in the sensory deprivation syndrome in infants. J Pediatr 70:332–339, 1967.

Lampe RM, Kagan A: Detection of clubbing: Schamroth's sign. Clin Pediatr 22:125, 1983.

Levy J, Reid M: Variations in writing posture and cerebral organization. Science. 194:337–339, 1976.

Mace JW, Goodman SI, Centerwall WR, Chinnock, RF: The child with an unusual odor: A clinical resume. Clin Pediatr 15:57–62, 1976.

McLaughlin G, Kirby RR, Kemmerer NT, DeLamos, RA: Indirect measurement of blood pressure in infants using Doppler ultra-sound. J Pediatr 79:300–303, 1971.

Park MK, Kawalion I, Gutheroth WG: Need for improved standard for blood pressure cuff size. Clin Pediatr 15:784–787, 1976.

Redlener I: Recognizing serious illness in small children. Hospital physician 8:42–43, 1972.

Robinow M, Roches AF: Low-set ears. Am J Dis Child 125:482–483, 1973.

Stoner EK: Evaluation of the Amputee. In Krusen FH, Kottke FJ, Ellwood PM (eds): Handbook of Physical Medicine and Rehabilitation, 2nd ed. Philadelphia, Saunders, 1971, pp 92–95.

Stuckey D: Palmar pulsation: A physical sign of patent ductus arteriosus in infancy. Med J Aust 2:681–682, 1957.

Weiner S, Nathanson M: Physical examination: Frequently observed errors. JAMA 236:852–855, 1976.

Zerfas AJ, Shorr IJ, and Neumann CG: Office assessment of nutritional status. Pediatr Clin North Am 24:253–272, 1977.

CHAPTER 7

Regional and System Physical Examination

7A. Head, Neck, and Sensory Organs

In this chapter, we deal with examination of the head and neck, and include the sensory organs. The sequence will follow the list given in Tables 2-1 and 2-2 on pages 8–11 in Chapter 2, "Defining Normality." Whenever appropriate, a list of characteristics that define normality for the organ or function under discussion will be given and will be followed by a description of the abnormalities to be looked for.

HEAD

Description of a normal head requires that the following descriptors be included:

- Size
  - Actual measurement (circumference)
  - Rate of growth
- Shape
- Abnormal swelling (extra growth)
- Abnormal depressions (continuity)
- Fontanels
  - Percussion
  - Auscultation
  - Transillumination

Size

The technique of measurement of head circumference is given on page 77. Normal values for various age groups given in Figures 6-24 and 6-25 (see page 82) should help determine whether the head size is normal or abnormal.

Abnormalities in the size of the head can be related to the *actual measurement* at the time of examination or to the *rate of growth.* The size (head circumference) can be large (macrocephaly) or small (microcephaly) and this can be determined by plotting the measurement in Figure 6-24 or Figure 6-25.

The rate of growth is another important factor, particularly in the first 5 years of life. Therefore, in addition to looking at the actual measurement at any one time, these measurements should be plotted in the graph and any unduly rapid growth in head circumference (as is seen in hydrocephalus) or lack of growth (as seen in craniostenosis) should be noted. This is particularly important in the first 2 years of life, since the brain reaches 50 percent of the adult size by 9 months of age and 75 percent of adult size by 2 years.

Shape

The various abnormal shapes may be described under three headings: flattened, prominent, and specific shapes. Flat occiput or parietal region may be seen in children who lie in one position for prolonged periods, as in children with mental retardation, and in severe muscle weaknesses. Prominent occiput may be seen in Dandy-Walker syndrome and Trisomy-18. Frontal bossing is seen in rickets, Crouzon disease, and Hurler syndrome. Biparietal bossing may indicate subdural hematoma. Some of the abnormalities of shape of the head with descriptive names are: oxycephaly (tower head) which is caused by premature closure of all the sutures resulting in the growth of the head in the region of the anterior fontanel as seen in Apert syndrome; turricephaly in which the top of the head is pointed; brachycephaly which is a short, wide, broad forehead as seen in Down's syndrome; plagiocephaly (one side rounded more than the other) due to unequal closure of cranial sutures as in craniostenosis; trigonocephaly in which the metopic suture is pointed (hyperphosphatasia—osteoectasia syndrome); scaphocephaly in which the head is elongated in the anteroposterior direction when seen in profile, as found in some normal children, in craniostenosis, and in certain syndromes (Soto).

Abnormal Swelling

Next, palpate for abnormal swelling (extra growth) which may be congenital (dermoid); traumatic, such as hematoma (both in newborn and in older children after trauma); infectious, such as abscess, or tumors. These conditions should be described using the standard descriptors for swellings: location, size, shape, characteristics of the margin and of the surface, consistency, color, heat, tenderness, pulsation (or absence of it), and attachment of the swelling to deeper and surrounding structures.

Abnormal Depressions

Next, one should look for depressions and defects (continuity) in the skull which may be abnormal (as in fracture) or normal (as in fontanel).

Fontanels

There are six fontanels at birth, each of which may or may not be palpable (Fig. 7A-1). The two most important are the anterior and posterior fontanels. The anterior fontanel usually measures 2.5 cm at 3 months of age. The size then diminishes, and the fontanel gets filled. Most anterior fontanels close between 9 to 18 months of age. In some normal infants, anterior fontanels may close as early as 4 to 5 months of age. Boys seem to have earlier closure than girls. The posterior fontanel is small even at birth (usually the size of a finger tip) and closes rapidly by 2 months of age.

The *characteristics of fontanels* to be described are: size, age at closure, fullness, and pulsation. Normal *size* has been described in the previous paragraph. An anterior fontanel that seems to *close too early* (before 4 months) is not abnormal per se, if the head circumference grows normally. In microcephaly and craniostenosis, the fontanel may be small or close early. The fontanels are of larger than normal dimension, or remain open for abnormally longer periods, in conditions such as hypothyroidism, hydrocephalus, rickets, and Trisomy-18 syndrome. An abnormally full, tense and elevated fontanel signifies increased intracranial pressure, whereas a depressed fontanel in a child with diarrhea and vomiting is a good indicator of severity of dehydration. Normally, the anterior fontanel is pulsatile,

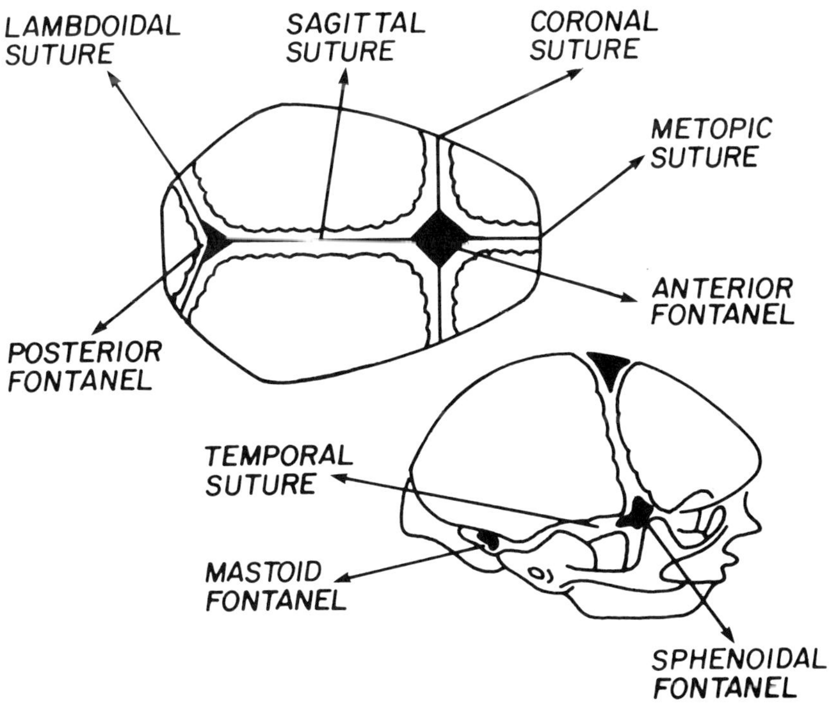

Figure 7A-1. Position of fontanels and cranial sutures.

but absence of *pulsation* may be normal. In the presence of increased intracranial tension, the fontanel may be tense without pulsations.

Additional Procedures

The next step in the examination of the head is to palpate the *mastoid bones* behind the ears. Normally, these bones are not well developed until the child is 2 or 3 years of age. Palpate for swelling, heat, and tenderness (evidences of mastoiditis). Remember also that the skull can be collapsed like a table tennis ball behind the ears in rickets.

Examine for characteristics of the *cranial sutures* (Fig. 7A-1). The sutures normally tend to overlap during the newborn period due to intrauterine molding. In some older children, some of the suture lines may appear prominent (particularly the metopic suture). On palpation, the suture line should not be palpable after 6 months of age. Unusually wide suture lines after 5 to 6 months of age may indicate a disease process such as hydrocephalus.

Three other procedures to be completed during the examination of the head are percussion, auscultation, and transillumination.

Percussion. In children with increased intracranial pressure and closed fontanels, percussion of the skull with a finger may produce a resonant sound. It is called Macewen's sign.

Auscultation. Auscultation of the skull, particularly over the occipital and frontal region may be of value in infants with congestive heart failure of unknown etiology. Cranial bruit has been described in association with A-V fistula or aneurysms of cerebral vessels, brain tumors, and coarctation of the aorta. However, cranial bruit is very common even in normal children, particularly in the very young. Therefore, routine auscultation of the skull is not necessary.

Transillumination. Transillumination of the skull should be performed in children with suspected subdural hematoma, hydrocephalus, and poor growth of the brain. The examination should be conducted in a dark room. A special ring is fitted to a flashlight,* and the ring is applied firmly against the scalp. The flashlight should be moved to examine the back, the side, and the front. Normally a small ring of light is seen around the rubber attachment. If the ring of light is over 0.5 cm wide, it denotes abnormality (e.g., subdural hematoma). In anencephaly and hydrocephalus, light may be transmitted directly across to the opposite side.

SCALP

When examining the head, examine the scalp for *abnormalities of the skin* under the following headings: (1) congenital defects, (2) congenital masses,

*Transdapter cuff for a flashlight may be obtained from Medical Department, Ross Laboratories, Columbus, Ohio 43216.

such as hemangioma, (3) infection such as folliculitis and abscess; and *scalp hair abnormalities.*

The scalp hair can give many clues to diagnosis. The characteristics of hair to be observed are:

- Quantity (generalized increase, localized increase, generalized decrease, localized decrease)
- Color
- Texture
- Surface characteristics (straight, curled, or beaded)
- Strength (brittle)
- Pattern of distribution/parietal whorl

Quantity

The *quantity of body hair* may be increased (hypertrichosis) in Cushing syndrome, in deLange syndrome, and many other conditions described on page 175. Scalp hair does not observably increase abnormally in quantity, but facial hair may be more than usual in prematures, in steroid toxicity, in porphyria cutanea tarda, and in various syndromes such as deLange and Hurler. There may be sparse but uniformly distributed scalp hair (*hypotrichosis*) as in hypothyroidism, drug toxicity, and cartilage-hair hypoplasia. Areas of total loss of hair in the midst of normal hair are *alopecia* and may be seen in congenital conditions and in fungal infection or may be due to psychological hair-pulling (trichotillomania). In all of the acquired conditions with alopecia, stubs of hair may be seen in the area of hair loss.

Color of hair is determined genetically, and there are all variations from dark, brunette, and redhead, to blonde. If there are abnormalities of color, determine whether the hair color is uniformly abnormal, abnormal only in certain areas, or whether there are alternating normal and abnormal colors. The color of all the scalp hair may be uniformly abnormal, such as the blonde hair suggesting, phenylketonuria, and albinism, or abnormal color may be seen only in certain areas such as the white forelock seen in Waardenburg syndrome and Chédiak-Higashi syndrome, or *alternate* pigmented and depigmented areas as in pili annulati.

Texture. Dry coarse hair is common in hypothyroidism and fetal alcohol syndrome, whereas fine thin hair is seen in homocystinuria, Weaver syndrome, and many other syndromes.

Surface Characteristics. Curled hair is a normal racial characteristic (black) but twisted shape of the hair along its long axis (associated with increased fragility) is known as pili torti and is seen in Menkes syndrome. A beaded appearance of the shaft may be due to constriction at regular intervals (as in monilethrix) or caused by nodular swellings along the shaft (as in trichorrhexis nodosa). Also remember to look for lice and their nits, which may give a beaded appearance to the hair.

Strength. Fragile hair is characteristic of many congenital syndromes and fungal infections.

Aberrant *scalp hair pattern* is indicative of abnormal brain development in early fetal life. A grossly abnormal scalp hair pattern often indicates severe brain damage and indicates mental deficiency. The normal pattern is characterized by a parietal whorl that is located anterior to the position of the posterior fontanel and from which the hair stream goes progressively outwards, sweeping anteriorly to the forehead. The whorl is usually unilateral and is to the left of the midline. Rarely, it is to the right of the midline or bilateral. The frontal and upper face has a facial hair stream that seems to start from the ocular puncta and flows outward (affecting the direction of the eyebrow hair) and converges with the parietal hair stream of the forehead.

One should look for abnormalities of hairline in the front, back, and the sides. The hairline may be abnormally low or high in each of these areas: (1) low hairline in the back often related to a short neck (Klippel-Feil syndrome) or webbed neck (Turner syndrome); (2) absence of hair on the sideburn area (as in anotia); (3) excess projection of hair into the sideburn areas as in Treacher Collins syndrome; (4) low beaked frontal pattern (widow's peak) as in nasal dysplasia; (5) frontal upsweep (cowlick) as in microcephaly; or (6) abnormal hair over lateral forehead associated with defective eye development.

Finally look at the whorls on the scalp. Unruly hair over the scalp is often associated with various mental retardation syndromes. Parietal whorls may be absent or located centrally or posteriorly in microcephaly.

FOREHEAD

The characteristics to be described are:

- Size
- Shape
- Extra growth
- Hair pattern

The vertical height of the forehead is increased in hydrocephalus, Crouzon disease, and Apert syndrome. It is prominent in rickets, osteogenesis imperfecta, and Hurler. The forehead is pointed in Apert, trigonocephaly, and midline brain defects. Extra growths in the form of dermoid cysts are located near the angles of the eye. Occasionally an encephalocele or meningocele may present in the forehead. The frontal hairline is low in Hurler syndrome, deLange syndrome, and in many cases of mental retardation. It has an inverted peak (widow's peak) in frontonasal dysplasia.

NECK

The points to look for in the neck are:

- Size

- Shape
- Position at rest
- Range of movement
- Anatomic structures:
  - Cervical glands
  - Muscles
  - Thyroid
  - Veins
  - Arteries
- Swelling and defects

Size and Shape

Normally, the neck is distinctly visible between the thorax and the head and face, and there are wide variations in its size. In obese individuals there is practically no neck! In addition, severe diphtheria (bull-neck type), subcutaneous emphysema, and infection of the floor of the mouth can lead to severe swelling of the neck, obliterating all details. These conditions can be recognized easily, since the history of the swelling will be of short duration. The neck may be *short* due to vertebral anomalies or may *appear to be short* due to webbing of the neck as in Turner syndrome or obesity.

Position

Normal position of the midline structures of the neck is perpendicular to a line drawn between the acromion processes. If the head is tilted, determine whether it is due to torticollis or tilting of the neck. This is best determined if the child is on his or her back, and the examiner stands at the head of the table. In torticollis, the occiput is tilted to one side and the chin tilted to the opposite side. The child looks to one side all the time and cannot turn his or her neck to the opposite side. In long-standing torticollis, there is atrophy of facial structures leading to facial asymmetry. In head tilting, both the occiput and the chin are deviated to the same side.

In severe atlanto-axial subluxation, the child sits with the chin supported by the hand. In caries of the spine, the neck is held stiffly, and the child walks very carefully to avoid jarring movements. In severe decorticate rigidity, meningeal irritation, and muscle spasm (as in tetanus) the occiput is tilted markedly backward, burrowing into the pillow (opisthotonus).

Range of Movement

The range of movement of the cervical spine and testing for muscles are described on pages 185 and 192. Flexion and extension take place in the atlanto-axial joint. They are tested by first asking the child to touch the chest with the chin and then to put the head back to look up at the ceiling. Rotation also occurs at the atlanto-axial joint and is tested when a child looks over the shoulders. Lateral bending occurs in all the points along the cervical spine and is tested by asking the child to touch the shoulder with the ear.

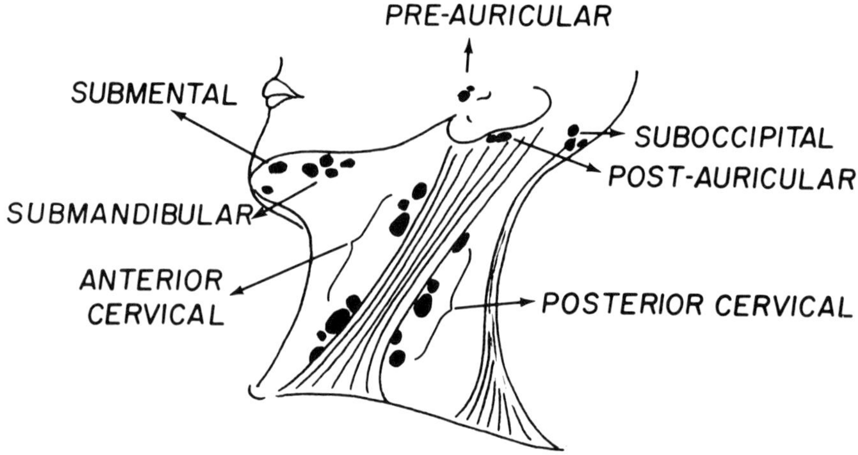

Figure 7A-2. Lymphatic glands of the neck.

Various Anatomic Structures in the Neck

The *cervical glands* can be grouped into the horizontal and vertical groups (Fig. 7A-2). The preauricular, postauricular, and suboccipital glands belong to the horizontal group. The suboccipital glands are particularly important, since they are enlarged in rubella and in scalp infections. The submandibular glands are also part of the horizontal group and are best felt with the examiner standing behind the patient and feeling the neck along the floor of the mouth while the patient is standing or sitting. The vertical groups of glands are felt along the anterior and posterior margins of the sternomastoid muscle and most of them belong to the superficial groups of cervical lymph nodes. Deep cervical nodes are hard to palpate under normal circumstances.

One should describe the characteristics of the palpable glands under the following headings: location of the glands; size; shape; consistency; temperature; tenderness; edge; pulsations; discreteness. Warm and tender glands indicate infection. Soft fluctuant swelling indicates suppuration. Matted glands indicate chronic inflammation. Discrete hard nodes (particularly a large hard node on one side only) may indicate malignancy.

The *thyroid gland* should not normally be visible except during adolescence. One should inspect for thyroid swelling from in front. Ask the child to swallow a drink of water or juice, since the thyroid is particularly visible when the child is swallowing. Palpation is best done with the examiner standing behind the patient and the neck flexed slightly. Ask the patient to swallow and feel the gland as it moves upward. The examiner should evaluate both lobes for the following characteristics: swelling, symmetry, surface characteristics (smooth or nodular), and consistency. In addition, remember to auscultate for a bruit (often present in thyrotoxicosis).

The *jugular vein* gives a good indication about pressure changes in the right atrium during the cardiac cycle. The neck vein should be examined with the child at an angle of about 45° (not sitting erect) and in good light. In a healthy person, the level of the column of blood in the jugular vein should be invisible, since it is never above the level of the manubrium sterni. In the presence of heart failure, however, the column of blood distending the vein is visible above the level of the manubrium at any position—even in an erect position (Fig. 7A-3).

In addition to observing the height of the column of blood in the jugular vein, one should look for the characteristics of venous pulsation. These waves are harder to observe in children because of problems with cooperation and shortness of the neck. The various arrhythmias and heart blocks in which the jugular venous pulse is very helpful in diagnosis are not common in children. It is however, good to watch for the "a" wave, which is prominent with increased right ventricular pressure (pulmonary stenosis, pulmonary hypertension) and is absent in auricular fibrillation.

It is often hard to differentiate between the jugular venous pulse and the carotid arterial pulse. The differentiating points are: (1) the jugular venous pulse has a clear upper level (absent in arterial pulse), (2) venous pulse is more visible than palpable (unlike the arterial pulse which is more palpable than visible), and (3) pressure on the liver may increase the fullness in the vein and accentuate the venous pulse but will not alter the arterial pulse.

Swelling and Defects

In children, the common causes of masses in the neck are lymph nodes, dermoid cysts, thyroglossal duct cyst, branchial cyst, thyroid gland, and lymphangioma (cystic hygroma). The common defects are: draining lymph nodes (in certain parts of the world tuberculosis is still common), thyroglossal cyst sinus, and branchial sinus. All the *swellings* should be described as suggested in Table 2-1: location, size, rate of growth, shape, margin, surface, consistency, color, temperature, pulsation, and adhesion to surrounding structures. In addition, transillumination should be performed, when appropriate, to define whether a mass is cystic or solid.

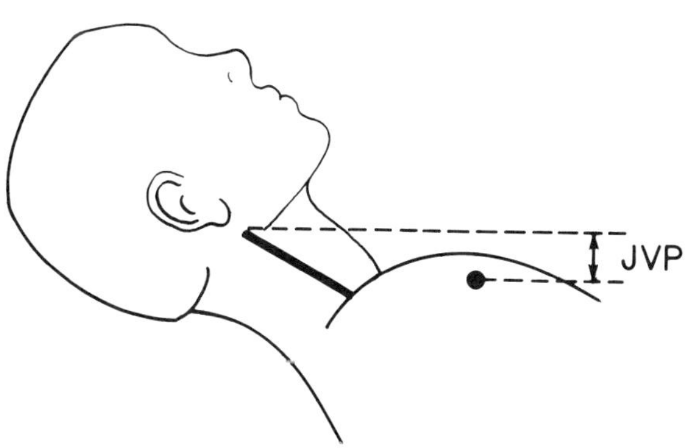

Figure 7A-3. Jugular venous pulse.

A thyroglossal duct cyst is located usually in the midline anywhere between the tongue and the hyoid bone, though occasionally it may be located just off the midline in either direction. It feels soft, feels like half a sphere, and moves upward with swallowing. If infected it may feel warm, look red, and be tender to palpation.

A dermoid cyst may be mistaken for a thyroglossal duct cyst since it also is midline and moves upward with swallowing. The points of difference are: (1) a dermoid cyst may be located anywhere on the midline of the neck—not confined to the upper part, (2) a full spherical shape is palpable, unlike a thyroglossal cyst which feels like half a sphere.

Branchial cleft cyst is rare but when it occurs it is seen high in the neck along the sternocleidomastoid muscle.

Cystic hygroma is lymphangioma of the neck. It is usually located over the anterior triangle of the neck and less commonly over the posterior triangle. It does not cross the midline. It feels cystic and it transilluminates.

Bronchogenic fistula (which is a sinus tract) is rare and is located in the lower portion of the neck; thyroglossal fistula is located in the upper part of the neck close to the midline.

EYES

Features of the eyes in relation to the rest of the head are discussed in this chapter. Neurologic evaluations are discussed in Chapter 7F. In this section, we will discuss only some general clinical features. *Always be certain to examine both eyes.*

Supraorbital Ridge

Abnormalities to be described are:

- Prominent ridges—as in fronto-metaphyseal dysplasia
- Shallow ridges—as in Apert syndrome

Eyebrows

Abnormalities to be described are:

- Quantity of hair—excessive, loss of hair, absence of hair
- Shape of the hair pattern
- Normal separation between the two eyebrows
- Infections
- Masses, growths

The quantity of brow hair may be *excessive* as a familial characteristic or as part of a generalized hypertrichosis, as seen in Hurler syndrome or de-Lange syndrome. *Loss* of hair may be part of generalized hair loss, as in hypothyroidism. Localized hair loss over the lateral end of the brow is seen in psychological hair pulling. Localized *absence* of hair over the medial third is seen in ectodermal dysplasia. Abnormal upsweep of hair over the medial third of the eyebrow is seen in Waardenburg syndrome. The eyebrows meet occasionally in normal people (synophrys); this is also seen in certain syndromes such as deLange syndrome. Various skin infections and parasitic infections, including tinea, may affect the eyebrows. If any swelling is present (such as dermoid cyst commonly noted at the outer edge of the eyebrow) it should be described using the standard descriptors: size, shape, surface, edge, consistency, temperature, and tenderness.

Eyelids

The characteristics to be described are:

- Size
- Shape
- Position in relation to the lower (or upper) eyelid (palpebral fissure)
- Position in relation to the eyeball
- Color
- Continuity, which may be disturbed by a defect or a growth
- Hair along the lid margin
- Muscle movement

There are no abnormalities of size and shape of the eyelids that are of clinical significance except that the lower lid may have a double pleat (Morgan's fold) in allergic children.

Palpebral Fissure. The relation between the lower and upper lid defines the palpebral fissure. The vertical height of the fissure may be unusually narrow (as in ptosis, fracture of the orbit, edema of the eyelids) or wide (as in exophthalmos, hyperthyroidism). The horizontal length of the palpebral fissure may be short, as in Trisomy-18, or appear short because of lateral displacement of inner canthi, as in blepharophimosis syndrome. The palpebral fissure may be slanted upwards (so that the inner canthus is at a lower level) as in Down syndrome, or slanted downwards (anti-Mongolian slant–outer canthus at a lower level) as in Treacher Collins syndrome.

There are certain differences between the palpebral fissure of a person belonging to the Mongolian race and patients with Down syndrome (Trisomy-21). In the Mongolian race the upper and lower lids become continuous with each other, giving a fold; whereas in Down syndrome, upper and lower lids meet medially behind a veillike fold (Figs. 7A-4 and 7A-5). The highest point of the palpebral fissure in the Mongolian race is at the junction of the outer two thirds with the inner third of the upper eyelid. The highest point of the palpebral fissure in Down syndrome is seen at the center of the upper eyelid.

Position in Relation to the Eyeball. Drooping of the eyelid is called ptosis and may be unilateral or bilateral. Patients with bilateral ptosis appear to have narrow palpebral fissure and often tilt their heads back and furrow

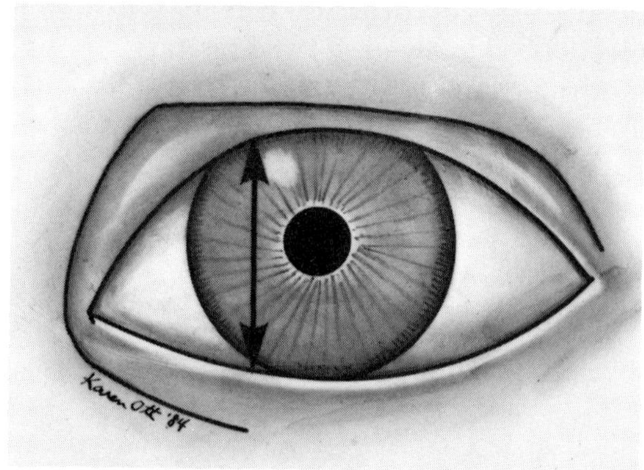

Figure 7A-4. Left eye of a normal male—Mongolian racial characteristics. Note that the upper and the lower eyelids are continuous. Maximum height of the palpebral fissure is closer to the inner canthus.

the forehead to see in front of them. Ptosis may be unilateral, as in third cranial nerve palsy or Horner syndrome, or bilateral, as in myasthenia gravis. Ectropion is outward-turning of the lid (as in burns), and entropion is inward-turning of the lid, as seen in severe infections of the eye.

Color. The heliotrope coloration of the upper eyelid is characteristic of dermatomyositis. Bluish coloration of lower lid is common in allergic children (allergic shiner).

Continuity. Interruption of the continuity of the lid margin is called coloboma. Coloboma of the upper lid only is seen in Goldenhar syndrome, whereas coloboma of both upper and lower lids is seen in Treacher Collins syndrome. The most common extra growth in the lid is: (1) stye-hordeolum externum, which usually points along the edge of the eyelid at the root of one of the hair follicles or, (2) chalazion, which is seen on the inner aspect of the lid. Generalized swelling of the lid may be due to edema, as in

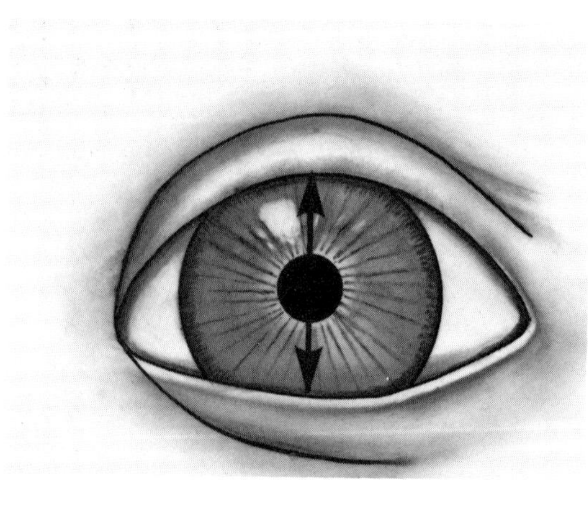

Figure 7A-5. Left eye of a child with Trisomy-21 syndrome (Down syndrome). Note the epicanthic fold behind which upper and lower lids meet. Also, the maximum height of the palpebral fissure is closer to the middle of the eye.

any generalized disease associated with edema or allergy, or due to emphysema, as seen after a fracture of the orbit.

Hair along the Lid Margins (Eyelashes). The commonest condition affecting the area of the hair follicle is blepharitis, as seen by redness, scaliness, crusting, and ulceration. It is often associated with skin allergies and seborrhea. The eyelashes are unusually long in certain normal children (one of the features of an attractive child) and in children with any chronic illness. Occasionally, lice may be seen along the eyelashes.

Muscle Movement. The upper eyelid may droop because of edema or because of paralysis of the levator palpebrae superioris. Paralysis of upper eyelids with drooping is called ptosis and may be seen in third nerve paralysis, in Horner syndrome, and in myopathies.

Excess closure of eyelids due to tonic spasm of the orbicularis oculi muscle is called blepharospasm and is seen in the presence of a foreign body in the eye, or corneal irritation, or photophobia from whatever cause. When examining small children, it is better not to force open the eyelids, since this is sure to make them close the lids even tighter. One can make newborns open their eyes by tilting them back and forth or by alternately turning them toward and away from a lighted window. Inability to close the eyelids is seen in seventh cranial nerve injury resulting in everted lids, widened palpebral fissure, and dryness of eyes.

Eyeballs

The appearance of the eyeball may be described as prominent or recessed. Proptosis and exophthalmos are words used interchangeably when describing *prominent* eyeballs. Both mean an abnormal protrusion of the eyeball. This is most easily appreciated when the examiner looks at the patient's eye from above the top of the head with the patient seated or lying down. There is a widened palpebral fissure and a larger proportion of the eyeball is seen than in normal individuals.

If the eye is prominent, the next question to ask is whether the eye is large in relation to the orbit (as in high myopia and buphthalmos) or the eye has been pushed forward (as in trauma). But physical examination of the eyeball alone may not give clues.

One should note whether the prominence is bilateral or unilateral. Bilaterally prominent eyeballs may be a racial or familial characteristic (caused by a shallow orbit). True bilateral protrusion (exophthalmos) occurs in thyrotoxicosis and many syndromes.

Unilateral true exophthalmos usually indicates serious disease, such as orbital cellulitis or rhabdomyosarcoma. It may be rarely pulsatile. Asymmetry of the palpebral fissure, facial palsy, and unilateral problems with closure of cranial sutures may make one eye appear more prominent than the other, but this is not true exophthalmos.

An eye may appear *recessed* either because it is truly small (microphthalmia), such as in "STORCH" complex, various congenital malformation syndromes, and after severe ophthalmic infections with phthisis bulbi (as seen in severe vitamin A deficiency) or because of the contour of the orbit (enophthalmos), as in Horner syndrome.

Tearing. Excessive tearing is seen in a local irritation of the eye, or allergies, or during crying. Dry eyes with lack of tears are seen in Riley-Day syndrome and Sjögren syndrome. Even in the absence of excess production of tears, one may see tears running down the cheeks if the lacrimal puncta are closed or if the eyelids are everted. The eyes may look dry in the presence of normal production of tears if the eye is never closed, as in a comatose patient.

Conjunctiva. Examination of the palpebral conjunctiva is difficult in small children. Unless absolutely essential, there is no need to pull on the eyelids and lose a child's cooperation. In cooperative children, the lower lid can be examined by pulling the lower lid down with the patient trying to look up. To evert the upper lid, one can gently grasp the lid close to the lashes, and roll the lid up over a thin pencil or cotton-tipped stick held horizontally over the lid. Characteristics to look for in describing the conjunctiva are: color, vessels, and secretion (described earlier under "Tearing"). The *color* of the conjunctiva is pale in anemia. Marked injection (redness) with purulent discharge is seen in conjunctivitis. Marked injection with watery secretion is seen in allergy and corneal irritation. Bacterial thrombi may cause purpuric lesions (as in subacute bacterial endocarditis). Pallor, edema, watery discharge, together with follicles in the conjunctiva of lower lids, may be seen in allergic conjunctivitis. Pterygium is a membranous growth over the bulbar conjunctiva along the palpebral fissure, often seen in allergic children. Follicles in the conjunctiva of upper lids occur in trachoma. In conjunctivitis, the redness is maximal at the junction of bulbar and palpebral conjunctiva and the circumcorneal area is clear. Circumcorneal injection is seen in injury and inflammation of the cornea or iris. Telangiectasis of the conjunctiva is seen in ataxia telangiectasia syndrome. Subconjunctival hemorrhage may indicate trauma, violent cough, or a bleeding disorder.

Sclera. The *color* of the sclera is normally white. Blue sclera is seen in some normal people, in osteogenesis imperfecta, and in Ehlers-Danlos syndrome. Black patches on the sclera may be caused either by nevi or by a thinning of sclera, which allows the color of the choroid to show through. Yellow coloration of the sclera indicates jaundice.

Intraocular *pressure* is estimated by asking the child to close the eyes and palpating the eyeball over the closed eyelids with the index fingers. This gives only a rough indication. To measure intraocular pressure accurately, tonometers are needed. Since local or general anesthesia is needed to use this instrument, it is obviously in the ophthalmologist's domain.

Cornea. The cornea's *size* may be relatively large compared to the rest of the eye (megalocornea) in certain normal individuals and in newborns. The transverse diameter is 10 mm at birth and about 12 mm at age 1; this is about the size in adults. A large cornea is seen as part of an enlarged globe of the eye in glaucoma. A small cornea (microcornea) is seen in many malformation syndromes. Normal *shape* of the cornea is characterized by its roundness and slight anterior curvature. Increased anterior curvature (Keratoconus) is seen in Down syndrome, osteogenesis imperfecta, and Ehlers-Danlos syndrome.

The *edge* of the cornea is usually clear. Occasionally, a patch of thickened conjunctiva (a pterygium) may grow over the edge of the cornea along the palpebral fissure. A phlycten is a small vesicle characteristically located on the corneal edge and is indicative of recent exposure to tuberculosis. Small vesicles that coalesce to form crescentic lesions along the corneal edge are seen in allergic children (limbal vernal conjunctivitis). Circumcorneal injection is an evidence of injury or infection of the cornea. Kayser-Fleischer ring is a greenish-gray ring along the outer margin of the cornea, seen in Wilson disease. Corneal *opacity* may be due to old injury, to severe infection complicating a vitamin A deficiency, to local inflammation (JRA), or may also be seen in certain syndromes (e.g., Hurler). Generalized haziness of the cornea is seen in glaucoma and early exposure keratitis. A salmon-pink batch of cornea is seen in acute interstitial keratitis.

The *continuity* of the cornea is disrupted by the presence of ulcers, which may only be visible as opacities or grayish infiltrates. If corneal injury, or ulcer, or infection is suspected, a damp litmus paper impregnated with fluorescein or drops of fluorescein should be applied to the conjunctival side of an everted lid. Areas of injury will show up as green stained marks. Perforation of the cornea is seen following injury caused by sharp objects or following severe eye infection.

Corneal *deposits* are not easily visible to unaided eyes. Slit-lamp examination is essential to rule out corneal deposits (as seen in storage disease and chronic inflammation), and this is best done by an ophthalmologist.

Iris. Complete absence of the iris is called aniridia and may be associated with Wilm's tumor. The iris has different *colors* in different races (dark brown, blue, green). The pale iris of albinism and the salt-and-pepper iris of Down syndrome are very evident. Loss of *continuity* of the circular iris is called coloboma (defect) and is seen as part of congenital malformation syndromes and after surgery. Coloboma of the iris has a high correlation with the presence of Wilm's tumor. The *margin* (pupillary) should be smooth. Irregularity with serrated edge suggests adhesions due to iritis. If the edge of the pupillary margin is visualized using the +8 or +10 lens of the ophthalmoscope, this irregularity can be easily visualized. Nodular lesions of the iris may be seen in neurofibromatosis.

Pupil. A dark pupil in the middle of the dark iris is hard to visualize, therefore, examining the pupils of children with a highly pigmented iris is often difficult. Shining the light obliquely facilitates visualization, and the use of a yellow light is ideal for visualizing the pupil of children with dark eyes. Use the +8 or +10 lens of an ophthalmoscope to visualize the pupillary margin clearly.

The normal pupil is *round* and is *centrally located,* though occasionally it is oval. Coloboma of the iris makes the pupil irregular. The pupil may not be located in the center even in normal children (eccentric pupil). Normally, the *edge* should be smooth. Look for irregularities and adhesions (synechiae).

Normal *size* varies from pinpoint to wide dilatation. Pinpoint pupils give the person a beady-eyed, suspicious look, whereas, wide pupils are characteristic of children who elicit a pleasant response. If the pupils are too large or too small, find out if the abnormality is unilateral or bilateral. Anisocoria means *inequality* of pupil size. This can arise from lesions causing a small or large pupil on one side, but it may also be a normal variant.

Bilateral constricted pupils may be normal or suggest conditions such as pontine lesions and poisoning with opiates. Unilateral constricted pupil should suggest Horner syndrome or carotid artery occlusion. If a pupil is fixed-dilated, find out if it is bilateral (atropine poisoning, deep coma) or unilateral (third nerve paralysis). Spasmodic variations in size is called hippus and is caused by tremors of the iris, and is seen in midbrain lesions.

To determine the pupil's *response to light* shine a bright pocket light (use a yellow light if the pupil is hard to see), first on one side and then the other. Normal response is for the pupil on the side of the light stimulus to constrict and then slightly redilate. This is called the direct light reflex. The pupil of the opposite side also constricts and this is called consensual light response. Both direct and consensual light reflex may be absent on one side only (efferent parasympathetic lesion) or absent on both sides (midbrain lesion). If light reflex is absent but consensual reflex is present, the lesion is in the optic nerve.

To test for the *accommodation reflex,* have the child look at a distant object. Ask the child to now look at a finger held very close to the face. Observe the pupils carefully when the eyes converge to look at the close object. Pupils should constrict to accommodate for the near object. When the accommodation reflex persists, though light reflex is absent, it is called an Argyll-Robertson pupil (syphilis, diabetes).

To test for the *response to a cutaneous stimulus* pinch the skin of the neck. Normally this should produce pupillary dilatation. Absence of this reflex indicates brain-stem damage.

When you shine a light through the pupil, you get a red flare. This is particularly visible if you look at the pupil through an ophthalmoscope. Absence of this *red reflex* requires immediate expert attention, since this is the most important clue to the diagnosis of retinoblastoma, infestation with Toxocara, retrolental fibroplasia, or cataract. In many of these conditions the normal red pupillary reflex is replaced by a white reflex and is termed the "cat's eye reflex" (first described by a father on his infant in 1765).

Lens. The normal lens should fill the entire pupillary area. Microphakia (small lens) is seen as part of microphthalmia of many of the congenital infections (STORCH). The normal lens is biconvex, and abnormalities of *shape* are hard to recognize. Look for the edge of the lens to find out if it is abnormally located, suggesting *dislocation* of the lens (trauma, Marfan syndrome). Finally look for *opacities* of the lens. The best way to look for this is through the +10 lens of an ophthalmoscope from a distance of 10 cm from the patient's eye. Breaks (dark areas) in the midst of the light reflex or absence of red reflex suggest the presence of cataract. Be certain to examine both lenses.

NOSE

The "pug nose" of the newborn is well known and may be an adaptation for breast-feeding. When examining the nose look at the following features:

- Size
- Shape
- Position in relation to face
- Position in relation to mouth
- Nasal bridge
- Rash
- Alae nasi
- Mucosa
- Septum
- Conchae
- Patency of nostrils

Size, Shape, Nasal Bridge

The size and shape of the nose may give many clues to diagnosis. A small or short nose is seen in various conditions, such as Apert syndrome, Trisomy-18, and Down syndrome. A relatively large nose is seen in Seckel dwarf and 13-q syndrome.

Rash

Among the rashes in the nasal area, the two most important to remember are: (1) the butterfly rash of systemic lupus erythematosus (SLE); (2) the allergic transverse crease that is a dark transverse line running at the junction of the bony and cartilaginous portion of the nose. Hypoplasia of the nares is seen in cleft lip and cleft palate.

Alae Nasi

The movements of the alae nasi are minimal during normal respiration, but, in the presence of respiratory obstruction, the alae nasi flare visibly, particularly in infants.

Interior of the Nose

While examining the interior of the nose, one should always remember to look for foreign bodies, particularly if there is a unilateral swelling, unilateral purulent or bloody discharge, or unilateral nasal obstruction. Tilting the tip of the nose upwards is all that is needed to get a good view of the vestibule of the nose in most children.

Mucosa, Nasal Septum

Hyperemia of the mucosa with mucopurulent discharge indicates infection, and pale mucosa with watery discharge denotes allergy. The nasal septum should be in the midline and should be examined for ulcerations (SLE), perforation (syphilis, trauma), bleeding points, and deviations. Look also for the pseudomembrane of diphtheria (particularly if the child has unilateral serosanguinous nasal discharge).

Conchae

On either side of the vestibule are the inferior conchae. They may be pale and boggy in allergic children. Above the inferior concha, part of the middle concha may be seen. Look for nasal polyps between these two conchae. Polyps are mobile and painless when touched, whereas the normal middle concha is firm and tender to the touch.

Patency

Examine older children by holding the lips together and finding out if they can breathe. Inability to draw in a breath obviously suggests bilateral nasal obstruction. In infants, persistent mouth breathing or cyanosis, when at rest with the mouth closed, should suggest bilateral nasal obstruction (e.g., choanal atresia). In newborns with suspected choanal atresia, pass a firm catheter first through one nostril and then through the other to demonstrate the obstruction. To look for unilateral nasal obstruction, hold the lips together and also block one of the nostrils to see if the child can draw in a breath through the other nostril.

EARS

Always be certain to examine both ears and describe abnormalities under the following headings:

- Size
- Shape
- Location: vertical, horizontal, coronal
- Abnormalities of surface characteristics
- Postauricular area
- Heat, warmth
- Pain, tenderness
- Discharge
- Use of otoscope

Surface Characteristics

The size, location, and position of the ear in relation to the rest of the head has already been discussed (pages 66–68). The normal appearance of the ear is depicted in Figure 7A-6. Look for fusion of antihelix with helix, cup-shaped ears, thickened large earlobes, absent superior crux of antihelix, failure of antihelix to fold posteriorly, and flared crux of helix. All of these malformations have been found associated with middle ear abnormalities and hearing loss. In addition, many congenital malformation syndromes are associated with ear anomalies. A crumpled ear is seen in arachnodactyly syndrome. Microtia (varying degrees with total absence labeled as anotia) may be an isolated anomaly with middle ear and hearing problems. Look also for preauricular pits and tags that may be associated with various anomalies.

Postauricular Area

It is important to look behind the ears, not only for the proverbial evidence of cleanliness, but for various types of rashes such as those of seborrheic dermatitis, eczema, measles, and rubella. Also, palpate the mastoid process, since mastoiditis is still a common condition in various parts of the world.

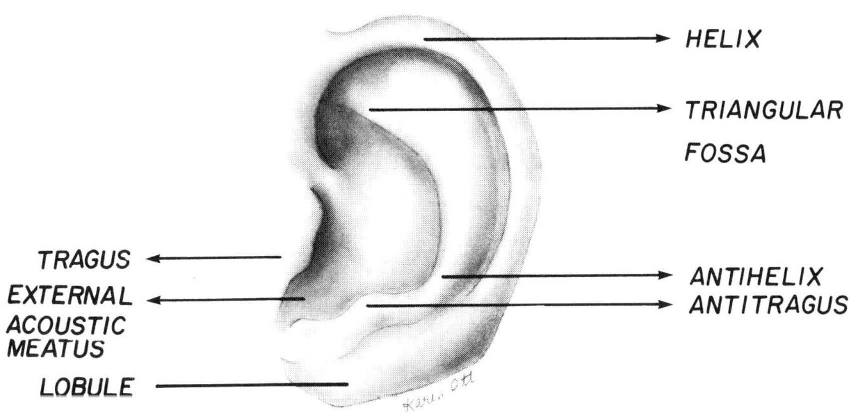

Figure 7A-6. Anatomic landmarks of the external ear.

Feel also for enlarged postauricular lymph nodes. These nodes are characteristically enlarged in rubella and scalp infections.

Temperature, Pain

A feeling of heat and warmth over the ear (as if it is on fire) is a common complaint of children with severe poison ivy dermatitis. A markedly swollen, nontender lobe is usually secondary to an insect bite. Tenderness on touching the earlobe or moving the pinna or tragus usually indicates otitis externa or a boil along the external auditory meatus. The pain of middle ear disease is not aggravated by manipulation of the ear, though the child may fight the examination.

Discharge

Look at the characteristics of the discharge. It may be watery (CSF), purulent (external otitis or otitis media), or bloody (external otitis, otitis media, foreign body, trauma). Look also for foreign bodies in the ear such as peas, parts of toys, and insects. (Insects will crawl out if 1 to 2 drops of ether are instilled into the ear. Of course, beware of the danger of fire and of ether in the eye.)

Examination with an Otoscope

Proper positioning of the child's ear and the otoscope are essential steps in examining the ear. There are many ways of immobilizing the child. The direction of the ear canal in newborns and infants is upward and in older children downward and forward. To visualize the tympanic membrane, the pinna of the ear is held by fingers of one hand and gently pulled *up and back* in older children and *downwards* in infants and newborns. The other hand holds the handle of the otoscope as in holding a pen. The knuckles of the fingers are steadied on the cheek of the child, and the handle of the otoscope is held horizontally (Fig. 7A-7). These two steps avoid any injury of the ear if the child should move. Actually this position allows continuous visualization of the membrane even if the child moves.

If the canal and the membrane are not visible, possible causes are: (1) secretions or a foreign body along the canal; (2) weak batteries of the otoscope; (3) faulty setting of the light bulb; (4) abnormal direction of the ear canal. Secretions and foreign body can be removed with an ear curette. The secretions of the ear may be dry and hard. If so, softening agents should be used before curetting the material. Occasionally, one may have to gently syringe the canal with warm (not hot) water to remove the cerumen. Hard, dry cerumen is a genetically determined, dominant characteristic in many Orientals.

The normal anatomy of the tympanic membrane as seen through an otoscope is diagrammed in Figure 7A-8.

The points to look for are:

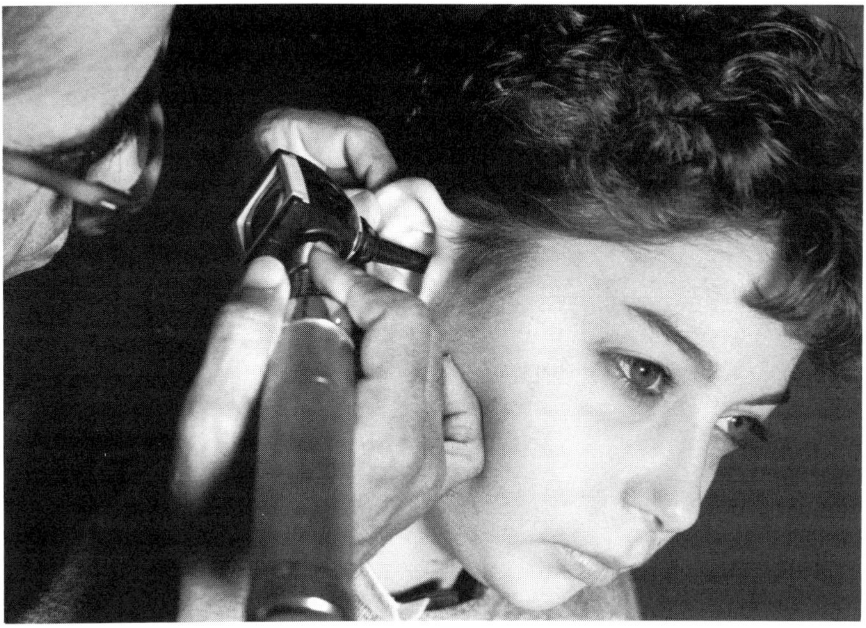

Figure 7A-7. Proper method for holding the otoscope.

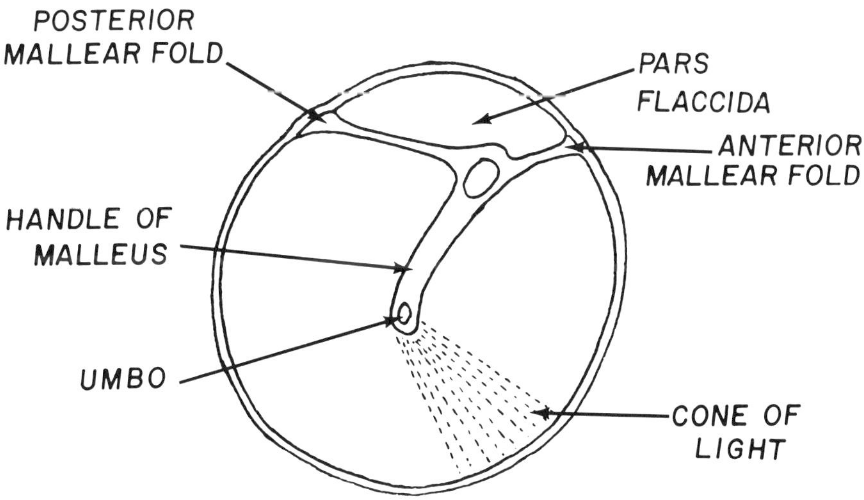

Figure 7A-8. Normal anatomy of the tympanic membrane of the ear.

1. Continuity of the membrane: is it intact or perforated?
2. Color: is it a normal pink? Is there only peripheral redness (crying child)? Is it red all over (inflamed)? Is it dull and purulent (infection)?
3. Is the cone of light reflex present? Absence of this reflex indicates loss of luster of the membrane because of inflammation.
4. Is the membrane bulging and convex, indicating pus, blood, or air in the middle ear; or is it retracted, indicative of eustachian tube obstruction?
5. Are there bubbles and an air-fluid column behind the membrane (serous otitis, allergy)?
6. The use of air tympanometry is recommended. While visualizing the membrane, gentle blowing of air through the tube should indicate whether the membrane moves as easily as it should. A thickened membrane in children with chronic otitis will not show the normal excursions. Normal movements of the membrane are also interfered with when there is fluid in the middle ear. Some of the more recent methods that use an electroacoustic impedance-bridge measure the compliance of the tympanic membrane more accurately. Use of this method is recommended in evaluating children with recurrent otitis media, allergies, and hearing difficulties.

MOUTH

The following characteristics of the mouth should be described:

- Size
- Appearance
- Continuity
- Color
- Movement of muscles
- Lips

Size and Appearance

The size of the mouth is assessed in relation to the size of the face and other structures. As mentioned earlier, the angles of the mouth should touch a vertical line dropped from the midpupil. If the angle of the mouth is external to this line the mouth is probably large and if the angle lies medial to the line, the mouth is small. A relatively large (broad mouth) is seen in certain syndromes, such as Marquio syndrome and Beckwith syndrome. A small mouth is seen in Hallermann-Streiff syndrome. "Fish mouth" (downturn of corners of the mouth) is seen in idiopathic hypercalcemia. Downturned corners of the mouth are also seen in Russell dwarfism. The continuity of the lips is broken, of course, in cleft lip. In addition, small pits in the lower lip may be seen in certain syndromes.

Color

The color of lips may be pale, as in anemia, blue as in cyanosis, or cherry red as in carbon monoxide poisoning. Circumoral pallor is seen in scarlet fever. Pigmented areas of the lips are seen in Peutz-Jeghers syndrome.

Movement of Muscles and Joints

Ask the patient to smile or open the mouth to show the teeth and look for uneven movements of the angles of the mouth, as seen in facial nerve paralysis. Congenital unilateral absence of depressor of the angle of the mouth may be evident when the child smiles or tries to purse the lip. The outer lower quadrant (on the affected side) of the face does not move normally. This defect may be associated with congenital malformations of the heart. In juvenile rheumatoid arthritis, the patient may not be able to open the mouth adequately due to temperomandibular joint involvement. Measurement of the distance between the upper and lower central incisor is a useful way of quantitating these problems. Older children usually have an inter-incisor distance of 2 cm. Closing of the eyelids when asked to open the mouth is called Marcus Gunn phenomenon. Spasm of the muscles of mastication with inability to open the mouth is called trismus (lockjaw).

Lips

The lips may be large (racial, Hurler, angioneurotic edema) or unusually pursed (whistling face). The philtrum may be long (Williams), short (DiGeorge), broad (Aarskog), flattened (geleophysic dwarf), or absent (cleft lip). Normal values for the height of the philtrum are available.

Salivary Glands

The major salivary glands are the parotids, submaxillary, and sublingual glands. In addition, there are many minor salivary glands in the mucous membrane of the mouth visible only under the microscope. The parotid glands are located below and in front of the external auditory meatus. The inferior end is below and behind the angle of the mouth. In true enlargement of the parotid, this portion is enlarged, resulting in fullness of the angle of the mandible and lateral deviation of the earlobe. This is best appreciated when the patient is seen from behind. Swelling can be due to infection (mumps) or tumor (mixed). The parotid duct (Stenson's duct) opens into the oral cavity opposite the upper second molar tooth. The submaxillary gland is located along the base of the mouth in relation to the posterior half of the base of the mandible. It is rarely palpable. The duct opens on the floor of the mouth under the tongue on either side of the base of the tongue. The sublingual gland is located under the sublingual fold of the floor of the mouth.

Examine these glands by inspection and palpation. Also look inside the mouth at the openings of the ducts. If there is evidence of obstruction to the duct, feel along the ducts for calculus or tumor. Look also at the discharge from these ducts (pus or blood) and redness at the opening.

Examination of the glands should include: all three glands on both sides; ducts of parotid and submaxillary on both sides; characteristics of the swelling (such as size, rate of growth, shape, recurrence); characteristics of saliva.

Excess salivary flow with drooling may indicate difficulty in handling normal secretion (as in mental retardation, painful lesions of the mouth, or neuromuscular paralysis of pharynx) or excess secretion (as in iodine and mercury poisoning). Normal children drool in the first year of life, but most children do not continue to drool after 18 months of age. Dryness of the mouth may be due to decreased secretion, as in atropine poisoning or a block in the duct.

Tongue

Normal characteristics of the tongue should be described under the following headings:

- Size
- Shape
- Continuity (cleft, furrows)
- Moisture
- Color
- Rash
- Ulcers
- Swelling
- Position in relation to mouth
- Movements
- Abnormal movements
- Appearance of papillae

Size, Shape, and Continuity. The tongue may be large, as in certain congenital malformation syndromes (Beckwith, hemangioma or lymphangioma of the tongue), angioneurotic edema, or infections in the floor of the mouth. A small atrophic tongue is seen usually in a nuclear lesion of the twelfth nerve and is unilateral.

Cleft tongue is seen in a number of malformation syndromes. Large furrows, giving the appearance of a "scrotal tongue," are seen in Down syndrome.

Moisture, Color. Next look for moisture. A dry tongue is a good indicator of the severity of dehydration, particularly in infants. Atropine poisoning and Sjögren syndrome are also characterized by dry tongue.

A pale tongue is seen in anemia. The tongue is blue in central cyanosis (not in peripheral cyanosis). Remember that the commonest reason for a pigmented tongue is recent ingestion of colored food and candies. A raw beefy-looking tongue with prominent fungiform papillae is called "strawberry tongue" (later stages of febrile illness and scarlet fever). A magenta-colored tongue which is edematous is seen in riboflavin deficiency. A scarlet-colored tongue with atrophic papillae is seen in niacin deficiency. A pale salmon-colored tongue with atrophic papillae is seen in sprue.

Rash. Various types of rashes may be seen on the surface of the tongue. Geographic tongue is commonly seen in normal children and is characterized by migrating areas of red patches with irregular white edges. This gives the appearance of a map and hence the name. There is a questionable association of geographic tongue with psoriasis.

Milk patches are white and easily removable. Thrush is a white patch which is hard to remove and leaves a bleeding spot underneath. Generalized coating of the tongue may be moist or dry and furry and is seen in any febrile condition.

Ulcers. Aphthous ulcers are the commonest ulcers in the tongue and are seen usually along the edges. They are usually few in number, are shallow and round. Herpetic gingivostomatitis is also characterized by ulcers on the tongue and can be located anywhere on the surface. They are grouped in clusters and the surrounding tissues are red. Vasculitic ulcers of SLE and periarteritis are extremely painful, with a dark spot in the center. Ulcers at the tip of the tongue usually indicate the presence of a severe cough from any cause (e.g., pertussis).

Swelling. Isolated swellings of the tongue are rare—except hematoma (as in hemophilia) and accessory thyroid at the base of the tongue (very rare). Look for masses at the base of the tongue. Small masses at the base of the tongue in the midline may be due to lingual thyroid or thyroglossal duct cyst. Look also for ranula, which is a cystic mass under the tongue which does not extend to the floor of the mouth.

Ask the child to open the mouth and see whether the tongue is deviated to one side. If so, observe jaw movements and exclude deviation of the jaw to one side which can also give the appearance of deviation of the tongue. The other possible explanation for deviation of the tongue is paralysis of one half of the tongue, so that the normal side pushes the tongue to the weaker side.

Movements. It is good to remember that some children suck the tongue instead of sucking the thumb. This is easy to identify if you notice movements of the floor of the mouth with the tip of the tongue held between the incisor teeth.

Some of the abnormal movements of the tongue are tremors (seen in thyrotoxicosis) and trombone tongue (seen in chorea). To elicit this finding, have the child stick his tongue out and keep it out as long as possible. In chorea, the tongue will involuntarily go in and out of the mouth giving the appearance of a trombone.

Appearance of Papillae. The papillae may be *hypertrophic* (strawberry tongue of scarlet fever), or *atrophic* as in various anemias and pellagra, or *absent* (as in familial dysautonomia). *Black hairy tongue* is characterized by the presence of a V-shaped brown to black area, anterior to the location of circumvallate papillae. This is due to hypertrophy of the filiform papillae and is often seen in hemophilia and purpura.

Gums and Alveolar Ridges

The normal gum has three characteristics: (a) pinkish-bluish color; (b) only a potential space between the marginal gingiva and the teeth, and (c) the area of gum that arches between the teeth does not extend through the entire height.

Color. In gingivitis due to any cause (vitamin C deficiency or herpetic gingivostomatitis) and in periodontal disease, the gum is reddish and bleeds easily. In dilantin hypertrophy, the gum is reddish, and there is true hypertrophy of gum overhanging the teeth. There is space between the gum and the crown of the teeth as can be demonstrated by passing the edge of a paper between the tooth and the gum. There is also gum arching between the teeth, giving the appearance of a curtain on the stage.

Children with bruxism (grinding of teeth while awake or asleep) also show arching of the gum between the teeth since the teeth are ground down and there is relatively more gum than teeth. The gum is not red, however, and there is no space between the teeth and the overhanging gum.

A black line along the margin of the gum may be normal as a racial characteristic. It is also seen in heavy metal poisoning.

Continuity. Ulcers and vesicles on the gum are seen in herpetic gingivostomatitis. Vesicles and pustules along the alveolar ridges in a child with fever may be the only clue to pneumococcal septicemia. Hemorrhage in the gum is related to trauma, purpura, and leukemia.

Alveolar Ridge. Hypertrophied alveolar ridges are seen in Hurler syndrome. A small swelling along the junction of the gum and tooth may be due to alveolar abscess, eosinophilic granuloma, or epulis. Epulis is a pearl-like tumor in the alveolar-buccal margin near the incisor teeth on the floor of the mouth, usually on one side only. An oral frenulum, attaching the upper lip to alveolar margin, is seen in Ellis-van Creveld syndrome.

Mucous Membrane of the Cheek

Important clinical clues to be looked for on the mucous membrane of the mouth are:

1. Small bluish-white spots surrounded by reddish zone opposite the molar teeth (Koplik spot) during the prodromal stages of measles

2. Reddish elevation around the orifice of parotid duct in mumps
3. Small, thick, white plaques that are hard to remove and may leave bleeding points if removed (thrush-candidiasis)
4. Whitish patch that is painful and friable because of healing areas of thermal burn, or laceration, or abrasion
5. Vesicular lesions as in herpes simplex or coxsackie virus infection
6. Bullous lesions as in erythema multiforme
7. Fewer numbers (less than three) of painful, round, shallow ulcers as in aphthosis stomatitis
8. Large numbers of deep ulcers of varying sizes as in granulocytopenia
9. Severe gangrene of the buccal mucosa leading to perforating ulcer of the cheek (called "noma") as in severe malnutrition
10. Pigmentation of the mucosa as in heavy metal poisoning or Addison's disease

Palate and Fauces

Characteristics to be considered include:

- Shape
- Surface
- Excess growths, rash, tumors
- Continuity
- Movements of the soft palate
- Uvula

Shape, Surface, and Continuity. The normal palate is smoothly curved in all directions but "gothic arch" (highly arched palate) is associated with various congenital malformation syndromes. Cleft palate should be easily visible. But to recognize a small posterior cleft, one has to look carefully at the back of the mouth. Findings that may suggest the presence of submucosal cleft are: (1) bifid uvula; (2) a membrane in the midline of the soft palate; and (3) forward movement of the groove of the soft palate during gagging.

Swelling. Swelling along the alveolar ridges may be due to epulis or eosinophilic granuloma or alveolar abscess or, if it is in the midline, a dermoid. Small cystic pearllike lesions on either side of the median raphae of the palate in the newborn is called Epstein's pearls.

Rash. Petechiae on the roof of the palate are seen in infectious mononucleosis, idiopathic thrombocytopenic purpura, leukemia, and severe pharyngitis. Vasculitic ulcers on the palate are seen characteristically in SLE and other vasculitides. Ulcers of the palate are seen in agranulocytosis and leukemia. In the normal newborn, abrasion of the palatal mucous membrane is caused by efforts at clearing the air passages and is called Bednar's aphthae. Thrush may produce white patches over the hard and soft palates. Intense redness and white patches should also arouse the suspicion of chemical burns. Intense soft red palate with edema is seen in dermatomyositis. Vesicles and ulcers over the anterior pillar of the fauces are seen in herpangina. In severe diphtheria, one may see yellowish or grey membrane over the anterior pillar of the fauces and particularly over the uvula.

Uvula. The uvula is normally seen in the midline and hangs in the midline when the child opens the mouth and says "ah." A large uvula may lie on the back of the tongue, tickling it and producing a cough. In the presence of paralysis of the soft palate, the uvula does not move at all when the patient says "ah" and it moves to one side (uninvolved side) in unilateral paralysis of the soft palate. Bifid uvula may indicate a submucosal cleft.

Tonsils

When examining the tonsils, the following characteristics should be described:

- Presence or absence
- Size
- Surface color, vesicle, ulcer, membrane
- Color

Technique of Examination. To look at the tonsils, proper positioning techniques and lighting are essential. A good clinician should be able to get all the information he wants in one quick glimpse.

One major warning: If you suspect epiglottitis, *don't try to have a look at the tonsils or the pharynx.*

The technique for immobilizing the child is the same as for examining the ears. The fingers of the hand holding the tongue blade should be steadied on the chin so that if the child moves or coughs, there is no damage to the throat. While the child says "ah" look at the tonsils, pharynx, fauces, uvula, soft palate, and hard palate. In some children visualization of the pharynx is easier if they make the sound "eh" instead of "ah."

Presence and Absence. Make sure the tonsils are present. If they are absent, very often it is due to past surgery (tonsillectomy) but may also indicate immune deficiency syndromes.

Size. Tonsils may appear large and meet in the center. If so, find out whether it is due to hypertrophy of the tonsils or due to pressure from peritonsillar tissue pushing one tonsil past the midline, as seen in quincy (peritonsillar abscess). Occasionally, the large tonsil may be the initial manifestation of lymphoma. Partial upper airway obstruction may occur as the result of grossly hypertrophied tonsils and adenoids (Pickwickian syndrome).

The color may be intensely red in viral pharyngitis or streptococcal infection. Areas of exudate are noted on the surface of the tonsils in streptococcal pharyngitis, infectious mononucleosis, and occasionally with viral infections. Grey or yellowish membrane may indicate diphtheria, particularly if it spreads to pharynx, uvula, and fauces. Similar membrane formation may also be noted in agranulocytosis from any cause. Vesicular lesions evolving into ulcers may be seen in herpangina; ulcers of the tonsils may indicate trauma and granulocytopenia.

Pharynx

The pharynx may also be intensely red in various types of viral and bacterial pharyngitis. Granular swellings along the posterior surface of the pharynx are seen in chronic pharyngitis and in allergic individuals. Postnasal drip can be visualized usually when the pharnyx is examined as described above. Retropharyngeal abscess may be visible in the posterior pharyngeal wall. If such a mass is visible, palpate gently to find out whether it is fluctuant. During this procedure make sure the patient is in Trendelenburg position, and be prepared for suction if the abscess should rupture. (A child with retropharyngeal abscess appears acutely ill with fever, dysphagia, drooling, and retracted neck.)

In chronic tonsillitis and adenoiditis, the child may have the following characteristics of "adenoid facies": an open mouth, "shiners" under the eyes, characteristic nasal voice, or snoring at night, and inability to pronounce sounds which end with "ng" (e.g., "talking").

TEETH

Describe the characteristics of *(milk) primary teeth* and *permanent teeth* under the following headings:

- Number
- Sequence and time of appearance
- Alignment within themselves and between upper and lower sets
- Color
- Texture
- Continuity
- Surface

Normal

The milk teeth are 20 in number and should be present by 24 months of age. There are wide variations in the timing of eruption of teeth. This is not a good indicator of developmental milestones. But lack of any primary teeth after 2 years is distinctly abnormal. Milk teeth are white in color and have a smooth edge in contrast to permanent teeth which have an ivory (off-white) color and serrated edge. If the characteristic of the edge is not visible, gently palpating the edge with the index finger will help determine whether there are fine serrations.

There are 32 permanent teeth. The "sixth-year molar" is the first permanent tooth to erupt. Though the sequence of appearance of permanent teeth is definite, their timing is indefinite. The last molar—which in man is probably unnecessary—may not erupt until adult life. The time of eruption and of budding of primary teeth is given in Table 7A-1, and the time of eruption of permanent teeth is given in Table 7A-2.

Abnormality of Numbers of Eruptions

Complete absence of all teeth (anodontia) is seen in congenital ectodermal dysplasia. Complete absence of a few teeth is often related to local conditions, such as cleft palate, impaction, and dentigenous cysts. Supernumerary teeth interfere with eruption of other teeth and therefore need attention.

Premature eruption of *deciduous* teeth may result in certain babies being born with teeth (natal teeth). Their significance is in relation to feeding and the danger of aspiration and early appearance of the corresponding permanent teeth. If you see *premature* eruption of *permanent* teeth, look for evidence of hyperpituitarism.

Delayed eruption of *deciduous* teeth (compare with normal values in Table 7A-1) is seen in conditions such as hypopituitarism, hypothyroidism,

TABLE 7A-1. CHRONOLOGY OF HUMAN DENTITION: PRIMARY OR DECIDUOUS TEETH

	Calcification		Eruption		Shedding	
	Begins at	***Complete at***	***Maxillary***	***Mandibular***	***Maxillary***	***Mandibular***
Central incisors	5th fetal months	18–24 months	6–8 months	5–7 months	7–8 years	6–7 years
Lateral incisors	5th fetal months	18–24 months	8–11 months	7–10 months	8–9 years	7–8 years
Cuspids (canines)	6th fetal months	30–36 months	16–20 months	16–20 months	11–12 years	9–11 years
First molars	5th fetal months	24–30 months	10–16 months	10–16 months	10–11 years	10–12 years
Second molars	6th fetal months	36 months	20–30 months	20–30 months	10–12 years	11–13 years

(Reproduced with permission from Behrman RE, Vaughan VC III (eds): Textbook of Pediatrics, 12th ed. Philadelphia, Saunders, 1983, p. 25.)

TABLE 7A-2. SECONDARY OR PERMANENT TEETH

	Calcification		Eruption	
	Begins at (months)	***Complete at (years)***	***Maxillary (years)***	***Mandibular (years)***
Central incisors	3–4	9–10	7–8	6–7
Lateral incisors	Max. 10–12 Mand. 3–4	10–11	8–9	7–8
Cuspids (canines)	4–5	12–15	11–12	9–11
First premolars	18–21	12–13	10–11	10–12
Second premolars	24–30	12–14	10–12	11–13
First molars	Birth	9–10	6–7	6–7
Second molars	30–36	14–16	12–13	12–13
Third molars	Max. 7–9 years Mand. 8–10 years	18–25	17–22	17–22

Adapted from chart prepared by PK Losch, Harvard School of Dental Medicine, who provided data for this chart.
(Reproduced with permission from Behrman RE, Vaughan VC III (eds): Textbook of Pediatrics, 12th ed. Philadelphia, Saunders, 1983, p. 25.)

cleidocranial dysotosis, and rickets. Delayed eruption of a single tooth occurs more commonly with *permanent* teeth and is due to factors such as retention of the primary tooth or hereditary traits.

Size and Shape

Next, look for the size of the teeth. Microdontia and macrodontia are difficult to define. A localized form of microdontia is often seen in the maxillary lateral incisor and the third molar and is caused by genetic factors. Localized macrodontia of maxillary incisors particularly in adolescents leads to cosmetic problems.

Color

Black teeth are seen in children taking oral iron preparations. Yellowish to yellowish-green discoloration is seen in children who were given tetracycline during infancy. In hypoplasia of enamel, the teeth look yellow to yellow-brown. Early lesions of caries appear brown, and established lesions are black and easy to identify. Other conditions that can be diagnosed from the color of the teeth are given in Table 7A-3.

Look for mottling or pitting of enamel. This may be seen involving only a single tooth (trauma), or groups of teeth (severe febrile illness, malnutrition), or all teeth (amelogenesis imperfecta). Pitting and mottling of enamel also occur in fluorosis. Excess plaque formation over the teeth is due to poor oral hygiene.

TABLE 7A-3. CONDITIONS ASSOCIATED WITH DISCOLORED TEETH

Color	Diagnosis
Brown to black (portions of crown)	Caries
Yellow to yellow-brown to yellow-green	Enamel dysplasia Tetracycline therapy Excess fluoride
Dark grey to black	Oral iron therapy Pulp decay
Green	Erythroblastosis
Red	Porphyria
White	Poor enamel

Continuity and Surface

Broken front teeth are common in children and are characterized by a chipped cutting edge. A chipped tooth associated with hemorrhage from the gum line should suggest fracture of the crown and of the root. If the tooth is also dislocated, it needs immediate attention. Caries cause dark holes on the biting surfaces but may also occur on the medial borders of the central maxillary incisors particularly in babies who are constantly sucking bottles with sugar, whether from milk, juice, or sugar water (Fig. 7A-9). Some caries cannot be detected by clinical examination alone. Special lighting, instruments, and a knowledge of tactile feel of small lesions are required to detect early lesions. Normally, the edge of incisors is serrated and is usually broader than the root. However, the crown may be narrower than the root (peg-shaped) with a lobular occlusal surface in congenital syphilis. Hutchinson incisor teeth are characterized by rounded shape and notching along the biting edge. This is also seen in congenital syphilis. Dens invaginatus, which usually involves the maxillary lateral incisor and is seen as a linear depression or defect in the continuity, is a common variation.

Alignment

Have the child bite down as hard as possible. Separate the lips and examine the bite. The occlusal surface of the teeth should appose with good alignment, with the posterior mandibular teeth interdigitating slightly ahead of the corresponding maxillary teeth. In malocclusion of class III variety, the posterior mandibular teeth are placed one or two teeth anterior to the corresponding maxillary teeth. A pronounced malocclusion of this type is called prognathism and is seen as a racial and familial characteristic and in acromegaly. When the posterior mandibular teeth are aligned posterior to the corresponding maxillary teeth, it is called class II oral occlusion. Hypognathia results in severe class II oral occlusion and is seen as a familial

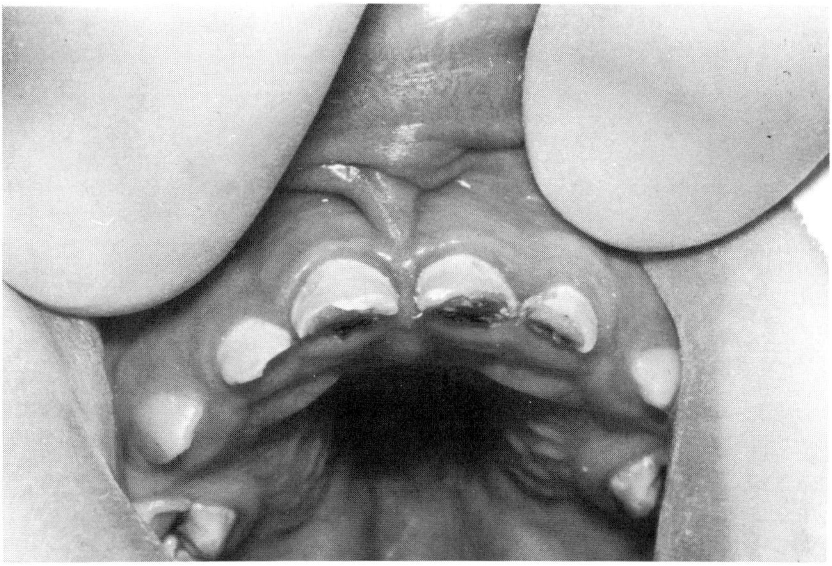

Figure 7A-9. "Bottle" caries. (*Photograph courtesy of RD Harshaw, DMD.)*

characteristic and in conditions such as Pierre-Robin syndrome and juvenile rheumatoid arthritis.

In addition, teeth may erupt in abnormal positions because of crowding or delayed shedding of deciduous teeth.

BIBLIOGRAPHY

Burech D, Koranyi K, Haynes RE, Kramer RN: Pneumococcal bacteremia associated with gingival lesions in infants. Am J Dis Child 129:1283–1284, 1975.

Jolley HM, Pless IB: Dental health and pediatrics. Pediatrics in Review 3(1):13–22, 1981.

Matson, D: Unilateral exophthalmos in childhood. Clinical Neurosurgery. Proceedings of the Congress of Neurological Surgeons, Washington, D.C. Baltimore, Md. Williams & Wilkins, 1958, Vol 5, pp 116–126.

Paradise JL: Testing for otitis media: Diagnosis ex machina. N Engl J Med 296: 445–448, 1977.

Polson AM: Gingival and periodontal problems in children. Pediatrics 54:190–195, 1974.

Smith DW: Recognizable patterns of human malformations. In Major Problems in Clinical Pediatrics, 3rd ed. Philadelphia, Saunders, 1982, Vol 7, pp 579–584.

Smith D, Gong BT: Scalp hair patterning as a clue to early brain development. J Pediatr 83:374–380, 1973.

7B. Chest (including heart and lungs)

GENERAL EXAMINATION OF THE CHEST

The sequence of examination of the chest will vary depending on the cooperation of the child. In many situations, a cursory examination may be all that is possible. Auscultation of the chest for heart sounds and for normal and abnormal breath sounds is possible even with a crying child. If one waits for each inspiration during the cry, one can hear all the adventitious sounds, except expiratory wheeze. Similarly, if one concentrates on the heart sounds during the expiratory phase of the cry, one should be able to pick up important findings. Thorough examination of the heart, however, requires a quiet child and a quiet environment. Examination of the chest will be described under the traditional headings of inspection, palpation, percussion, and auscultation.

Inspection

- Size
- Shape
- Visible abnormalities
- Movement with respiration

Size

The size of the chest is measured at midinspiration using a plastic or cloth tape which runs horizontally around the chest at the level of the xiphisternum. The child should be lying down during this measurement in the first 5 years of life. After this age, the measurement is made with the child standing. The chest circumference is 33 cm at birth (30 to 36 cm), 48 cm at 1 year of age (45 to 51 cm), and 52 cm at 3 years of age (50 to 56 cm).

The chest circumference is smaller than that of the head in the first 9 to 12 months of life. After 1 year of age, the chest circumference should be larger than the head circumference. Persistence of the infantile proportion should suggest hydrocephalus (see also page 92). A small thoracic cage is seen in Ellis-van Crevald syndrome.

Shape

The next item to observe is the shape of the chest. In infancy, the transverse diameter and the anteroposterior diameter of the chest are equal, resulting in a chest that appears round. After 2 years, however, the transverse diameter increases so that the appearance is transversely oval. A round chest in an older child is due to chronic obstructive lung disease, such as asthma.

Visible Abnormalities

Other abnormalities of the structure of the chest and thorax to be looked for are:

1. Absence of clavicle, as seen in cleiodocranial dysostosis.
2. Presternal edema, as seen in association with mumps.
3. Prominence of one side of the chest anteriorly, suggesting rib anomalies, scoliosis, or cardiac problems.
4. Hypoplastic nipples, as seen in Down syndrome and Turner syndrome.
5. Supernumerary nipples (may be associated with renal anomaly).
6. Shield-shaped chest, as seen in Turner syndrome. Normal values for distance between the nipples are available for various ages and indicate that the distance is normal in Turner syndrome.
7. Depression of the sternum (pectus excavatum) seen as an isolated congenital anomaly and with chronic nasal obstruction due to adenoidal hypertrophy.
8. Protrusion of the sternum (pigeon breast) as seen normally or in rickets, osteomalacia, and pectus carinatum.
9. Swelling of the costochondral junctions giving the appearance of rosary beads ("rachitic rosary") as seen in rickets.
10. A deep groove running along the sides of the chest parallel to the lower ribs seen normally in some children, particularly prematures. This corresponds to the attachment of the diaphragm. Unless it is very pronounced, it has no clinical significance. Deep grooves (Harrison's sulci) are seen in rickets and in any chronic obstructive pulmonary disorder.
11. Absence of pectoralis muscle leading to flattened upper part of the chest on one side. This may be associated with absence of nipple, absence of breast development, and pleural herniation.
12. Position of the scapula: one or both scapulae may be located in a high position with the lower angle turned toward the spine, as seen in Sprengel's deformity.

Movement with Respiration

Inspection of the movement of the chest should include description of normal movements and of abnormal movements.

In newborns and young infants, respiration is mostly abdominal. A relatively flat abdomen with diminished abdominal excursions in a new born should suggest diaphragmatic abnormalities. Inflamed peritoneum will also shift the emphasis to intercostal spaces in this age group. After 4 to 5 years of age, most of the respiration is due to intercostal muscles.

Normally, the chest moves evenly with each inspiration and expiration. Splinting of the chest with reduced total excursion during inspiration or cough should suggest pleural irritation. A short grunt during each expiration should suggest a painful condition of the chest (but children with pain anywhere seem to do this). Remember that avoidance of deep inspiration and cough may also indicate irritation of the central nervous system and increased intracranial pressure.

Unequal movement of the chest should suggest unilateral lung pathology. In children, the most important condition to remember is obstruction of the air passage due to a foreign body, and one should get a careful history of chewing on a foreign body or choking and coughing during a recent meal.

During normal respiration, both the chest and abdomen move, and the abdominal movements are more easily visible than the thoracic movements, particularly in infants. During inspiration, the abdomen bulges (caused by the downward movement of the diaphragm) and the thoracic cage moves upward and outwaı d (chest expansion). During expiration, the abdomen gets flatter, and the thoracic cage returns to the resting position. In diaphragmatic paralysis, the abdomen becomes prominent during expiration and flat during inspiration, and this is called paradoxical respiration. Fluoroscopy is essential for actual demonstration of paradoxical respiration. Diaphragmatic paralysis (from whatever cause—congenital, poliomyelitis) and pneumothorax may be associated with paradoxical respiration.

Accessory muscles of respiration include the scalenii, the sternomastoids, the trapezii, the latissimus dorsi, and the abdominal muscles. In the presence of upper airway obstruction (as in croup, diphtheria) or in lower airway obstruction (asthma), accessory muscles of inspiration (scalenii, sternomastoids, and trapezii) come into play, resulting in supraclavicular and suprasternal retraction. In moderate lower airway obstruction, retraction of the lower intercostal spaces and epigastrium is also seen. Accessory muscles of expiration (abdominal muscles and latissimus dorsi) are active in the presence of respiratory airway obstruction as in bronchial asthma. By their posture, patients with bronchial asthma fix the shoulder joint, so that the latissimi can act on the ribs and augment the expiratory effort.

The most standardized method for measuring *chest expansion* is one used by rheumatologists, since restriction of chest expansion is a major feature of ankylosing spondylitis. A conventional tape measure is used. Measurements are taken at the fourth intercostal space. The tape should not be pulled too tightly. The difference between the circumference at the height of maximum inspiration and at the height of maximal expiration expressed in centimeters is the measurement of chest expansion (see also page 78).

Palpation

- Obvious swelling and tenderness
- Trachea
- Cardiac impulse
- Movements
- Vibrations (fremitus)

Swelling and Tenderness

Any obvious swelling should be palpated for its texture, temperature, tension, and tenderness. Particularly note tenderness along the ribs, intercostal muscles, costochondral junctions, and manubrium. Sternal tenderness is noticed in leukemia. A prominent xiphoid process may cause a normal protrusion at the distal end of the sternum.

Trachea

With the index finger and the ring finger on the sternal attachment of the sternomastoid, feel with the middle finger on the suprasternal notch for the position of the trachea. A shallow suprasternal notch with a trachea that is easily palpated may indicate anterior displacement of the trachea, as in mediastinitis; or the notch may be deep and the trachea not easily palpable, as in the presence of anterior mediastinal tumor. Very slight deviation of the trachea towards the right is normal. Marked deviation of the trachea to one or the other side may indicate either a pulling force on the lungs toward the side of the deviation of the trachea (e.g., collapse or fibrosis of the lung on the ipsilateral side) or a force pushing the trachea away from the affected side (e.g., pneumothorax or pleural effusion on the contralateral side). Take care to exclude scoliosis before interpreting tracheal deviation as secondary to lung disease (see page 195). Look for pendular movement of the trachea, moving to one side during inspiration and to the opposite side during expiration. This can be appreciated with the same maneuver as for palpation of the trachea. Pendular movement of the trachea is seen in obstruction to a large bronchus or in a large pneumothorax. Also palpate for rhonchus or thud over the trachea. If present, it indicates tracheal or laryngeal obstruction.

Cardiac Impulse

Next, locate the point of maximum cardiac impulse, which is usually located over the fifth left intercostal space on or just inside the midclavicular line. In the absence of obvious heart disease or scoliosis, a change in position of the apical impulse of the trachea should suggest deviation of the mediastinum because of lung disease or, in infants, congenital defects in placement of the organs (dextrocardia or large diaphragmatic hernia).

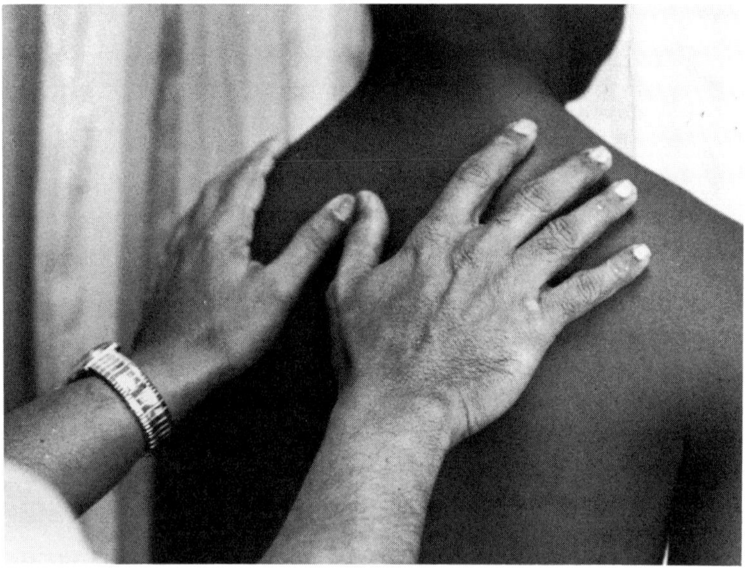

Figure 7B-1. Method for estimating the equality of expansion of the two halves of the chest.

Chest Excursion

The next step is to estimate the excursions of the two halves of the chest with respiration. The palms of the hand are laid on the posterior surface of the chest symmetrically with the thumbs touching each other in the midline (Fig. 7B-1). The fingers are spread over the sides of the chest. The arms of the examiner are steadied against the examinee's chest wall. Now, the excursions of the palm are noted with each inspiration. Normally, the palms move equally, as demonstrated by symmetrical movements of the thumbs going away from the midline with each inspiration and coming back together during expiration. When the two sides do not move symmetrically, the excursions are limited on one side and the thumb does not move away from the midline on the affected side, or the movements of thumbs are asymmetrical. This asymmetry should suggest the presence of effusions or collapse or consolidation of the lung on the side with reduced excursions of the chest.

Vocal Fremitus

Palpating for vocal fremitus may also help in recognizing changes in the conducting capacity of the lung. The child is asked to repeat the word "one" or "ninety-nine" while the examiner palpates all areas of the chest. The hand should detect distinct vibrations of equal intensity on corresponding areas of two sides of the chest. This is vocal fremitus. The intensity of the fremitus is diminished over areas where there is collapse of the lung (as in foreign-body obstruction of bronchus) or in pleural effusion. Vocal fremitus is increased over areas with consolidation or over a large cavity near the surface of the area being palpated.

Occasionally, a to-and-fro *rub* may be palpable over an area of pleura which is inflamed. This is palpable pleural rub. A palpable thud over the chest usually indicates a foreign body in the trachea.

Percussion

Observation made by percussion and auscultation of the chest should be described following the anatomic landmarks of the chest shown in Figure 7B-2. The anterior aspect of the chest is divided into the presternal area and the right and left anterior portions. Each side is divided from above downward into supraclavicular (above the clavicle), infraclavicular (up to the level of the second rib), mammary (up to the fifth rib), and inframammary regions. On the lateral aspects, there are two areas: the axillary region (up to the level of the fourth rib), and the infraaxillary region. In the back, on either side, the regions from above downward are suprascapular, interscapular, and infrascapular. Description of physical findings using this anatomic surface landmark gives clinical precision. For example, a statement such as "stony dullness over right infrascapular area" is more precise than "dullness over right base." In these days of laboratory precision, why not be equally precise about clinical descriptions?

One needs a cooperative patient to perform this procedure properly. It is preferable if the child is sitting or lying flat on the back so that observations on both sides of the chest can be compared. If there is scoliosis, percussion findings between the two sides cannot be truly compared.

The purpose of percussion is to make a comparison of the percussion note between corresponding areas of the two sides of the chest. Areas of altered resonance give clues to the presence of collapse of the lung, cavitation of the lung, consolidation of the lung, and fluid in the pleural cavity. Auenbrugger, who was also a musician, got his idea for percussion of the chest from listening to the sounds when tapping barrels of beer to find out how full or empty they were.

Direct percussion with one finger over the chest wall is easily done on smaller infants and gives valuable information. This requires experience.

The indirect, two-finger technique is the commonly used method for percussion of the chest (Fig. 7B-3). The middle finger (pleximeter finger) of the left hand is placed on the chest wall so that it rests firmly, but not hard. The other fingers should not touch the chest wall since they may dampen the resonance. The middle phalanx of the middle finger (pleximeter finger) is then struck with the tip of the index or middle finger (plexor finger) of the right hand. The plexor finger should be bent in such a way that the strike lands perpendicularly—not at an angle. The striking

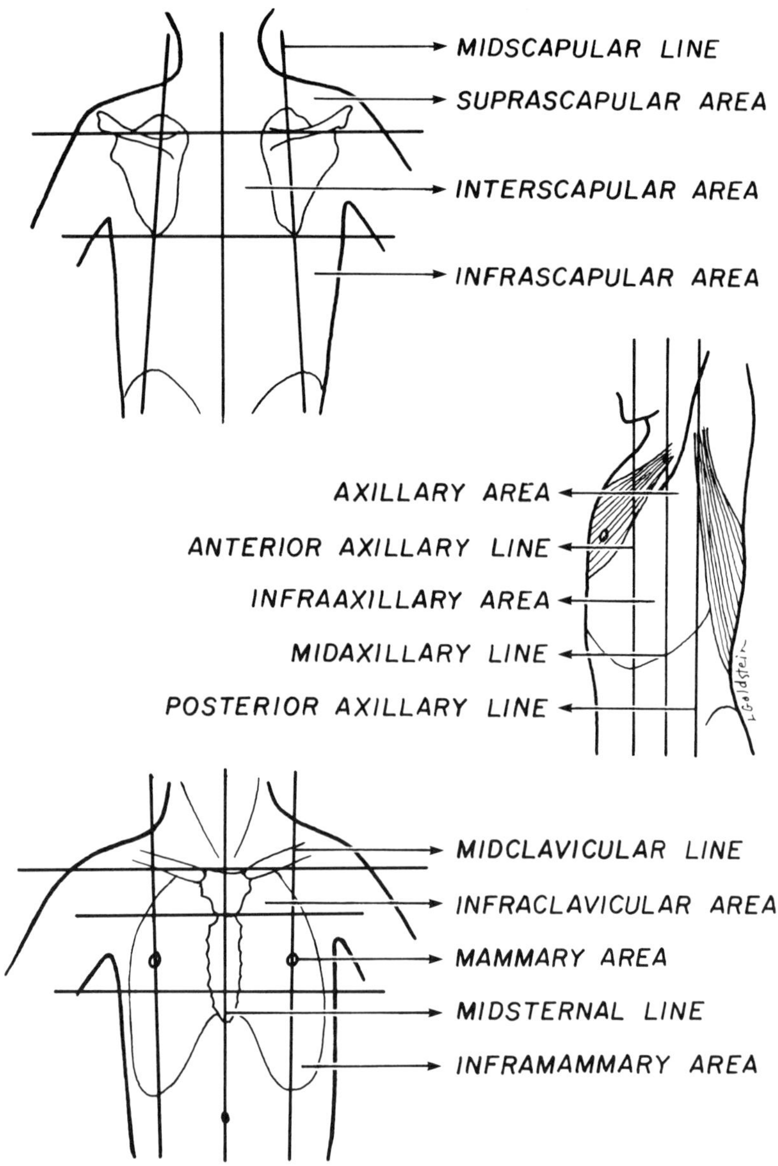

Figure 7B-2. Surface anatomy of the chest used to describe location of abnormalities on percussion and auscultation.

finger should strike and spring back quickly so that it does not dampen the resonance that is created. The movement of the striking finger should originate at the wrist—not at the elbow, which is likely to produce heavy percussion. Proper technique of percussion comes with experience, and experience comes from repeated practice—not with aging!

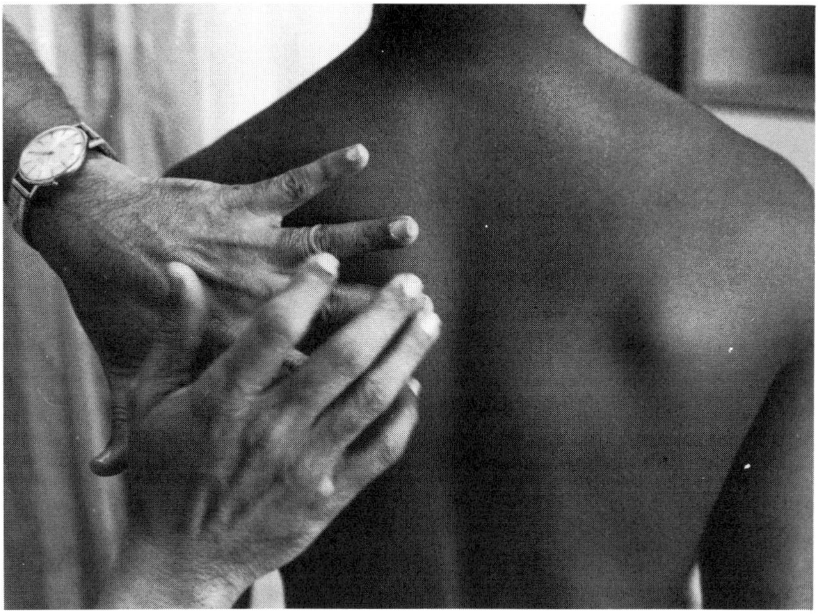

Figure 7B-3. Two-finger method of percussion of the chest.

It is best to start at the top (supraclavicular area) and proceed downward, systematically covering the front, sides, and back of the chest. Since the resonance is meaningful only in comparison to the opposite side, the percussion is done on the left infraclavicular area, right infraclavicular area, left mammary region, right mammary region, left inframammary region, right inframammary region—and so on. Remember to place the pleximeter finger parallel to the expected line of dullness. For example, in order to determine the upper edge of liver dullness, the finger is laid parallel to the ribs. But to percuss the right border of the heart, the finger is placed vertically on the chest, parallel to the right border of the sternum.

Dullness on percussion is noticed normally over the liver on the right side (at about the tenth intercostal space on midclavicular line, eighth rib on midaxillary line, and at the tenth rib posteriorly).

What is normal *resonance?* This is best explained by first explaining something else. Percussion over a hollow viscus such as the stomach gives a tympanic note. Percussion over a firm (not solid-hard) organ like the liver, gives a dull note. A lung is a hollow organ but is divided into a number of air-filled bags packed together. The percussion note over the normal lung is in between the two notes described above.

The chest is rather hyperresonant in normal infants, in those with a thin chest wall, in emphysema (as in asthmatics), and in the presence of pneumothorax. On the left side of the chest, when one proceeds downward anteriorly, an area of hyperresonance is expected because of the underlying stomach. This is easy to note in comparison to the dull note on the right side over the liver. If one finds dullness on the left and resonance on the right one should suspect tranposition of the viscera. It is a lot more fun making the diagnosis of situs inversus, clinically and by yourself, than to be told by a radiologist!

Normally one expects *dullness* over the heart. Though percussion of the chest is not reliable in determining the heart size during percussion of the chest, one has to be aware of the normal dullness over the precordium. Also, dullness over the right mammary region should alert one to the possibility of dextrocardia. Increased dullness on either side of the sternum over the second space should suggest widened mediastinum from whatever cause.

The dullness over effusions is absolute and is termed stony dullness. Other conditions in which dullness is noted include consolidation of portions of the lung, fibrosis, collapse of the lung (without air in the pleura), and pleural thickening. But this dullness is not absolute. With experience, one learns to feel for the resistance to the pleximeter finger and interprets this resistance, as well as interpreting the sound generated.

Auscultation

Recently we came across a clinical note that stated "Coarse rhonchi over the right base due to bronchospasm—order X-ray chest!" What is a coarse rhonchus? What is the right base? Is it the base of the lung? If so, is it the base of the upper lobe or of the lower lobe? Since the upper and lower lobes of the lung overlap, how is one sure that the sounds come from the base of either of these lobes? Finally, bronchospasm does not produce "rhonchus"—it produces a wheeze. Bronchospasm is an interpretation of a physical finding and not a physical finding. The original statement would have been clinically more precise if it read as follows: "Wheeze over the right infrascapular area." The emphasis in this section therefore will be on recognizing normal and abnormal sounds and defining them with clinical precision—as precisely as is possible.

Certain general points to remember during auscultation are as follows: (1) Listen directly over the chest wall without intervening clothes; (2) In young infants one has to catch what is available in whatever position they are lying or sitting. But in cooperative youngsters, have them sit comfortably without any portion of the chest being dampened. Auscultation of a toddler is best conducted while the child is being held by a parent. Examining children while they are lying prone or supine is acceptable, but not when they are lying on one side; (3) Use the bell of the stethoscope in younger infants, since the diaphragm will pick up sounds from too large an area; (4) Make sure the chest piece is not too cold, because that will be the end of any cooperation! (5) Make sure the child is not shivering—one can

TABLE 7B-1. BREATH SOUNDS BY AUSCULTATION

Normal Breath Sounds	Voice Sounds	Adventitious Sounds
Vesicular	Bronchophony	Crackles (rales)
Bronchial	Whispering pectoriloquy	Wheezes (rhonchi)
Bronchovesicular		Rub

hear many adventitious sounds in a shivering child; (6) The child's face should be in a neutral position, because a face turned to one side may cause variations in intensity of breath sounds on corresponding areas of both sides of the chest; (7) Examine the child in a methodical fashion to include all parts of the chest, as described earlier on page 131.

LUNGS

The main goals during examination of the lungs with the stethoscope are: (1) to listen to the characteristics of breath sounds in various areas, and (2) to compare these characteristics on one side of the chest with those on the corresponding area of the chest on the opposite side.

The characteristics of breath sounds (Table 7B-1) are best described under three headings:

1. Normal breath sounds
2. Vocal resonance (voice sounds)
3. Adventitious sounds

All these sounds should be described in relation to the location, intensity, pitch, and the timing (inspiration or expiration).

Normal Breath Sounds

Normal breath sounds are of two types: vesicular and bronchial. They have an inspiratory and expiratory phase and are due to movement of air in and out of the chest during the respiratory cycle.

Vesicular breath sounds are the common normal sounds heard over the entire chest, particularly over the axilla and infrascapular areas. They are produced by the transmission of sounds through alveoli and alveoli can best be compared to mufflers in the car. The characteristics of the vesicular sounds are diagrammatically represented as follows:

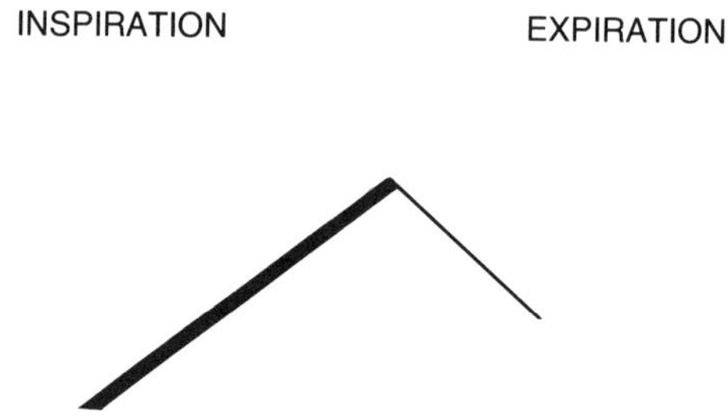

The inspiratory sound is a high-intensity rushing sound with a low pitch. It is heard through the entire period of inspiration. Expiratory sound is heard immediately following the inspiratory phase, without a pause, and is heard only during the earlier part of expiration. The three most important clinical points about normal breath sounds are: (1) the duration of the inspiratory phase is twice as long as the expiratory phase, (2) there is no pause between inspiration and expiration, and (3) the end of the expiratory phase is silent.

Bronchial breathing is heard normally when the stethoscope is placed over the trachea and above the midline of the upper anterior chest. In small infants, bronchial breath sounds are heard normally on either side of the second thoracic spine over the posterior aspect of the chest. Bronchial breath sounds heard over the rest of the chest are abnormal and are due to conditions that remove the muffler effect of the alveoli. In other words, bronchial breath sounds are heard when patent bronchi communicate sounds to the chest wall through a uniform sound-conducting medium, such as consolidated lung, a large cavity, or occasionally a small effusion.

The characteristics of bronchial breath sounds are diagrammatically represented as follows:

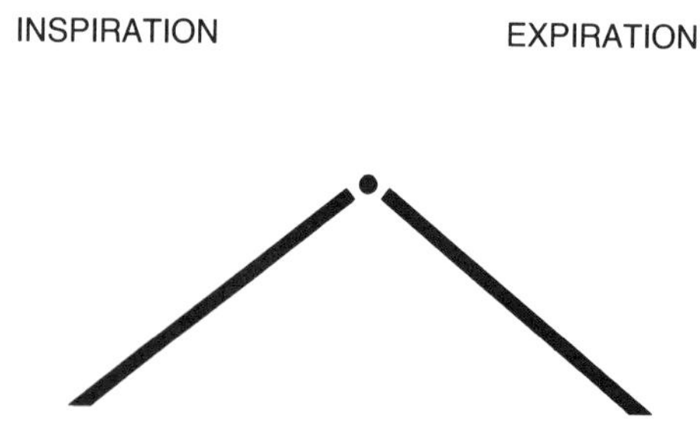

The inspiratory sound is of higher pitch and has an aspirate quality. It is heard throughout the inspiratory phase. There is a pause between inspiration and expiration. The expiratory sound is harsher than the inspiratory sound and is heard throughout expiration. The two most important qualities of bronchial breath sounds are: (1) prolongation of the expiratory phase so that it is equal to or longer than the inspiratory phase, and (2) a distinct pause between inspiration and expiration.

The intensity of breath sounds is diminished over areas with reduced air entry, as for instance in bronchopneumonia or in collapse of the lung due to foreign body obstruction. The breath sounds may be totally absent or the intensity of breath sounds diminished over areas of a lung with fibrosis, thickened pleura, pleural effusion, and pneumothorax. Obstruction of a bronchus will result in reduced breath sounds over the area of the lung supplied by that bronchus.

Vocal Resonance

Ask the child to repeat words such as "one" or "ninety-nine," and listen to the chest with the stethoscope. Normally, the sound is transmitted through the lung and is heard over the chest wall with a resonant quality. The words, however, are indistinct. The main point in listening to vocal resonance is comparison of corresponding areas of the two halves of the chest.

Vocal resonance is diminished or absent when air cannot pass through air passages, as in foreign body obstruction, or when it cannot be conducted to the chest wall, as in massive pleural effusion or pneumothorax. Vocal resonance is diminished also in the presence of emphysema and pleural thickening. Vocal resonance is said to be increased when the sounds are heard as if they are close to the ears or when the words are heard distinctly. When it is heard as if originating in the ears rather than at the chest wall, it is called bronchophony. Under this situation, even a whisper by the patient is heard distinctly and it is called whispering pectoriloquy.

Vocal resonance is increased in consolidation of the lungs. Bronchophony and whispering pectoriloquy are heard in massive lobar pneumonia, in the presence of a large cavity as in tuberculosis, or just above the level of fluid in pleural effusion.

Adventitious Sounds

The nomenclature of adventitious sounds is chaotic. Laennec, the originator of the words *rales* and *rhonchi,* used them interchangeably. The French word *rales* meant "to breathe with noise." But to the lay Frenchman in those days the term *rales* was upsetting since it meant "death rattle." In the presence of patients, therefore, Laennec used the term *rhonchus* which is the Latin translation of the French word *rales.* (An analogy is the use of the word, *TB* for the case sheet and the word, *PT* for pulmonary tuberculosis when talking in the presence of patients.) The definitions of the words *rales* and *rhonchi* became confusing when they were translated into English usage.

Some elegant works by Forgacs correlating clinical findings with pulmonary functions and pathology has shown a way out of the chaos. The preferred terms for adventitious breath sounds are: *crackles* for discontinuous, interrupted sounds and *wheezes* for uninterrupted continuous musical sounds. The word *crackles* should include the following two terminologies: rales and crepitations. The word *wheeze* should include the following terminologies: rhonchus and wheeze.

Crackles are explosive, nonmusical sounds. They occur in bursts and resemble popping of bubbles and thus are classified as discontinuous sounds. Crackles may be coarse, medium, or fine. Coarse crackles are louder and slightly longer in duration than fine crackles.

If you hear crackles, listen carefully to find out whether they are heard early in inspiration or at the end of the inspiratory phase. Early inspiratory crackles are characterized by very few bubbly sounds, heard usually in the lower portions of the chest and independent of the position of the patient. They are heard in diseases associated with airway obstruction. End-inspiratory crackles are characterized by their profuse nature and are better heard with the patient in a sitting position. They are indicative of restrictive disease.

Wheeze is a continuous musical sound and may be high-pitched with a whistling quality, as in asthma, or low-pitched with a snoring quality, as in emphysema.

If you hear wheezes, listen carefully for the following characteristics: (a) pitch: high or low; (b) complexity: monophonic, as in asthma, or polyphonic, as in chronic obstructive bronchitis; (c) duration: long, as in incomplete occlusion of a bronchus, or short, as in fibrosing alveolitis, and (d) timing: inspiratory, as in croup, or expiratory, as in asthma.

Pleural *friction rub* is associated with both inspiration and expiration and is a rubbing leathery sound. This has both discontinuous sounds and continuous sounds. A tugging sound heard in the trachea indicates a foreign body. A crunching sound over the left chest close to the pericardium indicates pneumothorax.*

HEART

Examination of the heart should include arterial pulse, venous pulse, and blood pressure. These are discussed in Chapter 6 on pages 85–87, Chapter 7, page 98, and in Chapter 10 on page 318.

Chest Landmarks

Before examining the precordium, certain landmarks on the chest have to be learned. The junction of the manubrium with the body of the sternum

*For teaching purposes, an excellent recording of normal and abnormal breath sounds on cassette tape is available from Dr. Raymond L. H. Murphy, Jr., Pulmonary Service, Samuel Shattuck and Faulkner Hospital, Boston, Massachusetts. Note that Dr. Murphy prefers the term *rhonchus* for all uninterrupted musical sounds.

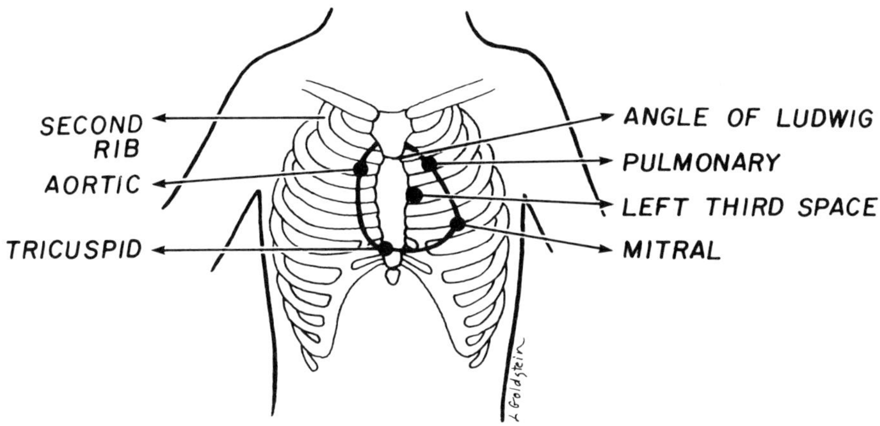

Figure 7B-4. Surface anatomy of the chest to describe heart sounds and murmurs. Name of the location refers to the area at which sounds originating from the corresponding valves are best heard. Note that this area is located away from the true anatomic location of the valve.

corresponds to the costo-chondral junction of the second rib and is called the angle of Ludwig. Therefore, in defining the location of impulses or murmurs on the horizontal axis, feel for the angle of Ludwig (Fig. 7B-4). The space below this angle is the second intercostal space. From this definitive location, other landmarks can be easily identified. The xiphisternum starts at the level of connection of the sixth rib to the lower end of the sternum.

On the vertical axis, points of reference are midsternal line, lateral sternal line, and midclavicular line anteriorly. These are self-explanatory (Figure 7B-2). Anterior-, mid-, and posterior-axillary lines on the lateral aspect of the chest and midscapular line over the posterior aspect of the chest are the other landmarks. In Figure 7B-4, note that the anatomic location of the valves of the heart is different from the location at which sounds originating from that valve are best heard.

Inspection

For proper examination of the chest, one has to undress the patient fully. Observe for visible pulsation over various parts of the chest and in the epigastrium. If visible pulsations are seen on the right side, consider the possibility that the patient has dextrocardia, provided there is no scoliosis or massive pulmonary problem pushing or pulling the mediastinum. In coarctation of the aorta, collateral arterial circulation may develop, giving rise to visible pulsation of intercostal arteries of the chest wall. These are more visible over the posterior aspect of the chest wall and are more apparent when the patient with untreated coarctation becomes older (also see page 317).

Pulsations in the epigastrium can be seen normally in thin children or when they become excited. Occasionally, pulsations in the epigastrium are due to enlarged right ventricle or pulsatile liver as in tricuspid regurgitation.

Palpation

Apex beat corresponds to the lowermost and outermost point of the cardiac impulse. In normal older children it is visible at or inside the midclavicular line on the fifth intercostal space. If it is not felt near this location, find out whether it is felt elsewhere over the anterior chest wall or is obscured. Apex beat is obscured in pericardial effusion, emphysema, and in obesity. It is hyperdynamic in children during fever, in hyperthyroidism, in hypertension, and in impending heart failure. Apex beat may be displaced due to disease of the lung or scoliosis. If these causes are excluded, the common cause of displaced apex beat is dextrocardia or cardiac enlargement.

Next, feel for the quality of the palpable *cardiac impulse.* A sensation of lifting of the palm on palpation of the precordium close to the sternum, indicates right ventricular enlargement. The impulse hits the palm and stays with the palm. Left ventricular impulse is more forceful, stays only temporarily with the palpating palm, and is maximal farther to the left. In conditions of systolic overload (as in aortic stenosis), a forceful sustained heave is felt, but in diastolic overload (mitral regurgitation), the impulse is less forceful.

The pulmonary artery, if enlarged, can be palpated over the second left interspace at the lateral sternal line. An intense second pulmonary sound also can be palpated.

Thrill is a "purring" sensation under the palm over the precordium in the presence of certain organic heart diseases. If a thrill is felt, locate its point of maximum intensity and its relationship to the cardiac cycle. Use the diagram on page 137 (Fig. 7B-4) to recognize the location of the thrill. Time the thrill in relation to the maximum cardiac impulse.

Thrill over the pulmonary area may be systolic (pulmonary stenosis) or diastolic (pulmonary regurgitation). A to-and-fro thrill over the left infraclavicular area should indicate a patent ductus. A systolic thrill over the left parasternal line may indicate pulmonary stenosis, ventricular septal defect, or auricular septal defect. A diastolic thrill along the left parasternal line is indicative of aortic regurgitation. A systolic thrill over the mitral area indicates regurgitation, whereas a diastolic thrill over this area indicates mitral stenosis. Aortic stenosis is characterized by a systolic thrill over the aortic area and aortic regurgitation is characterized by a diastolic thrill best appreciated along the left parasternal line. Functional murmurs are almost never associated with a thrill except in children with a very thin chest wall. A palpable thrill over blood vessels may indicate the presence of aneurysm or arteriovenous fistula.

Percussion

Percussion is a very poor method for determining heart size, but there are two methods for percussion of the chest with which to make a rough estimate:

Direct percussion: Percuss with the plexor finger parallel to the heart border. In other words, the finger should be held parallel to the sternum on the right and left sides and parallel to the ribs at the first and second interspaces. Start away from the heart and move toward the heart at ¼ inch intervals till the percussion note changes.

Indirect scratch method: Keep the stethoscope over the heart. Scratch over the chest wall with a finger vertically along the right anterior axillary line. Repeat scratching the chest vertically at ¼ inch intervals, starting medial to the anterior axillary line and proceeding toward the right sternal border till the quality of the sound heard through the stethoscope changes.

In children, the only important condition for which percussion will be useful is pericardial effusion. In this condition, the dullness is absolute.

Auscultation

Auscultation should be performed in a systematic fashion starting over the mitral area and moving clockwise or counterclockwise to each of the four major areas (Fig. 7B-4) corresponding to the four major valves. Other areas which should not be forgotten are: (1) the second left intercostal space (murmurs of patent ductus arteriosus are heard best over this area), and (2) the back and neck. Murmurs transmitted to the back and neck are organic murmurs. Murmurs heard over the neck and back are more likely to be associated with valvular stenosis; softer murmurs, as in septal defects, do not transmit as well. Functional murmurs do not spread so far away from their point of maximum intensity. Both the bell and the diaphragm of the stethoscope should be used. *High frequency* sounds (second sounds) and murmurs (diastolic of aortic or pulmonic regurgitation) are best heard with the *diaphragm,* and *low frequency* sounds (first, third, and fourth) and murmurs (of atrial defect) with the *bell.* Children should be examined both in sitting and in supine positions because the characteristics of murmurs may vary with change of position.

The auscultatory findings for each of the major areas of the precordium are to be expressed under the following headings:

- Heart Sounds: First and second sounds
Splitting and spacing of heart sounds
Third heart sound
Opening snap
Ejection click
Triple rhythm

Gallop rhythm
Fourth heart sound

- Adventitious Sounds: Murmur
  Rub
  Pleuropericardial

HEART SOUNDS

The normal first and second heart sounds are produced by events in the normal cardiac cycle. The first sound is short and sharp (best described with the sound of "lup") and is caused by the simultaneous closure of mitral and tricuspid valves. The second sound has been characterized by the sound of "dub" and is caused by the closure of pulmonary and aortic valves. It is normally split because of the slight delay in the closure of the pulmonary valve as compared to the aortic valve.

The intensity of the sound may not be valuable by itself as an aid to diagnosis. But it is good to remember that heart sounds are faint and distant in obese individuals, in pericardial effusion, and in emphysema. The sounds may be faint and weak in shock and in myocarditis. The intensity of the aortic first sound is increased in fever, in thyrotoxicosis, systemic hypertension, and in mitral stenosis. The pulmonary second sound is accentuated in pulmonary hypertension.

Splitting

Splitting of the second sound is normal and is best appreciated over the pulmonic area. Splitting of the first sound is rare. These sounds have to be distinguished from the third heart sound heard normally in many children (Table 7B-2).

Splitting of the first sound is hard to detect. Even if detected, it is no indication of heart disease. Its importance is that it can be confused with systolic ejection click.

The split second heart sound is best heard over the pulmonary area.

TABLE 7B-2. DIFFERENCES BETWEEN SPLITTING OF FIRST AND SECOND HEART SOUNDS AND THE THIRD HEART SOUND

	Split	Third Sounds
Location	Usually pulmonary area	Usually apex
Intensity (of the components)	Equal intensities	Different intensities
Interval (between the components)	Very short	Longer interval
Variation with respiration	Interval between A2 and P2 varies with respiration	Interval between A2 and S3 does not vary with respiration

Listen to the heart in a quiet room and listen for the split during the peak of inspiration and at the end of expiration. Normally, the split is more marked and clearly recognized during the peak of inspiration. Ask yourself the following questions while listening to the split:

1. Is splitting present or absent? If absent, consider aortic stenosis and extremely severe pulmonary stenosis.
2. If present, is it normally split?
3. If it is split widely with prolongation of the interval between the aortic and pulmonic component, does the wide split appear to be fixed (without any difference during inspiration and expiration)? If so, consider a large atrial septal defect.
4. Is the split paradoxical (aortic component coming after pulmonary component)? If it is paradoxical, the split narrows during inspiration (instead of widening). This occurs in aortic stenosis, left bundle branch block, and patent ductus arteriosus.

Third Heart Sound (S3)

A third heart sound may be heard normally during diastole over the apex (mitral area) in many healthy children, including adolescents. It is caused by the rapid flow of blood to the ventricles early in diastole. Third heart sound is best heard when the patient is in the left lateral position. It is loudest during expiration. Though the presence of third heart sound is not abnormal in the pediatric age group, increased intensity of this sound is often associated with a hyperdynamic heart, as in anemia or a large left-to-right shunt.

The third heart sound has to be differentiated from splitting of the first and second sounds, opening snap, and gallop rhythm. The differences between the third heart sound and normal splitting are listed in Table 7B-2.

Opening Snap

The opening snap is a clicking sound heard in diastole almost immediately after the second sound and is indicative of a stenotic mitral valve with mobile anterior leaflet. This may occasionally be mistaken for a widely split second heart sound. The differentiating points are: (1) the opening snap is heard best over the precordium at the fourth intercostal space over the left lower sternal border whereas the split second sound is heard over the pulmonary area, and (2) the opening snap is best heard in expiration or shows no variation with respiration, whereas the split is best heard in inspiration.

Opening snap also has to be differentiated from the third heart sound which is heard over the apex, low pitched and muffled. Opening snap has a sharp quality and occurs earlier than S3 but later than split S2.

Ejection Sounds and Clicks

Unlike opening snap, ejection sound is heard during systole. It is a high pitched sound and is produced by an abnormal semilunar valve (pulmonary or aortic) or conditions leading to sudden dilatation of the pulmonary artery or the aorta. These sounds may be associated with a murmur.

The characteristics of the ejection sound heard over the aortic and pulmonary area are:

	Aortic	Pulmonary
Location	Entire precordium	Upper left sternal border
Relation to heart sounds	Separated from first sound by a few milliseconds	Close to or on top of the first sound
Relation to respiration	No relationship to phase of respiration	Better heard during expiration, diminishes in intensity during inspiration
Intensity	Not sharp	Sharp

The term *systolic click* is applied to sounds heard during mid or late systole. These sounds have a clicking quality and may or may not be associated with murmur. An apical midsystolic click is always abnormal and is indicative of a "prolapsed mitral valve." Occasionally clicks may be associated with a small pneumothorax. These clicks will be associated with respiratory movement.

Triple Rhythm

Triple rhythm may be caused by a normal third heart sound or a gallop rhythm. Both are heard mainly over the mitral area. The differences are: (1) the third component of gallop rhythm may be palpable, and (2) gallop rhythm appears in the presence of other serious heart disease.

Gallop Rhythm

Gallop rhythm is the name given to heart sounds that resemble the sound of galloping horses rather than the "tick-tack," "lup-dub," to-and-fro characteristics of normal heart sounds. There is a third or fourth component with each cardiac cycle. A third sound gallop, also called protodiastolic gallop, is located over the apex of the heart and is often a sign of heart failure. A fourth sound gallop is called a presystolic gallop. A summation gallop is produced in the presence of tachycardia when these two components fuse. It is often hard to differentiate between these subtypes of gallop rhythm.

Fourth Heart Sound (S4)

The characteristics of the fourth heart sound are similar to those of the third heart sound. It is best heard over the apex of the heart with the patient in the left lateral position and with the bell of the stethoscope. It is accentuated during expiration. Fourth heart sound is said to be caused by atrial contraction and is heard just before S1. Many authorities consider the presence of S4 abnormal.

ADVENTITIOUS SOUNDS

Adventitious sounds are not heard in normal individuals (except the functional murmur) and are heard in addition to the heart sounds. These may be classified as murmurs, rubbing sounds, and cardiorespiratory sounds. The characteristics of the precordial murmur, if heard, should be discussed under the following headings: (1) location; (2) relationship to cardiac cycle; (3) intensity; (4) change in intensity in relation to respiration; (5) direction of spread; and (6) change in intensity in relation to posture.

Murmurs

Location. Examples of certain murmurs in relation to the location of maximum intensity are listed in Table 7B-3.

Relationship to Cardiac Cycle. (Table 7B-3) Heart murmurs are classified as *systolic* (when they occur with or immediately following the first heart

TABLE 7B-3. HEART MURMURS: LOCATION AND RELATIONSHIP TO CARDIAC CYCLE

Location	Systolic	Diastolic
Mitral area	Functional murmur	
	Mitral regurgitation	Mitral stenosis
Pulmonary area	Functional murmur	
	Pulmonary stenosis	Pulmonary hypertension
	Atrial septal defect	Pulmonary regurgitation
Lower left sternal border	Ventricular septal defect	Aortic regurgitation
	Functional murmur	Pulmonary regurgitation
	Aortic stenosis	
Aortic area	Aortic stenosis	Aortic regurgitation
	Coarctation of aorta	
Tricuspid	Tricuspid regurgitation	Tricuspid stenosis
Left second intercostal space	Patent ductus arteriosus	Patent ductus arteriosus
Neck	Venous hum	
	Aortic stenosis	
	Pulmonary stenosis	
Back	Usually a valvular stenosis	

sound and before the second sound), *diastolic* (when they occur after the second but before the first sound), or *continuous* (when they occur through systole and diastole). To recognize this relationship, concentrate your attention on the first sound and keep saying "one, one" as the first sound is heard, for five or six cardiac cycles. Then try to locate the relationship of the murmur to the first sound. Repeat the same steps now with your attention on the second sound, to recognize the characteristics of the diastolic murmur.

If you heard systolic murmur over any area, try to determine whether it is heard very early in systole, in midsystole, or throughout systole. Systolic murmur may be:

- *Holosystolic*—occurring throughout systole, beginning with the first heart sound and ending with the second sound. Murmurs of ventricular septal defect and mitral regurgitation are holosystolic.
- *Early systolic murmur*—occurring very early, beginning with the first sound and ending in midsystole. These are also called ejection murmurs. These murmurs are usually short and soft. Murmurs of aortic stenosis and functional murmurs belong to this class. The location, mild intensity, lack of spread, and absence of thrill will help differentiate the functional murmur.
- *Midsystolic*—starting a few milliseconds into the systole (not at the very beginning), peaking in midsystole, and ending before the second heart sound. These are also called flow murmurs. Examples of this type of murmur are: functional murmurs, murmurs of mild aortic and pulmonary stenosis, and murmurs of atrial septal defect. (A beginner may find it hard to recognize these characteristics. During the training sessions, listening to sounds in combination with phonocardiograms should help.)

Diastolic murmurs are always organic. They may be early diastolic, as in pulmonary and aortic regurgitation, or middiastolic as in early mitral stenosis.

Continuous murmurs are heard in patent ductus arteriosus and in arteriovenous fistula.

Intensity. The intensity of the murmur is not necessarily related to the seriousness of the disease. For example, the small ventricular septal defect can produce a very rough harsh murmur, whereas the diastolic murmur of aortic regurgitation may be hardly audible. Murmurs due to obstruction of flow through a narrowed valve are rough, whereas murmurs due to leakage of blood through incompetent valves are soft and blowing in character.

The murmurs are usually graded from I to VI with Grade I being the softest that can be heard and Grade VI being the one that is heard even without the stethoscope.

Grade I	Soft, not heard in all positions, no thrill
Grade II	Soft, heard in all positions, no thrill
Grade III	Loud, no thrill
Grade IV	Loud, thrill present
Grade V	Louder murmur with thrill
Grade VI	Loudest heard even without a stethoscope; thrill present

Intensity in Relation to Respiration. Murmurs originating on the right side of the heart increase in intensity during inspiration caused by an increase in stroke output of the right side during inspiration. Conversely, murmurs arising on the left side are accentuated during expiration. Hence the technique of listening to the parasternal area during expiration to listen for aortic diastolic murmur. The Still's type of functional murmur may also vary in intensity with the respiratory cycle.

Ask the patient to hold his or her breath for a few seconds and listen to the intensity of the murmur. After the patient starts breathing normally, keep listening to the intensity of the murmur for 10 to 12 more cardiac cycles. Murmurs originating on the right side of the heart (atrial septal defect, pulmonary stenosis) tend to return to control-intensities very quickly, whereas murmurs originating on the left side of the heart (ventricular septal defect) return to control-intensities slowly.

Direction of Spread. The murmur is said to radiate if it is heard with equal intensity some distance away from the point of maximum intensity. *Presence of a thrill and radiation of murmur away from the point of origin indicate that the heart murmur is an organic murmur.* Innocent murmurs are not associated with thrill and do not radiate to the back. The innocent murmur of the pulmonary ejection type may radiate down along the parasternal line to the fourth intercostal space.

A list of heart lesions with their characteristic murmur and the direction of the spread of the murmur are given in Table 7B-4.

Relationship to Posture. Next determine the effect of posture on the murmur. For example, if you hear a murmur over the root of the neck on the right side with the patient sitting, listen to the same area with the patient supine. If the murmur disappears, it is obviously cervical venous hum. On the other hand, the ejection type of functional murmur heard over the pulmonary area is heard best in the supine position. The murmur of aortic regurgitation is heard better when the patient is sitting up leaning forward (and is holding the breath in expiration).

Murmurs of mitral regurgitation and aortic stenosis decrease in intensity when the patient goes from a recumbent to a sitting position.

Asking the patient to sit up from a lying down position for 10 to 15 times may bring on the soft systolic murmur of acute rheumatic fever, which may not be heard in a patient resting in bed. This murmur is best

TABLE 7B-4. CHARACTERISTICS OF RADIATION (SPREADING) OF HEART MURMUR

Lesion	Murmur	Radiation to
Mitral regurgitation	Mitral systolic	Lateral and posterior aspect of the chest
Mitral stenosis	Mitral diastolic	Lateral and posterior aspect of the chest
Pulmonary stenosis	Pulmonary systolic	Left side of neck, left infraclavicular area and the back
Pulmonary regurgitation	Pulmonary diastolic	Left parasternal line
Aortic stenosis	Aortic systolic	To the neck along carotids; may transmit to apex
Aortic regurgitation	Aortic diastolic	Along the left lateral sternal border
Patent ductus arteriosus	To-and-fro over left infraclavicular area	Second and third left intercostal spaces, parasternally
Atrial septal defect	Second and third left intercostal spaces, parasternal line	Poor transmission
Ventricular septal defect	Third to fifth left intercostal spaces, parasternal line	To the right of the sternum, to entire precordium

heard if the patient turns to the left side after the exercise. Repeatedly going from standing to squatting position may also accentuate the systolic murmur of mitral valve prolapse.

Innocent Murmurs (Functional Murmurs, Physiologic Murmurs). During his favorite routine of listening to murmurs over various areas of the body, Dr. Donald Cassels (1957) of the University of Chicago mentions seven areas where *functional murmurs* can be heard: (1) Systolic murmurs can be heard over the head of young children particularly before the closure of the fontanel. It is a systolic murmur and is heard symmetrically above both ears and over parietal areas; (2) A murmur near the tip of the mastoid close to where the vessels enter the base of the skull. This is also symmetrical; (3) Cervical venous hum (continuous murmur) heard over the right side of the neck; (4) A murmur at the root of the neck but only in systole; (5) Murmurs originating at sites above the clavicle (items 3 and 4) but radiating below the clavicle; (6) Basal systolic functional murmur; (7) Still's murmur.

Innocent or physiologic murmurs are so common in the pediatric age group that they deserve some explanation. The commonest of these are: (1) the "twanging-string" murmur of Still; (2) basal ejection murmur; and (3) the venous hum (items 7, 6, and 3 of the preceding paragraph).

"Twanging-string" murmur of Still has a musical quality and is best heard over the midprecordium to the left of the lower sternum. It is heard in the first one-third of systole and has crescendo–decrescendo characteristics. It is heard best when the patient is supine. The intensity is variable and may increase with exercise.

Basal systolic murmur is heard over the left second interspace and is best heard in the first one-third of systole. It has a harsher quality and therefore may be mistaken for the murmur of pulmonic stenosis. Absence of thrill and absence of transmission to posterior chest wall differentiate this from an organic murmur.

Venous hum is a low pitched continuous murmur (systole and diastole) heard best at the base of the neck. Cervical venous hum is commonly heard on the right side of the neck, may be accompanied by a thrill, and is often transmitted to the second right intercostal space. It is accentuated when the patient is sitting. It disappears when the patient lies down and is obliterated by valsalva maneuver. Valsalva maneuver is performed by straining (as done during difficult bowel movement) in which the patient attempts forced expiration with the mouth and nose closed. Cervical venous hum is physiologic but is more common in the presence of high output states, such as anemia. Venous hum is obliterated in the presence of constrictive pericarditis or superior vena cava obstruction.

Rubs

A pericardial rub is a to-and-fro leathery, scratching sound heard with systole and diastole. It is very often heard for only a short duration of time, disappears, and reappears again. If there is effusion, the rub disappears. Pericardial rub is best heard with the patient sitting up and the chest piece of the stethoscope held over the left second and third intercostal space immediately to the left of the sternum.

Cardiorespiratory murmurs are usually heard at the apex or over areas where heart and lung are close together. They are heard as if they originate close to the chest piece of the stethoscope, vary with respiration, mid or late systolic, and have a high pitch. They are often heard in pericarditis and in emphysema.

SOME PHYSICAL PRINCIPLES OF AUSCULTATION

Immediate or direct auscultation by applying the ears to the chest was practiced by Hippocrates, Harvey, and Corvisart long before Laennec's description of the stethoscope.* Laennec was forced to think up a method for indirect auscultation when he encountered a 16-year-old obese girl with heart disease. Laennec described his two-part, 12-inch-long cylinder of wood with one funnel-shaped end in 1819. This was obviously monoaural. The first binaural stethoscope was described in 1843 by C. J. B. Williams. In this device, the chest piece and the earpiece were connected by a rigid lead tube. The prototype of the modern stethoscope with a flexible tube

*The word *stethoscope* means "to measure the chest" (scope to measure; stethos meaning chest).

was described by Dr. George Cammann in 1855. All these stethoscopes had a bell-type chest piece. The first diaphragm-type chest piece with a flexible membrane was invented by Dr. Marsh of Cincinnati in 1851. After many modifications, the modern bakelite chest piece was patented by Dr. R. C. M. Bowles of Brookline, Massachusetts, in 1901 and his name has since been used almost synonymously with the diaphragm-type chest piece.

During auscultation, vibrations set up inside the chest and transmitted through the chest wall are picked up by the chest piece of the stethoscope, transmitted through the column of air in the tubing and reach the ear. The ear is only the recording mechanism. The brain has to interpret these sounds. It is logical to conclude that the final interpretation of the sounds originating in the chest is subject to the following variables:

Variables related to the source of sound:	Origin of sound (heart or lung) The frequency of vibrations The sound pressure (energy) of the sounds The conducting medium of the chest
Variables related to the stethoscope:	Type of chest piece Tubing Earpiece
Variables related to the interpreter of the sound:	Age and experience of the physician The characteristics of the human ear and brain

The following is a summary of the characteristics of these variables so that you can understand why you do what you do with the stethoscope. The normal heart sounds originate from the closure and opening of atrioventricular valves and the closure and opening of the semilunar valves. The normal breath sounds are due to the passage of air to and from the alveoli through bronchi of varying sizes. The contents of the chest have an attenuating effect on the sound waves. Therefore, the sounds originating in the major four valves are heard best over that area of the chest wall which is reached via a path of minimum attenuation. This is the reason why the sound originating in the mitral valve is heard best over the apex of the heart though the valve itself is located more medially.

The frequency cycles of the heart and lung sounds range from 120 to 1000 cycles per second (cps). Most of these are below the 660 cps range. It is obvious therefore that an efficient transmitting mechanism is required to hear these sounds, though an occasional click or pericardial rub can be heard by the patient or observer without any aid. As a general rule, breath sounds have a higher pitch than heart sounds. The frequencies of various heart and lung sounds are listed in Table 7B-5.

During auscultation, we hear sounds of varying pitch and intensity. The human ear is a good detector of change in frequency cycles, if the change is gradual. But it is not adequate for detecting changes in intensity

TABLE 7B-5. FREQUENCY CYCLE OF VARIOUS HEART AND LUNG SOUNDS

	Sounds	Frequencies (cycle per sec)
Heart	Low pitched heart murmurs	400
	High pitched heart murmurs	660
	Systolic and diastolic murmurs	120 to 660 (up to 1000)
	Presystolic murmurs	140
	Pericardial rub	140 to 660
Lungs	Rales	120 to 1000
	Amphonic breathing	240 to 660
	Bronchial	240 to 1000

at the very low energy levels characteristic of the heart and lung sounds. Presence of sounds of varying pitch introduces the problem of masking. As the intensity increases, the low-pitched tones become more prominent, since the high-pitched tones are masked or attenuated. Obesity has a definite effect on the quality of the heart sounds. Another type of masking is seen when a first or second sound is very loud and is followed by a murmur of low intensity. The ear is fatigued after the loud sound and misses the murmur. A diaphragm-type of chest piece is capable of attenuating the loud sound and thereby makes the low intensity murmur more audible. This is the reason for using the diaphragm while listening for the aortic diastolic murmurs along the left sternal border.

The bell is capable of picking up all the sounds generated in the chest. Though there are differences of opinion, it is reasonable to assume that when a bell is applied to the chest wall, the skin under the bell acts as a diaphragm. By applying varying pressures on the bell, the skin can be made taut or lax, which in turn can alter the natural period of oscillation of the skin that is acting as a diaphragm. Therefore, when a bell is applied firmly on the chest, lower frequency sounds are attenuated. For example, the intensity of the first and second heart sounds is reduced. (A high pitched diastolic murmur may be better heard this way also.) Conversely, when the bell is applied lightly, low-pitched murmurs, third heart sounds, and gallop rhythm are heard more distinctly.

Since the pressure variations at the ear are inversely proportional to the volume of air in the bell, it is better to use bells with small volume. Very shallow bells, however, may get obliterated by flesh in obese patients. This is no problem with a diaphragm-type chest piece, and therefore one can use shallow chambers with the diaphragm-type chest piece. The diaphragm-type is particularly useful to detect high-pitched sounds, such as the aortic diastolic murmur and the bronchial respiratory sounds.

The length and rigidity of the tubing is another variable that can affect the acoustics of a stethoscope. It has been shown that at frequencies between 100 to 1000 cps, the efficiency decreases with the increasing length of the tubing. Since noise in the room can interfere with appreciation of the sounds heard through the stethoscope, it is obvious that a well-fitting earpiece which does not hurt should be an important feature of a good stethoscope.

The human ear itself is another variable, but it is not of major consequence. It is true that younger medical students hear sounds of higher frequencies better than older clinicians. However, the hearing loss of old age is for sounds of frequency cycles over 3000 cps which is above the level of the frequency spectrum of heart and lung sounds. Also, the experience of old age helps. After all, in final analysis, it is not the stethoscope but what is between the earpieces, that counts!

BIBLIOGRAPHY

Cassels D: Cardiovascular murmurs in infants and children. Med Clin North Am 41:75–88, 1957.

Cochran PT: Bedside aides to auscultation of the heart. JAMA 239:54–55, 1978.

Commey, JOO, Levison H: Physical signs in childhood asthma. Pediatrics 58:537–541, 1976.

Ertel PY, Lawrence M, Brown RK, Stern AM: Stethoscope and acoustics-1: The doctor and his stethoscope. Circulation 34:889–898, 1966.

Forgacs P: Lung Sounds. London, Bailliere Tindall, 1978.

Friedman S: The innocent (functional) cardiac murmurs of childhood. Clin Pediatr 4:77–81, 1965.

Hardison JE: Cervical venous hum: A help and a hindrance. N Engl J Med 292:1239–1240, 1975.

Leatham A: An Introduction to the Examination of the Cardiovascular System. Oxford, Oxford University Press, 1977.

McNamara DG: Idiopathic benign mitral leaflet prolapse: The pediatrican's view. Am J Dis Child 136:152, 1982.

Moll JMH, Wright V: An objective clinical study of chest expansion. Ann Rheum Dis 31:1–8, 1972.

Nadas AS, Fyler D: Pediatric Cardiology, 3rd ed. Philadelphia, Saunders, 1972.

Nath AR, Capel, LH: Inspiratory crackles: Early and late. Thorax 29:223–227, 1974.

Poynter FNL, Keile KD: A Short History of Medicine: Science in Society Series 2. London, Mills and Boon, 1961, p. 47.

Rabin, CB: New or neglected physical signs in diagnosis of chest diseases. JAMA 194:546–550, 1965.

Rappaport MB, Sprague HB: Physiologic and physical laws that govern auscultation and their clinical application. Am Heart J 21:257–318, 1941.

Robertson AH, Coope R: Rales, rhonchi, and Laennec. Lancet 273:417–423, 1957.

Schwartz ML, Little RC: Physiological basis for the heart sounds and their clinical significance. N Engl J Med 264:280–285, 1961.

Tilkian AG, Conver MB: Understanding Heart Sounds and Murmurs with an Introduction to Lung Sounds, 2nd ed. Philadelphia, Saunders, 1984.

7C. Abdomen and Genitalia

ABDOMEN

Landmarks

The abdomen can be divided into quadrants (right-upper, left-upper, right-lower, and left-lower) or, using the old English method, into three areas horizontally and three areas vertically for a total of nine areas, as in this diagram:

RIGHT HYPOCHONDRIUM	EPIGASTRIUM	LEFT HYPOCHONDRIUM
RIGHT LUMBAR (FLANK)	UMBILICUS	LEFT LUMBAR (FLANK)
RIGHT ILIAC	HYPOGASTRIC OR SUPRAPUBIC	LEFT ILIAC

Inspection

Note whether the abdomen has normal full contour, is flat, or is protuberant. The causes of fullness can be described under 5 *F*'s: fat, flatus, feces, fluid, and fetus. Considering the frequency of teenage pregnancy and obesity, these are still the important five items to remember, even among the pediatric patients.

Abdominal distension due to laxity of the abdominal wall is seen in rickets, celiac disease, and hypothyroidism. Flat abdomen is seen in normal thin children, malnutrition, failure to thrive, and in anorexia.

In the newborn, the abdomen is normally full and often convex, and a flat abdomen should suggest diaphragmatic hernia. Complete absence of the muscles of the abdominal wall gives the skin a wrinkled appearance and is called the "prune-belly syndrome" (often associated with cryptorchidism and hydroureter).

Localized swellings should be looked for also. Massive hepatomegaly or splenomegaly may be easily visible and are easily identified by the location. Masses coming out of the abdominal wall, such as umbilical hernia, are easy to recognize. Masses in the inguinal region are usually due to hernia or hydrocele or undescended testis or inguinal nodes.

Next look for abnormal pulsations. Pulsations of the epigastric region may be seen in thin individuals, particularly if excited, but epigastric pulsations may also indicate pulsations of the liver or enlargement of the right ventricle.

Normally, the abdominal wall moves with the respiratory cycle, becoming more prominent during inspiration and collapsing during expiration. Movements of the abdominal wall during phases of respiration are reversed in diaphragmatic paralysis, collapsing during inspiration and becoming prominent during expiration. Movements of the abdominal wall with respiration are diminished or absent when there is guarding of abdominal muscles, as in peritonitis.

Next, examine the abdomen for peristaltic movements of the intestine. Have the patient lie supine and observe the abdominal wall in an oblique light. Peristaltic movements may be visible normally in thin individuals. Observe to see whether these peristaltic movements are excessive and also observe the direction of the wave. Peristaltic movements of the stomach are visible over the left upper quadrant of the abdomen in emaciated infants with pyloric stenosis. One can see the waves moving from left to right, particularly if the baby is fed some water. Peristalsis of the large intestine owing to obstruction is seen in the lower quadrants and the flanks. Movement is from right to left.

Purplish striae indicate recent weight gain or Cushing syndrome. With passage of time they turn white in color. Slate color discoloration of the abdominal wall is seen in Addison disease.

Distended veins seen in the epigastrium may indicate obstruction of the inferior vena cava. Prominent veins in the periumbilical area of the abdominal wall are more likely related to portal obstruction. This is demonstrated by pressing on the vein with two fingers held close together and emptying the vein in both directions by separating the fingers as pressure is applied along the veins. Now release one finger and see whether the vein fills. If it does not, release the other finger to see whether the emptied vein fills. In the presence of obstruction to the inferior vena cava, the direction of blood flow is from below upwards and can be demonstrated using the same method.

Diastasis of the rectus muscle is noticed along the midline and is seen as a linear protrusion. Though this may be a normal variant, occasionally it is due to weak abdominal musculature.

Exstrophy of the bladder is characterized by the presence of exposed urinary bladder in the midline just above the symphysis.

Umbilicus

- Defect/hernia
- Drainage
- Mass

Usually at birth, there is a small defect of the abdominal wall at the umbilicus leading to an insignificant hernia. The defect usually is less than 1 inch in diameter. Umbilical hernia is seen more commonly in black children up to 7 years of age. Surgical repair is indicated if there are associated lesions, such as persistent urachus, or if the skin over the sac has become too thin and atrophic. Examine the hernia for reducibility and for consistency. Uncomplicated umbilical hernia is soft and reducible. Strangulated hernia feels tense and does not reduce. A large hernia of the abdominal contents into the base of the umbilicus, particularly in the presence of poor abdominal musculature, is called an omphalocele.

Occasionally, in the neonatal period, there may be discharge from the umbilicus. Observe and see whether the discharge is watery (urine) or purulent or serosanguinous. This may be caused by an infected cord stump, or by persistent urachus, or urachal cyst, or patent omphalomesenteric duct, or it may be a normal finding.

The cord usually falls off in 6 to 18 days after birth, and the raw surface has healed by 12 to 21 days. Occasionally granulation tissue persists, resulting in granuloma. This has to be distinguished from polyp, which by definition should have a pedicle. Polyp is also bright red and has mucoid discharge. Polyps are related to urachal and omphalomesenteric ducts and therefore are associated with fecal or watery discharge. Look also for a small opening in the center of the lesion with a probe. If an opening is present, the lesion is not a granuloma but is related to urachus or omphalomesenteric duct.

Palpation

The technique of palpation of the abdomen is an art. Even the most cooperative children may tense up during this procedure. In small children, the abdominal wall tenses up when they cry. A cold pair of hands elicit a protective spasm, and the abdomen gets tight. Some children are so ticklish that you cannot even bring your hand near them without making the abdomen tense.

There are various techniques to relax the abdominal wall. The central theme is distraction. Some children distract easily if you engage them in a serious conversation. Others will relax with laughing and some standard jokes are in order. Some children have to be examined when they are sitting up or lying prone. Flexing the hips and asking the child to take a deep breath will relax the abdominal wall in most children. In some, asking the child to take deep breaths and palpating quickly during expiration will work. The same is accomplished in a crying child. Wait until the child relaxes the tension on the abdominal wall at the end of the expiratory phase of crying and, when the child takes a deep breath, press the fingers as the abdomen relaxes. In ticklish children, have your hand placed on top of the child's hand but with the index finger somewhat overlapping. Palpate the abdomen with the child's own hand, except your index finger can dip in a little just on the inside of the child's hand (Fig. 7C-1).

Note whether the tone of the abdominal wall is soft or firm or tense. A hard tense feeling usually indicates tender intraabdominal pathology. Boardlike rigidity indicates peritonitis. Diffuse firmness may indicate chest

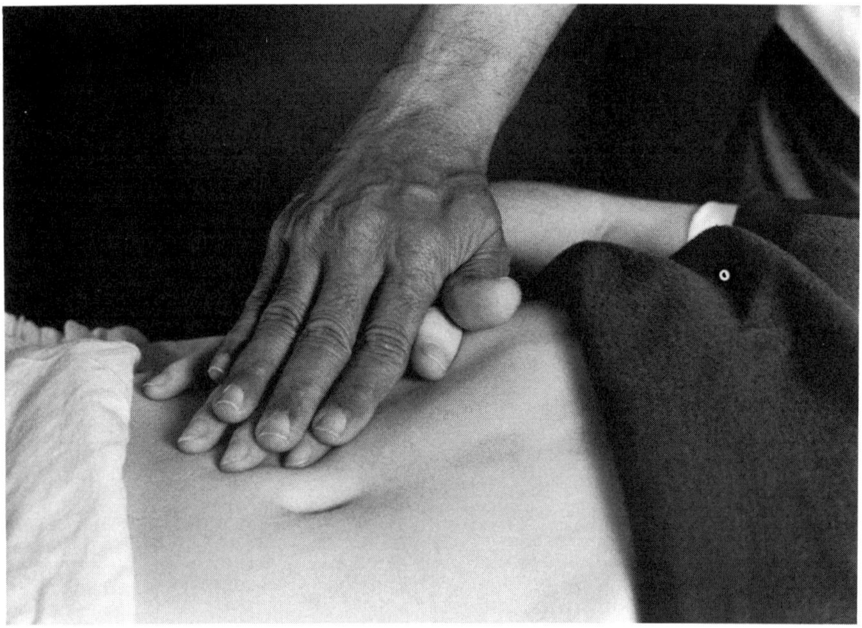

Figure 7C-1. Technique for palpation of abdomen in children who are sensitive to touch.

disease or muscle spasm, as in tetanus. Localized firmness indicates a mass (e.g., a midline firm mass may be a full bladder). Very soft texture of the abdominal wall is seen in prune-belly syndrome. A palpable mass in the right lower quadrant may be the cecum or the appendix. A mass in the right upper quadrant is usually related to the liver, and in the left upper quadrant is related to the stomach or the spleen. Flank masses are usually related to the kidneys.

Before palpating the abdomen, make sure the child has no area of pain in the abdomen. Ask the child to point to where it hurts and palpate the painful area last. Normally, abdominal palpation should cause no pain. If there is an area of tenderness, note its location and point of maximum intensity. Also, try to elicit rebound tenderness. Press firmly over one area of the abdomen. If there is no pain, suddenly release and remove the fingers from the abdominal wall. If there is tenderness on withdrawal of the fingers, it is called *rebound tenderness* and indicates peritoneal irritation.

Tenderness along the edge of the liver is seen in hepatitis. Tenderness over the right upper quadrant to the right of the midline is seen in duodenal ulcer. Tenderness of the right lower quadrant is seen in appendiceal infection. Left upper quadrant tenderness may be indicative of splenic rupture or infarct. Tenderness along the left upper and lower quadrants along the flanks is seen in ulcerative colitis and amebiasis. Loin tenderness is seen in perinephric abscess. Diffuse tenderness of the abdomen indicates peritonitis. Pain due to spastic bowel conditions is relieved by pressure and squeezing, whereas pain due to intraabdominal inflammatory conditions is aggravated by pressure.

Pyloric Stenosis. A few words about the palpation of the abdomen for the pyloric mass in congenital pyloric stenosis. It is best to examine the infant after the stomach has been emptied. Have someone hold the baby in a relaxed position. It will be helpful to give the baby some sugar-water to drink just before palpating for the mass. Sometimes it is necessary to feed the baby clear liquids until the baby vomits and than palpate the abdomen soon after the vomiting. The examiner should gently flex the hip with one hand to relax the anterior abdominal wall, then palpate the abdomen with the other hand at a point midway between the umbilicus and the costal margin along the lateral border of the right rectus muscle. The fingertips should be used with a kneading up-and-down motion. The pyloric mass is usually felt as a firm olivelike swelling.

Appendicitis. Appendicitis often starts in children with a history of persistent but vague and diffuse abdominal pain, often in the periumbilical area. Since this location for pain is common in children, it is not diagnostic. But soon it localizes to the right lower quadrant. The appendix may not be located in the classical location, so symptoms and signs may vary depending on the location. Flank pain may be seen with location of the appendix along the paracolic gutter. There may also be loss of appetite, low grade fever, and change in bowel habits. Constipation is the usual manifestation though diarrhea may occur with retrocecal or pelvic appendix.

The classical finding on examination is local point tenderness over the inflamed appendix. This may be located on the McBurney's point, which is a point midway between the right anterior superior iliac spine and the umbilicus. If the appendix is located along the paracolic gutter, the tenderness may be over the flank of the abdomen or felt only on deep palpation. If the appendix is in retrocecal or pelvic position, tenderness is elicited on a deep rectal examination. Cough may also aggravate the pain and cause the child to wince.

If the appendix has perforated, the child will appear toxic and pale, may have grunting respiration, and is often lying still. The abdomen is rigid with generalized guarding, and bowel sounds are absent. A mass may be palpable in the right lower quadrant, either on examination of the abdomen or on rectal examination.

Liver. The liver is normally located on the right side and its size varies with the age and size of the child. In addition, size of the liver as determined by palpation will be different from the size determined by percussion. Neither of these are as accurate as the size determined by roentgenograms. Good studies are available with normal data for total height of the liver and for the size of the liver palpable below the costal margin using clinical methods.

With the child lying supine without a pillow, stand on the right side of the child (if you are right-handed) and palpate starting from the lower right quadrant gradually moving up. If the liver edge is palpated, measure the size below the costal margin at the midclavicular line using a ruler or tape measure. Normal values are: 3.0 to 3.5 cm below the costal margin up to 6 months of age; 0 to 3 cm in children between 6 months to 4 years of age; less than 2 cm in children between 4 years and 10 years of age and less than 1 cm in children over 10 years of age.

To measure the total height of the liver, percuss along the midclavicular line anteriorly with the pleximeter finger held parallel to the ribs using heavy percussion. A mark is made at the intercostal space when dullness is first noted. To determine the lower border of the liver, percussion is started at the right lower quadrant and gradually moved toward the costal margin. Light percussion is used. The point at which the tone changes to dullness is marked, and this denotes the lower edge of the liver. The vertical height between the two points is now measured. Normal values for vertical height of the liver (liver span) at various ages are given in Table 7C-1.

Be sure to palpate the left lobe of the liver at the epigastrium. This is particularly important in the tropics, where amebic abscess of the liver and portal hypertension are common. In both these conditions, the left lobe of the liver is more prominent than the right lobe. It is good to auscultate over

TABLE 7C-1. EXPECTED LIVER SPAN OF INFANTS AND CHILDREN (in cm)

Males			Females		
Age/yr	*Mean Estimated Liver Span*	*SEM*	*Age/yr*	*Mean Estimated Liver Span*	*SEM*
6 months	2.4	2.5	6 months	2.6	2.6
1	2.8	2.0	1	3.1	2.1
2	3.5	1.6	2	3.6	1.7
3	4.0	1.6	3	4.0	1.7
4	4.4	1.6	4	4.3	1.6
5	4.8	1.5	5	4.5	1.6
6	5.1	1.5	6	4.8	1.6
8	5.6	1.5	8	5.1	1.6
10	6.1	1.6	10	5.4	1.7
12	6.5	1.8	12	5.6	1.8
14	6.8	2.0	14	5.8	2.1
16	7.1	2.2	16	6.0	2.3
18	7.4	2.5	18	6.1	2.6
20	7.7	2.8	20	6.3	2.9

SEM: Standard Error of the Mean.

(Reproduced with permission from Lawson EE, Grand RJ, Neff RK, and Cohen LF: Clinical estimation of liver span in infants and children. Amer J Dis Child 132:474–476, 1978. Copyright 1978, American Medical Association.)

the liver, since a hepatic rub can be heard in the presence of perihepatitis, liver abscess, and leukemic infiltration of the liver.

Spleen. The spleen is located normally on the left side. It is usually not palpable unless it is enlarged at least three times its size. If the spleen is not palpable with the patient in the supine position, try to feel for it with the patient in the right lateral position. The patient is asked to lie on his right side. The examiner's left hand is placed over the left lower ribs on the midscapular line pushing the spleen forward. Now, the right hand is used to palpate the spleen. This is called Short's maneuver. Remember to start over the right lower quadrant and proceed diagonally toward the left upper quadrant. Recognizing an enlarged spleen depends on feeling the edge of the organ. A very large spleen may cross the midline with the palpable edge on the right side, and the examiner can easily miss the edge if palpation is done only on the left side.

Castell described a percussion sign for determining an enlarged spleen. With the patient in the supine position, percussion of the lower intercostal spaces on the anterior axillary line should produce a resonant note both in inspiration and expiration. If the spleen is enlarged, the percussion over the lower intercostal spaces is resonant during expiration and dull during inspiration. Remember also to listen over the spleen with the stethoscope since a splenic rub may be heard in perisplenitis.

Other Intraabdominal Organs and Masses. Masses over the right lower quadrant are usually related to the appendix but may be due to cecal mass or to ovarian masses in the female. In intussusception, an ill-defined sausage-shaped mass is felt over the right upper quadrant. Associated with this, the right lower quadrant is found to be empty.

Palpation of the kidneys may be difficult in obese children. In normal children, one uses deep bimanual palpation to feel for the kidneys. With the patient supine and the abdomen relaxed, place the palm of one hand posteriorly at the flank, pushing the kidneys forward. With the other hand placed anteriorly below the costal margin, push the abdominal wall backwards and upwards. The kidney is felt best in deep inspiration.

After feeling for the liver and spleen and the urinary bladder, feel for any other intraabdominal masses. If any mass is felt in the abdomen describe its characteristics under the following headings:

1. Location
2. Upper and lower borders
3. Does it cross midline or is it in midline?
4. Is it attached to abdominal wall?
5. Is it firm, hard, soft, or cystic?
6. Does it move with respiration?

7. Is it movable?
8. Is there bruit or murmur? Is it pulsatile?

Percussion (for fluid)

Normally, the abdomen sounds tympanic on percussion except when percussed over solid organs such as the liver or a full bladder. A highly tympanic note is heard in intestinal obstruction or paralytic ileus. A dull note on an enlarged abdomen may indicate free fluid in the abdominal cavity or a tumor.

There are two methods to elicit signs of free fluid in the peritoneal cavity:

Fluid wave: With the patient supine, have another observer place the edge of the hand vertically on the midline of the abdominal wall (Fig. 7C-2). The examiner now places the palm of the hand on one side and taps

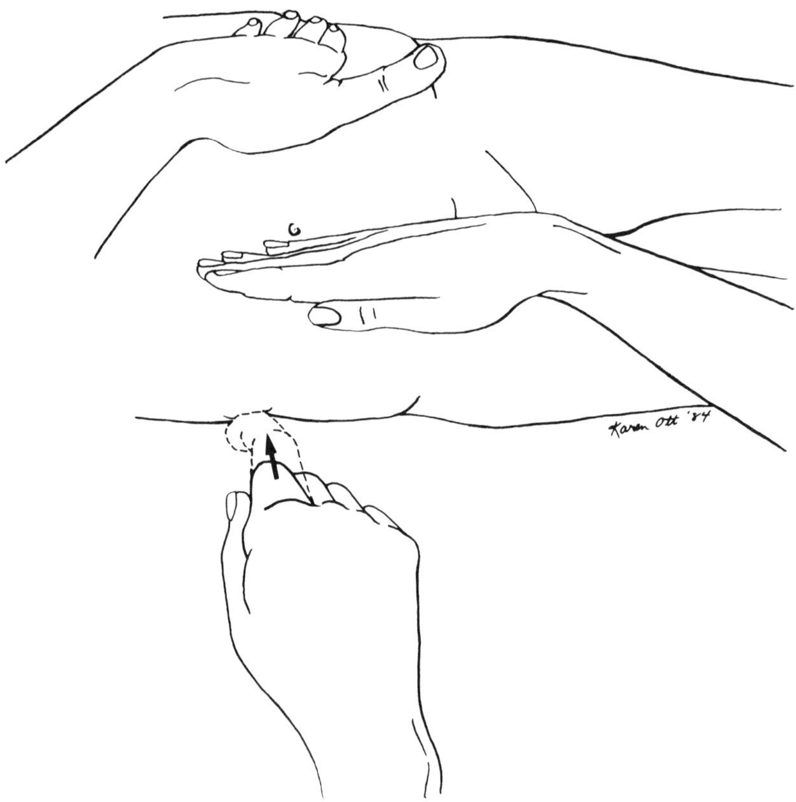

Figure 7C-2. Method used to elicit fluid wave in the abdomen. The examiner is palpating the flank of the abdomen with one hand and tapping on the opposite flank with fingers of the other hand. An assistant places his hand in the midline to obliterate the feeling of stretching of the skin which may interfere with appreciation of the fluid wave.

with the fingers on the opposite flank. If free fluid is present, one can feel a fluid wave created by the tap.

Shifting dullness: With the patient in the supine position, place a finger on the flank parallel to the midline. Percuss over an area of dullness. Now ask the patient to roll over and lie on the opposite side to the percussed dullness, while the examiner keeps the pleximeter finger in place. After the fluid has time to settle at the dependent position, percuss again. Percussion will now give a tympanic note over the same area where it was dull when the patient was supine.

To detect very small amounts of fluid, place the patient in a knee-chest position and percuss over the periumbilical area. Normally this area should not be dull on percussion.

Bowel Sounds (auscultation)

Normally, the bowel sounds are best heard along a diagonal line 6 inches long, starting 1 inch to the left and above the umbilicus and running toward the right lower quadrant. The sounds have a gurgling quality. These sounds are increased and have a higher pitch in the presence of gastroenteritis. The sounds have a metallic quality during early stages of intestinal obstruction. These sounds are absent in paralytic ileus and in late obstruction. In the presence of ascites and peritonitis, the sound may be distant.

In addition, listen to murmurs over the abdomen, particularly over the (loin) flank, since renal artery stenosis can produce a systolic murmur.

INGUINAL REGIONS

Hernia, hydrocele, undescended testicle, and lymph nodes are the common causes of swelling in the inguinal region. If a swelling is present in this area, describe the characteristics as outlined earlier (page 8, Table 2–1). In addition, describe whenever there are fluctuations in size, either spontaneously or related to coughing or crying.

Hernia

Indirect inguinal hernia is the commonest variety (direct inguinal and femoral hernia are rare). It occurs more often in boys. Classically, there is a bulge in the inguinal region extending into the scrotum. This enlarges and becomes tense when the child cries. Usually the swelling becomes smaller in size when the child is not straining, or it may be reduced by external manipulation. If the swelling cannot be reduced, one should suspect an associated hydrocele of the spermatic cord or the hernia may be incarcerated. To differentiate between these two conditions, palpate above the level of the hernia. If an empty hernial sac is palpable above this mass, it probably represents a combination of hernia and a hydrocele. If no empty hernial sac is palpable above the level of the mass, if the mass is not reducible, and if the child is in pain, it is probably an incarcerated hernia. Not infrequently, in a young female, an ovary may be palpated in the hernial sac.

Other subtle evidences of inguinal hernia can be looked for as follows: palpate the spermatic cord and compare with the opposite side and with what you have felt in normal children. A thickened cord is an evidence of indirect inguinal hernia. Also, palpate the cord gently and roll it along its longitudinal axis under your fingers. A silky texture to the cord may be suggestive of an indirect inguinal hernia. This is a very subjective sign, and surgical hernia repair should not be initiated on the basis of the "silky cord" sign alone.

Hydrocele

Hydrocele produces a swelling of the scrotum or along the spermatic cord. It is usually a fluctuant swelling, alters in size (if associated with a hernia), or gradually increases in size (if there is communication between the processus vaginalis and the hydrocele sac). A hydrocele may transilluminate, but hernias usually do not.

Hydrocele is often physiologic up to 3 months of age and the fluid is reabsorbed. If there is hydrocele after 4 months of age, it is not normal or physiologic and is usually associated with an indirect inguinal hernia. One should look for signs of hernia as described in the earlier paragraph.

A cystic mass along the inguinal canal in a girl is due to hydrocele of the tunica vaginalis and is called the hydrocele of the canal of Nuck. Such a swelling should also make one suspect a testis in a phenotypic female.

Undescended Testes

Will be described in the following section on genitalia.

Lymph Nodes

Inguinal nodes are located along the crease made by flexion of the hip lateral to the inguinal canal. Children normally may have palpable inguinal nodes, but they are relatively small to medium size, soft to firm in consistency, freely movable and tender.

In contrast, femoral nodes are located below the line of the inguinal ligament in the femoral triangle in a vertical direction. Palpable femoral nodes are not usually normal.

If nodes are palpable, describe the characteristics as outlined in Table 2–1, page 8.

GENITALIA

Male Genitalia

Normally, any full-term newborn should have a well-formed penis and scrotum. The length of the penis at this period is usually 4 cm. The shape is normally cylindrical (and it may be bent if there is aberrent location of the urethral opening). The urethra opens at the tip of the penis. The normal prepuce is easily retractable so that the meatal opening can be observed.

The scrotum is highly pigmented in the newborn. The testes are both located in the scrotal sac and measure about 1 cm in length. The left scrotum is at a lower level than the right, and there is no enlargement of the scrotum on straining or coughing. As the children grow older, the anatomy is about the same, except for reduction of pigmentation of the scrotum. During the preadolescent period, secondary sexual characteristics start appearing.

During physical examination, undress the child completely and examine under good light. The *abnormalities* to be looked for should be described under the following headings:

- Size and shape of penis
- Prepuce
- Urethral orifice
- Size of scrotum
- Color of scrotum
- Testes and secondary sexual characteristics

The *size* of the penis is variable. If a penis is large, determine whether it is a real increase in size or an appearance of large size due to priapism, as in sickle cell disease. True enlargement of the penis is seen in precocious puberty, lesions of the central nervous system, testicular tumors, and congenital adrenal hyperplasia. In adrenal hyperplasia the penis is large but not the testes, whereas in precocious puberty both the testes and penis are large.

If the penis is small, is it true hypoplasia or an apparently small penis? The penis may appear small in fat boys, and the true size not appreciated unless the prepubic fat tissue is pushed in to reveal the full length of the shaft. True hypoplasia may be seen in certain congenital malformation syndromes, hypopituitarism, and Klinefelter syndrome.

Next, look at the *shape*. The shape of the penis may be curved, as in hypospadias, or stiff and painful, as in sickle cell crisis.

Now examine the *prepuce*. If the preputial sac is very narrow and cannot be retracted, it is called phimosis. One good method to test for phimosis in doubtful cases is to have the child lie supine. Pick up folds of the prepuce with both hands and pull gently upward without hurting. If a good tunnel is formed by the preputial skin, with the meatal opening clearly visible at the end of the tunnel, it is normal.

The normal *urethral orifice* is located at the tip of the penis. If it is located on the under surface of the urethra it is hypospadias. The most important conditions associated with hypospadias are cryptorchidism and hermaphroditism. There are associations with many other syndromes. Epispadias is location of the urethral orifice on the dorsal surface of the penis.

This is less common than hypospadias but often associated with extrophy of the bladder.

Normally, there should be no urethral discharge at any age in a male. If it occurs, one should think of foreign bodies (less common in boys), balanoposthitis, gonorrhea, and Reiter syndrome.

Normally, the *scrotal sac* converges at the base of the penis on its ventral aspect. If portions of the scrotal skin come around the base of the penis over the dorsal aspect also (shawl scrotum), one should suspect incomplete masculinization or virilization syndromes.

Initially examine the scrotum without touching. Normally, the left side of the scrotum is at a lower level than the right. But one side is not larger than the other. If one side appears larger than the other, one has to decide whether the larger side is abnormal (due to swelling of the testes or swelling around the testes) or the smaller side is abnormal due to absence of testis in its usual location. Palpation of the testicle and the soft tissues of the scrotum should help decide this question. In addition, look at the wrinkles over the scrotum. If the distance between the wrinkles is narrower on the small side as compared to the larger side, most likely the testis has not descended into that scrotum.

The scrotum may be small if the testis has not descended. If the scrotum is empty, palpate along the inguinal canal between the anterior superior iliac spine and pubic tubercle for the testis. In many children when lying down, the testes may appear to be in a higher position. When they sit or stand, however, the testes descend into the scrotum. If on palpation a testicular mass is felt along the inguinal canal, try to gently push this into the scrotum with the thumb and index finger of the other hand through the scrotum. If this can be done, the testis is descended, even if it goes back up quickly. This is called a retractile testis. If the mass is felt along the inguinal canal but cannot be pushed down into the scrotum by the above technique, it is an undescended testis. If the testis is not felt anywhere, it is abdominal testis (provided, of course, it is a male; a penis with an absent testis, of course, should suggest the possibility of ambiguous genitalia).

Another useful technique to palpate the testis along the inguinal canal is as follows: moisten the finger tips with liquid soap and rub the fingers gently but firmly along the inguinal canal from above downward. If the testis is there, it will "plop" under your finger.

A large scrotum may indicate one of the following: (1) thickened skin (as in elephantiasis of the scrotum); (2) fluid in the sac (hydrocele); (3) intestines in the scrotum (hernia); (4) large testis; (5) large epididymis.

A large scrotum that becomes small when the child is lying down or when the child is relaxed but gets large from a cough or straining is probably a hernia. Masses that cannot be reduced may be normal structures within the scrotum, such as the testis, or they may be testicular tumors. Hydrocele, of course, cannot be reduced completely, though it may become smaller on pressure.

Normal color of the scrotum is darker than the rest of the body. Red color with tenderness should indicate inflammation (orchitis) or torsion of the testis. Blue lines along the scrotal sac indicate varicocele. Normally the scrotum is not tender to palpation, though the testis has a peculiar characteristic sensation. Tender scrotum may indicate inflammation of any of the tissues or torsion of the testis or a strangulated or incarcerated hernia.

Now look for the size of the penis, scrotum, testicular size, and pubic hair to determine the state of sexual development. Normal stages of sexual development are given in Tables 10-1, 10-2, and 10-3 pages 311 and 312.

Female Genitalia

Examination of the genitalia may be a traumatic experience for children of any age. Therefore proper preparation and good explanations are essential. One should be sensitive to the child's feelings and shyness. The examination should not be abrupt or threatening. While examining adolescent girls, make sure a female nurse or the mother is present. Examine under good light. Proper positioning is essential for a good examination of the genitalia. In young infants and children who cannot cooperate, examine the children sitting on their mother's lap in a semirecumbent position. Have the child's feet supported on your knees and ask the child to place the soles of the feet together. This diverts their attention and also fully abducts the thighs. Now, grasp the labia majora between the thumb and index finger and draw outwards, thus exposing the labia minora, urethral meatus, and vagina. Most of the findings can be easily observed on inspection alone. Bimanual palpation is possible if done cautiously. The finger cannot advance too far into the fornix, which is very short.

In the newborn, the genitalia are highly pigmented and edematous, particularly in breech delivery.

In older prepubertal children, the labia minora have receded in size with relation to the remainder of the external genitalia. The glans clitoris is no longer than 3 mm and is 2 mm wide. The hymen is seen just interior to the introitus. The vaginal mucosa is red and appears thin. If the older child is placed in the knee-chest position, the introitus will gape open, allowing a view of the vagina and cervix; foreign bodies may be seen in this position.

The points to be looked for on examination of the female genitalia (other than in newborns) are:

1. Normal secondary sexual development: look for the appearance and distribution of pubic hair. Tanner's classification of various stages of sexual development are given in Tables 10-1, 10-2, and 10-3.
2. Look at the general hygiene, smell, and staining of pants; don't forget to look for lice if pubic hair is present.
3. Urethral discharge is uncommon at any age. If present, it may indicate mechanical irritation (tight panties, foreign body, mastur-

bation), physiological (for 2 to 3 years before menstruation starts), or inflammation anywhere along the tract.

4. Look for cyst, caruncle, or prolapse around the urethral orifice.
5. Look for foreign bodies by separating the labia. A foreign body in the vagina is a common cause for vaginal discharge and bleeding. Occasionally, bimanual palpation with one finger in the rectum and one in the vagina is needed to palpate the foreign body.
6. Look for discharge and the characteristics of the vaginal discharge. Bloody vaginal discharge seen in the newborn period is often due to estrogen withdrawal and is physiologic. In older infants, a foreign body is a common cause for vaginal discharge. This is intermittent, blood stained, and foul smelling. In adolescent girls, bloody vaginal discharge is usually due to normal menstruation and rarely due to sarcoma botryoides. Watery discharge may be caused by local irritation or local infections. Purulent discharge, particularly in adolescent girls, should suggest gonococcal infection. Whitish cheesy discharge is associated with *Candida* infection.
7. Examine the clitoris. A large clitoris may be a normal variation or may indicate precocious puberty. In gonadal dysgenesis and hypopituitarism, the clitoris is small. If there is no tissue surrounding the superior aspect of what appears to be the clitoris, it is probably not a clitoris.
8. In prepubertal girls, synechiae may fuse the two sides of the labiae. These can be easily separated normally, and they will always separate spontaneously in association with the vaginal pH change in puberty.
9. Next examine the labia majora. They may be fused in congenital adrenal hyperplastia giving the appearance of a scrotum. Labia majora are hypoplastic and the clitoris appears large in Trisomy-18 syndrome.
10. Look for an imperforate hymen, particularly in the presence of what appears to be an enlarged uterus in an adolescent girl.

Ambiguous Genitalia

Ambiguity is suggested by the presence of:

1. Large clitoris
2. Small penis
3. Hypospadias
4. Undescended testis
5. Fused labia majora
6. Inguinal hernia with a mass in a "female" infant

If ambiguous genitalia are suspected in the newborn period, investigation is required prior to sex assignment.

When there is a discrepancy between the morphology of the gonads and of the external genitalia it is intersexuality. If in a XX female with ovaries the external genitalia are virilized, it is a female pseudohermaphrodite. If, in a XY male with testes, the external genitalia are ambiguous or female, it is a male pseudohermaphrodite.

ANUS AND RECTUM

Examination of the genitalia and anus can be traumatic to a child. Proper preparation and gentle methods are crucial for a good examination and future cooperation. It is best to examine these areas with the child lying on his or her left side (left lateral position).

On inspection, first look at the location of the anus. In certain congenital malformations of the rectum, the opening may be too far forward, close to the genitalia. There may be no opening at all or the opening of the rectum may be through a small fistula or into the vagina (female) or urethra (male). Passage of meconium through the vagina or urethra should suggest that recto-urethral or recto-vaginal communication exists.

Next look for pinworm or segments of tapeworm close to the anal opening. Presence of cracks and fissures in the mucocutaneous junction is called fissure-in-ano. This may be related to a variety of causes, such as pinworms, constipation, eczema, or other mechanical irritation. Painful fissure in turn causes constipation and blood streaks in the stools.

Conditions that cause nodular lesions in and around the anus are: (1) rectal tag; (2) polyps; (3) hemorrhoids; (4) prolapse of the rectum; and (5) anorectal abscess. Small rectal tags are of no clinical significance. If there are rectal polyps, remember to look for oral mucous-membrane pigmentation (Peutz-Jegher syndrome). Polyps are pedunculated and reddish in color. Hemorrhoids are uncommon in children and are characterized by solid dark protrusions. If they occur, look for some underlying cause such as vena caval or mesenteric obstruction. A true prolapse of the rectum is seen in chronic diarrhea, amebic dysentery, cystic fibrosis, severe cough (pertussis), or severe worm infestations. Also look for anorectal abscess which will be tender, warm, indurated, or fluctuant.

Fistulae are uncommon in children except in the presence of a congenital anomaly, in which case they open into the vagina or urethra. Acquired fistula are due to abscesses and open into the perianal skin. This is particularly common in ulcerative colitis and regional ileitis. A probe can usually be introduced into the fistula.

Rectal examination is done with the child in the left lateral position. In most children, particularly the small ones, it is better to use the examiner's little finger. In older children one may use the gloved index finger. The finger cot should be greased properly before entering the rectum.

As you enter, first feel for the sphincter tone. If the anal opening is tight, it may denote anal stenosis or an anxious child, but if the examining finger cannot be moved in at all think of agenesis of the rectum or imperforate anus. In conditions associated with spinal cord lesions (such as myelomeningocele and traumatic paralysis), the sphincter does not grip the finger since the sphincter tone is poor or absent.

Exquisite tenderness on entering the rectum may indicate anorectal abscess or acute prostatitis. Usually, fecal masses can be felt in the rectum. An empty rectum may suggest intestinal obstruction or megacolon. In megacolon, one may feel a sudden widening of the ampulla proximal to the line of agenesis of ganglia. If any mass (other than feces) is felt, determine whether it is part of the gut, or a polyp, or a mass in the pelvis. Bimanual palpation with one finger in the rectum and fingers of the other hand over the anterior abdominal wall or in the vagina will help determine the nature of the pelvic mass.

On bimanual palpation, the uterus (in girls) and the bladder (both sexes) may be felt usually on the midline. Foreign bodies in the vagina and rectum may be felt during this procedure.

Remember: (1) to look at the face of the child during the rectal examination to see whether there is tenderness; (2) to examine the stool obtained by rectal examination for ova, parasites, and blood.

BIBLIOGRAPHY

Castell DO: The spleen percussion sign: A useful diagnostic technique. Ann Intern Med 67:1265–1267, 1967.

Deligeorgis D, Yannakos D, Panayotou P, Doxiadis S: The normal borders of liver in infancy and childhood: Clinical and X-ray study. Arch Dis Child 45:702–704, 1970.

Emans SJH, Goldstein DP: Pediatric and Adolescent Gynecology, 2nd ed. Boston, Little, Brown, 1982.

Koop CE: Visible and Palpable Lesions in Children. New York, Grune & Stratton, 1976.

Lawson EE, Grand RJ, Neff RK, Cohen LF: Clinical estimation of liver span in infants and children. Am J Dis Child 132:474–476, 1978.

Redman JF, Bissada NK: How to make a good examination of the genitalia in young girls. Clin Pediatr 15:907–908, 1976.

7D. Skin

The skin is an ideal body system for observation and interpretation of clinical findings in a logical fashion. The major clinical findings in relation to the skin are to be described under three headings:

- Color
- Nature of lesion
- Texture (palpation)

COLOR

First observe the color of the skin in various parts of the body. Mottling of skin is not uncommon in the normal newborn and infants, particularly if the room is cold. This mottling will clear when the environmental temperature becomes warm. Mottling can also occur in the presence of shock at any age, giving a "crazy pavement" appearance.

Undue redness of the entire skin may be noted in the presence of fever, after exertion, exposure to the sun, early stages of scarlet fever, and atropine toxicity. Undue pallor of one extremity may be due to arterial occlusion. Sudden episodes of pallor of the fingers and toes, on exposure to cold, followed by sequential changes in the color of fingers to blue, red, and then to normal is called Raynaud's phenomenon. Cyanosis is blue color of the skin. Determine whether it affects only the distal parts of the body (peripheral) or affects the lips and tongue also (central).

Jaundice is yellowish discoloration of the skin and conjunctiva. The intensity of staining may vary from the very slight jaundice of Gilbert disease to the intense green-yellow of biliary atresia. Presence of associated itching and dark stool suggests biliary obstruction.

Next look at the *normal* pigmentation of the skin which varies among various ethnic groups. Even within each group there are variations. If there is *depigmentation,* find out whether it is *localized* or *generalized.* Also inquire about the time of onset. Congenital generalized absence of melanin pigment is seen in albinism, in which the scalp hair and eyebrows are also pale. A congenital form of localized hypopigmentation is partial albinism (piebaldism), in which the forehead, anterior scalp (white forelock), elbows, and knees are affected with areas of hypopigmentation.

Vitiligo is an acquired disorder causing localized areas of depigmentation. Areas commonly affected are the face around the eyes and mouth, hands, feet, elbows, and knees. Another important condition in which hypopigmented lesions occur is tuberous sclerosis. Patients with this disorder develop white macules shaped like an ash leaf, particularly over the trunk. These lesions are visible to the naked eye but may need examination under a Wood lamp.

Excess pigmentation may be due to racial characteristics or exposure to the sun. Determine whether it is generalized or localized in distribution. A generalized slate color is seen in Addison's disease and in congenital adrenal hyperplasia. This pigmentation of Addison's disease also involves the buccal mucosa. Localized areas of hyperpigmentation may be seen, as in a normal area of overproduction of melanin (freckles and moles), or as a result of chronic inflammation (as in eczema), or as in cafe-au-lait spots (Fig. 7D-1).

Alternate areas of depigmentation and excess pigmentation are seen in scleroderma and vitiligo.

NATURE OF LESIONS

Clinical diagnosis on the basis of the description of the lesions (rashes) becomes easy if we describe them under the following headings: primary lesion, secondary lesion, and distribution.

The *primary* lesions are:

1. Macules: these are flat lesions flush with the surface of the skin that blanch with pressure (petechiae do not).

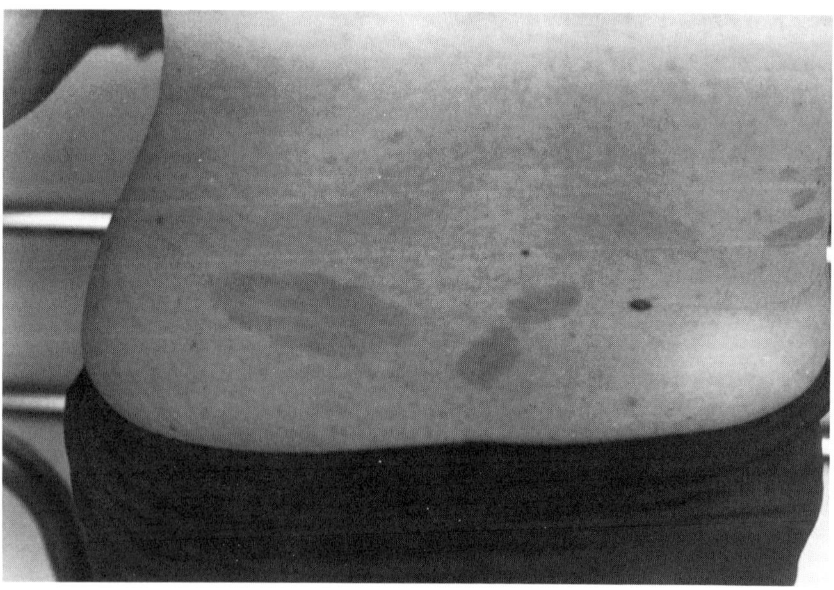

Figure 7D-1. *Cafe-au-lait* lesions. *(Photograph courtesy of Dr. PJ Koblenzer.)*

2. Papules: these are thickened, elevated lesions and are small in size (up to 1 cm). Papules, nodules, and tumors are different gradations of morphologically similar lesions except for variation in size and depth of involvement. Plaques are confluent papules.
3. Vesicles: these are also elevated lesions—projecting above the surface of the skin but having fluid in them. Small lesions are called vesicles and larger ones are called bullae or blebs.
4. Pustules: similar to vesicles but containing pus. Deeper lesions with pus are called abscesses.
5. Wheals: slightly elevated lesions of the skin with the central portion of the lesion paler than the periphery.
6. Petechiae and purpura: bloodstained spots in the skin. Petechiae are smaller (less than 0.2 cm) and purpura are larger (up to 1.0 cm).

The *secondary* lesions are:

1. Excoriations, caused by scratching, leaving nail marks. Lichenification is hyperpigmented dry plaques with accentuated skin markings.
2. Crust formation, the result of dried fluid (serum, blood, or pus) if the primary lesion is a vesicle or pustule (as in impetigo, Fig. 7D-2).

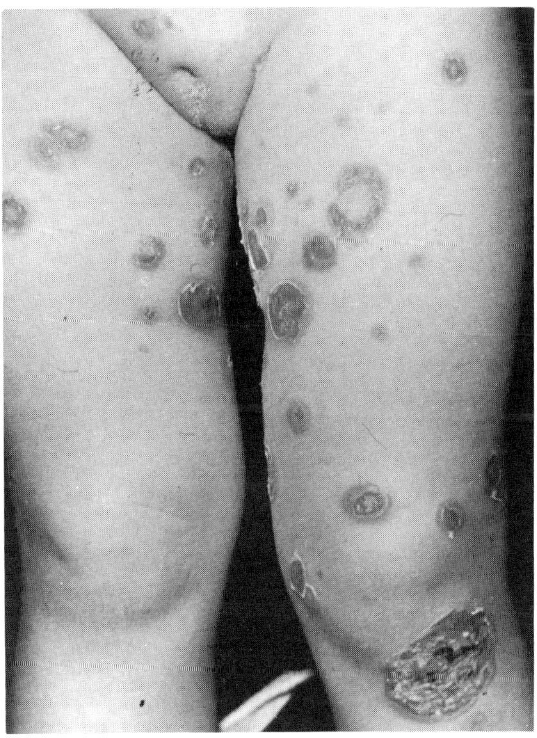

Figure 7D-2. Impetigo. *(Photograph courtesy of Dr. PJ Koblenzer and the Skin and Cancer Hospital of Philadelphia.)*

3. Desquamation, a scaling of the primary lesion with desiccated plates of cornified epithelial cells.
4. Increased pigmentation around the primary lesion, a common condition.
5. Ulceration, a depressed lesion due to loss of both epidermis and part of the dermis.
6. Scar formation, caused by replacement of dermis and subcutaneous tissue with fibrous tissue following injury (no normal skin markings, no hair follicles, no sweat pores, and no melanin).
7. Atrophy, characterized by an "ironed-out" appearance and increased translucency.

DISTRIBUTION OF LESIONS

In the differential diagnosis, one combines the characteristics of the primary and secondary lesions with the areas of distribution. When describing the lesion remember to include the following headings:

1. Primary lesion
2. Secondary lesion
3. Distribution
4. If elevated, is it rounded or pointed?
5. If vesicle, is it umbilicated?
6. Is there redness around it?
7. Is there pigmentation around it?
8. Does it "feel" more than it "looks"?
9. Is it superficial or deep?
10. If it is an ulcer, describe the base and the edge of the ulcer. Also look for induration under or around the ulcer.

The pattern of distribution of skin lesions gives valuable clues to diagnosis. For example, red pointed papules and pustules over the face and on the back of the upper part of the trunk in an adolescent are most likely caused by acne (Chapter 10, p. 313). Lesions of pityriasis rosea are seen mostly on the trunk (Fig. 7D-3). Lesions of scabies (grayish linear lesions with a vesicle or pustule at one end) are often seen over the palms, creases of the wrist (Fig. 7D-4), axilla, perianal area, and dorsum of the penis. Grouped vesicles along dermatomal distribution suggest herpes zoster.

Rash in the diaper area involving the groin folds is the result of retention of moisture in the area. Rash in the same area sparing the folds but involving the convexities is probably contact dermatitis. Rash in the diaper area with satellite lesions indicates secondary infection, either fungal or bacterial.

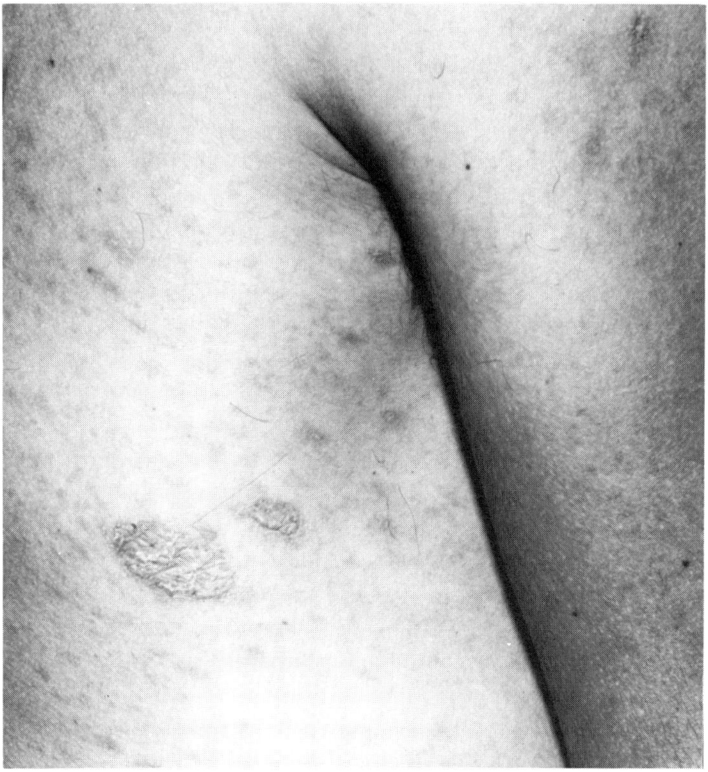

Figure 7D-3. Pityriasis rosea. Note the herald lesion and also the characteristic lesions along the lines of cleavage. *(Photograph courtesy of Dr. PJ Koblenzer and the Skin and Cancer Hospital of Philadelphia.)*

PALPATION OF LESIONS

Texture: Normal skin has a smooth, soft, moist feeling. Rough and dry skin come from a simple cause such as excess bathing or to a serious condition such as congenital icthyosis (collodion baby). A rough coarse skin is commonly seen in various allergies and hypothyroidism.

Edema: Pitting on pressure is a good sign of the presence of edema. Occasionally it may be firm and nonpitting. An area of skin may appear edematous in the presence of subcutaneous emphysema.

Elasticity: To test for elasticity pick up the skin and let go. Normally the skin should fall back to the original state quickly. In the presence of dehydration, the skin does not fall back quickly and remains in folds ("tented"). This is particularly well demonstrated over the anterior abdominal wall.

Excess elasticity of the skin demonstrated over the elbow, forearm and

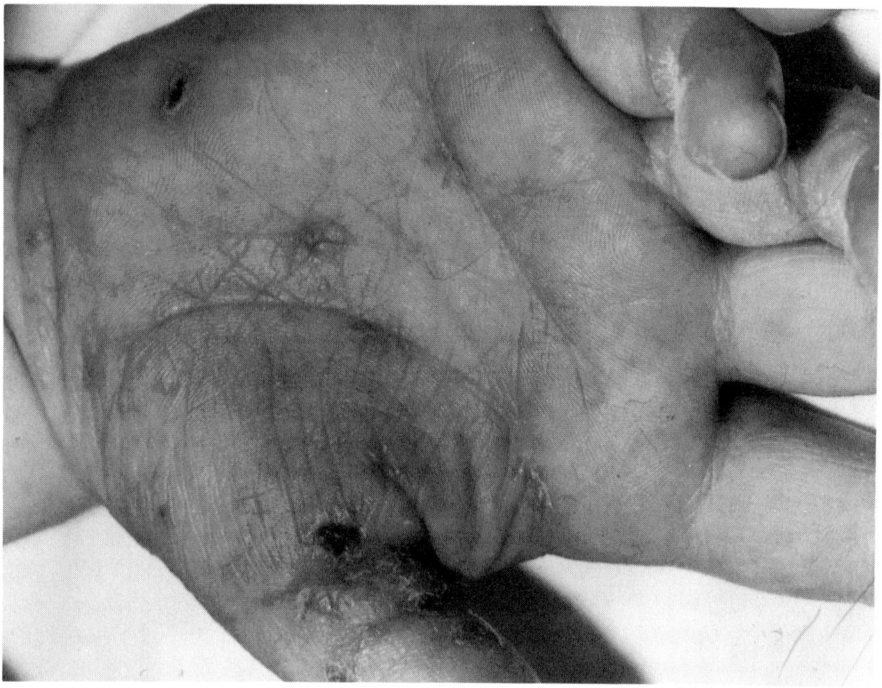

Figure 7D-4. Scabies. *(Photograph courtesy of Dr. PJ Koblenzer and the Skin and Cancer Hospital of Philadelphia.)*

interscapular areas, and the cheek is seen in variants of Ehler-Danlos syndrome.

Collections of pus, blood, lymph, or air under the skin can also be palpated during this stage of the examination.

HEMANGIOMAS

Vascular tumors (nevi) of the skin may be flat or nodular (tumorous). Examples of the flat type are: stork-bite lesion of the newborn (over the eyelids, glabella, or nuchal region), port-wine stain of Sturge-Weber syndrome, and spider nevus. The nodular type may be: strawberry hemangioma, red in color with a well-defined border, blanching on pressure, and firm in consistency; cavernous hemangioma with ill-defined borders and red-blue color. They feel like a bag of worms and do not fully collapse on pressure; mixed type, which has characteristics of a cavernous hemangioma and surface characteristics of port-wine stain.

Nevus Flammeus (port-wine stain) is present from birth, flat, well circumscribed, pink or purple, and varies in size. It often involves the neck and face. When present in the back of the neck it is called nevus of unna. When it is present as a feature of Sturge-Weber syndrome, it is seen over one half of the face. The color is purple. Port-wine stain may also be seen in association with other syndromes such as Klippel-Trenaunay-Weber and Trisomy-13.

Capillary Hemangiomata are also called strawberry nevi. They are bright in color, clearly circumscribed, slightly elevated above the surface of the skin, compressible, and blanch on pressure. They may be solitary lesions or multiple. When they are seen in the newborn as a flat lesion over the bridge of the nose and the nape of the neck, they are called stork-bite lesions. They may be present at birth, but they usually start during the first 2 months of life, gradually increase in size, and then regress. Most of the lesions spontaneously regress by the age of 9 years. The common locations are the face, scalp, back, and anterior chest.

Cavernous Hemangiomata are located deeper in the skin. Their margins, therefore, are not clear. The color is also more blue than red or purple. They may be nodular or cystic. These lesions also gradually grow bigger before regression, though the chances of spontaneous clearing are less than with capillary hemangioma.

NEVI

In popular usage, nevus is a word used to describe any birthmark or a pigmented skin lesion. Since pigmented lesions could be produced by either blood vessels or pigment from the melanocytes one can talk about vascular nevi and pigmented nevi.

Vascular Nevi were discussed in the preceding section. When describing these lesions, mention when they started (at birth or later), their location, size, increase or decrease in size, depth of lesion, margin, and compressibility.

Pigmented nevi originating from the nevus cells are different from the hyperpigmentation arising from mature melanocytes. The classification of these nevi as junctional, intradermal, or compound is based on the location of the nevus at the dermal-epidermal junction, dermis alone, or at both locations.

Junctional nevi are the commonest of these lesions, appearing most often in early childhood. They appear over any part of the body, are of varying shades of tan to brown, of various sizes, and are flat. Intradermal nevi are seen usually in adults. They can also be seen in any part of the body and are of varying sizes and shades of color. They are, however, usually dome-shaped or elevated, and coarse hair may be seen with this lesion. Compound nevi may be present at birth, but occur most often in older children. They are elevated lesions and flesh colored. Dark coarse hair may be seen with this lesion.

Occasionally a child may be born with a very large pigmented lesion that is often elevated above the surface and has an angular margin. These lesions are seen over the upper back, shoulders, and thighs, often in a dermatome distribution and they get descriptive names such as "bathing trunk," "coat-sleeve," and "stocking nevi." These are called the giant congenital pigmented nevi. Some of these lesions are associated with coarse brown hair. These giant hairy nevi may be associated with neurological problems.

Nevus of Ota is a bluish-gray lesion usually present at birth over the trigeminal area (face). These individuals may also have bluish discoloration of the sclera on the affected side.

Hyperpigmented lesions (freckles) are light or dark brown lesions which are seen usually over sun-exposed parts of the body such as the face. These lesions are not present at birth. In contrast, lentigines are also dark brown lesions but they can affect any part of the body and are present from birth.

Cafe-au-lait spots (Figure 7D-1) are hyperpigmented light tan macules of varying sizes which may be present at birth or develop during childhood. Normal children may have a few *cafe-au-lait* spots (fewer than three), but six or more lesions with a diameter of 1.5 cm or greater are considered to be characteristic of neurofibromatosis. Usually the border is regular, but large unilateral *cafe-au-lait* spots with an uneven border are considered characteristic of McCune-Albright syndrome (polyostotic fibrous dysplasia).

NAILS

A look at the nails can give many diagnostic clues. It was indicated earlier that curvature of the nail is not the same as clubbing. Many normal people (particularly women) have a longitudinal curvature of the nail. In true clubbing, the vertical height at the base of the nail is more than the vertical height of the distal interphalangeal joints (Fig. 6-11, page 71).

Fitzpatrick classifies the nail changes in a logical way, as follows:

Quantitative:	Area of nail—increased/decreased
	Thickness of nail—increased/decreased
	Nail bed changes—increased thickness
Qualitative:	Color
	Surface
	Consistency
	Adherence to nail bed

Quantitative changes. Acromegaly is the best example of a condition in which the total area of the nail is increased. In hyperparathyroidism the nails are large in surface area, broad and rounded, not clubbed.

Thickened nail plate is seen characteristically in chronic fungal infections. Thickened nail bed is seen in chronic inflammatory conditions or in the presence of fibrous tumors.

Decreased amount of nail is seen following accidental removal of nail, in nervous nail biters, and in epidermolysis.

Qualitative Changes. Color change to a red or blue area under the nail is most commonly caused by an injury resulting in subungual hematoma. The other important lesion to recognize is the subungual hemorrhage of subacute bacterial endocarditis. The nail beds will be blue in both central and peripheral cyanosis. Various other color changes have been noticed in chemical poisoning. In kala-azar and in Addison's disease fungus infections of the nail are associated with color changes—white flecks to yellow patches. Of course, one should not forget the nail polish!

Surface. Normally the surface should be smooth with slight convexity. Concave nails (koilonychia) are classically associated with iron-deficiency anemia though one sees such changes very rarely. Increased convexity of the nail surface is seen in many normal adults, but not so much in children. Loss of continuity of the surface with pits is seen classically in psoriasis and in eczema. Longitudinal and transverse ridges are common in adults and are seen rarely in children. Malnutrition and severe chronic inflammatory conditions such as eczematous dermatitis are the usual associated conditions.

Consistency. The nail may be excessively soft, as in chemical injury or malnutrition. It may be brittle, as in chemical injury. This is particularly seen after excess use of nail polish and polish removers. A very friable nail is seen in fungus infections and psoriasis.

Adherence. Partial separation of the nail from the nail bed is commonly due to trauma. It is also seen after severe dermatitis or exanthem, such as in erythema multiforme exudativum or exfoliative dermatitis. Look also for redness and swelling around the edge of the nail.

Nail fold infection is called paronychia, if acute. Though it is often caused by staphylococci, paronychia may also result from *Candida* and rarely from herpes simplex.

Pterygium is a layer of cuticle that grows over the proximal portion of the nail and is seen in dermatomyositis. Periungual erythema is seen also in dermatomyositis. Periungual telangiectasis is seen in scleroderma.

HAIR*

The characteristics of the hair to be observed are:

---

*See also Chapter 7A, page 95.

Quantitative:	Increase:	generalized
		localized
	Decrease:	generalized
		localized
Qualitative:	Color	
	Texture	
	Surface characteristics (straight, curled, or beaded)	
	Strength (brittle)	

Some of these items have been described under scalp hair (see page 95). The *quantity* of hair may be *increased generally* in Cushing syndrome, steroid therapy, deLange syndrome, dilantin therapy, and porphyria. Children with chronic illness also tend to show hirsutism. A localized area of hypertrichosis may be seen in association with a nevus (nevus pilosus). Areas of the body placed in a cast show hypertrichosis soon after removal of the cast.

Generalized *hypotrichosis* is seen in conditions such as hypothyroidism, congenital ectodermal defect, and drug toxicity (thallium, cytotoxic drugs, vitamin A). If the loss of hair is localized, consider alopecia areata, local infections (Fig. 7D-5), and psychological hair pulling (trichotillomania).

The *color* of hair is better appreciated in relation to scalp hair. If the color of body hair is abnormally pale, consider albinism.

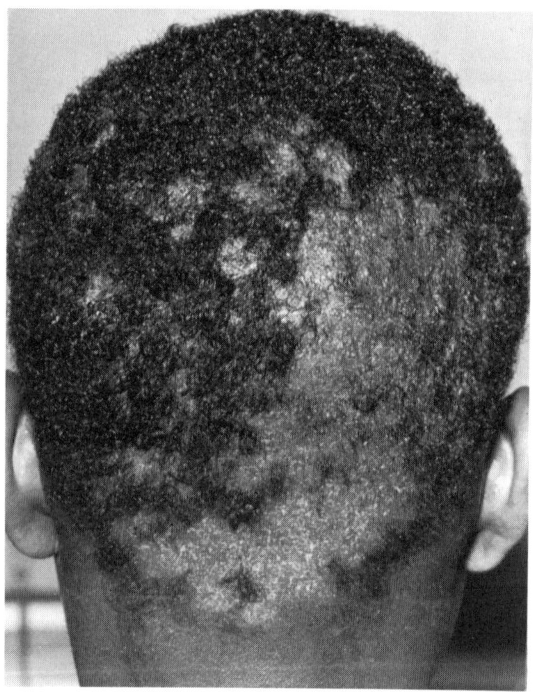

Figure 7D-5. Tinea capitis. *(Photograph courtesy of Dr. PJ Koblenzer and the Skin and Cancer Hospital of Philadelphia.)*

Texture also is better appreciated and listed with scalp hair. Dry coarse hair is common in hypothyroidism, whereas fine thin hair is seen in conditions such as homocystinuria.

Surface characteristics such as a beaded appearance of the hair (monilethrix) and nodular swellings (*trichorrhexis nodosa*) are also better appreciated with scalp hair. Lice and their nits have to be looked for in pubic hair of adolescent boys and girls. The hair is fragile in many congenital syndromes and in areas of fungal infections.

BIBLIOGRAPHY

Fitzpatrick TB, Walker SA: Dermatological Differential Diagnosis. Chicago, Year Book Med., Pub. 1962.

Hurwitz S: Clinical Pediatric Dermatology. Philadelphia, Saunders, 1981.

Jacobs AH: Eruptions in the diaper area. Pediatr. Clin North Am 25(2): 209–225, 1978.

Jacobs, AH: Birthmarks I: Vascular nevi. Pediatrics in Review 1:21–24, 1979.

Jacobs, AH: Birthmarks II: Melanocytic and epidermal nevi. Pediatrics in Review 1:47–50, 1979.

7E. Musculoskeletal System

Examination of the bones, joints, and muscles is a much neglected subject in pediatrics. Many common complaints such as limb pain, joint pain, limp, and swollen joints for which children are brought to the clinician are musculoskeletal in nature. One need not be aware of the mode of action of every muscle and the range of motion of every joint to perform an adequate musculoskeletal examination.

MUSCLES

Certain points in the history give important clues to the presence of muscle disease. In the perinatal period, they are: (1) reduced intrauterine movements; (2) neonatal respiratory distress; (3) poor suck; and (4) reduced activity of limbs.

In older infants and children the following points in the history may indicate existence of muscle disease: (1) floppy baby; (2) delayed milestones; (3) trouble walking or running; (4) frequent tripping and falling; (5) easily tired (fatigue); (6) double vision at the end of the day; (7) trouble climbing stairs and getting up from a sitting position; (8) muscle pain (spontaneous or after exercise); (9) swallowing difficulty; (10) garbled speech after eating cold food (myotonia?); (11) trouble letting go of objects.

Finally, family history is extremely important. The differential diagnosis of various muscle diseases is made easier when there is a family history of similar illness.

Physical examination should include: (1) inspection, palpation, and percussion of the muscle(s); (2) evaluation of the strength of individual or groups of muscles; (3) exclusion of nervous system disorders that have associated myopathy; (4) exclusion of joint diseases associated with disuse atrophy; (5) observation of gait, and (6) assessment of activities of daily living (ADL). Remember, of course, to examine all the other systems, looking for specific clues to diagnosis.

Inspection

Here one looks into the following characteristics of muscle:

- Size
- Shape
- Symmetry

Size can be small or large. Shape depends on the normality of each muscle. Symmetry refers to muscles with bilateral distribution.

Congenital absence of certain muscles is well known and easily recognizable. They may be present as an isolated abnormality (e.g., pectoralis major) or may be associated with a syndrome (e.g., depressor labii oris with congenital heart disease; pectoralis muscle with leukemia; temporalis with myotonia).

Certain muscles may be small due to wasting (best example, quadriceps wasting following injury to or inflammation of the knee). Wasting may be due to disuse, primary muscle degeneration, or secondary to anterior horn cell or peripheral nerve disease. These types of wasting are best identified in relation to the opposite side. If there is wasting, determine whether it is localized or generalized. Generalized wasting is easily recognizable in anyone with a chronic disease. It is often correlated with loss of weight. If the wasting is localized, determine whether it is related to one muscle, one group of muscles, one limb, or one half of the body. In long-standing hemiplegia, one side may be atrophic compared to the other. In peripheral nerve paralysis, only one group of muscles is involved.

If you find hypertrophic muscle, determine whether it is normal and healthy, as in an adolescent, or is suggestive of disease. Determine whether the muscle hypertrophy is localized or generalized. For example, congenital hemihypertrophy involves one half of the body and should always alert the physician to serious disease. Hypertrophy of an isolated muscle is seen classically in Duchenne dystrophy in which calf muscles are unusually large. Generalized hypertrophy of muscles is seen in congenital adrenal hyperplasia.

Fascicultation of muscle bundles is seen in conditions associated with irritation of the anterior horn cells (e.g., poliomyelitis or Werdnig-Hoffmann).

Palpation

A feeling of induration over the muscles is seen in dermatomyositis, infectious myositis, and in pyomyositis. Tenderness of muscles is seen in dermatomyositis and trichinosis. Temperature variations are not useful in diagnosis. When testing muscles with very little strength, palpating along the tendon when the patient is attempting a particular movement may help us recognize muscle movements not otherwise demonstrable.

Percussion

Contraction of percussed muscle with delay in relaxation is typically seen in myotonia congenita. This may best be tested on the biceps. This is demonstrable with tongue muscles also.

Muscle Strength

A series of screening tests will tell us about significant muscle weakness. Screening tests are as follows:

1. Ask the patient to get up from a supine position. (If anterior neck flexors are weak, the patient cannot lift the head off the pillow.)
2. Ask the patient to shrug the shoulders (this will demonstrate weakness of the trapezius).
3. Ask the patient to elevate the arms over the head (inability to do so indicates weakness of deltoids).
4. Ask the patient to flex the elbow with palm facing upward (this tests the biceps).
5. With the patient sitting at the edge of the table and with the popliteal space flush with the edge, ask the patient to extend the knee (tests the quadriceps).
6. With the patient lying on the right lateral side, have the patient flex the knee and abduct the hip on the left side (this tests the left gluteus medius). Repeat the test with the patient lying on the left side.
7. With the patient lying prone and the knees flexed, ask the patient to lift the hip off the table (this tests the gluteus maximus).
8. Ask the patient to push down on the examiner's palm with the sole of the foot; ask the child to walk on the toes (this tests gastrocnemius and soleus).

When examining for strength of various muscles, the usual method is to ask the patient to move in one direction and apply resistance to it. A better method is to let the patient move the joint to the maximum possible range with the muscle being tested and then have the examiner apply force to bring it back to neutral. For example, while testing for biceps, let the patient flex the elbow. Then ask the patient to resist the elbow being extended by the examiner.

If you need a more detailed evaluation of strength of various muscles, use the help of a physical therapist or a physiatrist. They try to examine muscles under ideal conditions actively and passively, with and without gravity, and with and without resistance. The physiatrists and physical therapists grade muscle strength as follows:

0	No movement of muscle
Trace (1)	No movement of joint Palpable contraction
Poor (2)	Full range, gravity eliminated
Fair (3)	Full range against gravity
Good (4)	Full range against gravity and moderate resistance
Normal (5)	Full range against gravity and normal resistance

If there is weakness of muscles, note the pattern of distribution. Proximal muscle weakness is seen in dermatomyositis; distal extremity weakness alone is seen in peripheral neuritis; one-sided weakness is seen in unilateral cerebral insult; unequal lower limb weakness is seen in myelomeningocele and equal complete lower limb weakness is seen in paraplegia.

Activities of Daily Living (ADL)

Evaluation of activities of daily living is important for helping children with physical handicaps, such as severe rheumatoid arthritis or neuromuscular disease. ADL evaluation is also used for functional classification of severely handicapped children. The functional categories are:

I. Fully independent
II. Mostly independent—minimal help required
III. Wheelchair-bound—but can take care of certain items
IV. Totally dependent on others

We have found certain simple functional tests to be very useful in following the degree of muscle weakness in dermatomyositis. They are as follows:

1. Elevation of neck from supine lying
2. Elevation of extended lower limb (in seconds)
3. Ability to get up from lying down without help
4. Ability to get up from sitting with arms folded in front

There are certain findings in other systems that, together with muscle weakness, suggest specific diagnoses. They are listed in Table 7E-1.

TABLE 7E-1. HELPFUL ASSOCIATED CLUES IN DIAGNOSING DISEASES OF MUSCLE WEAKNESS

Presence of	Suggests
1. Myotonia	Mental retardation
2. Exaggerated reflexes	Disease of central nervous system
3. Fasciculations	Anterior horn cell disease
4. Rashes	Collagen vascular disorders
5. Sensory changes	Peripheral nerve disease
6. Dark urine	Myoglobinuria

Gait

The importance of analysis of gait has been referred to already (Chapter 6, page 62). In relation to muscle weakness, certain characteristic gaits are:

- Waddling—proximal weakness around hip
- Toe walking—Duchenne/tight heel cord
- Slapping gait—peripheral neuropathy
- High-stepping gait—lesions of the posterior column

These gaits are easily tested by asking the child to walk and run. Also make the child walk on the toes (tests plantar flexors) and heels (tests dorsiflexors). Test the child also for the ability to stand on one leg (tests gluteus medius).

JOINTS AND BONES

The word *orthopedics* means "straight child." The word *pediatrics* came from the word *orthopedics*. It is sad, therefore, that pediatricians feel inadequate in examining bones, joints, and tendons.

Joints

The points to remember in examining joints are:

- History
- Inspection
- Palpation
- Auscultation
- Testing for range of movement
- Functional evaluation (including gait)
- Examination of bone, tendon, and periarticular tissues
- Examination of other systems

History. Points that suggest joint problems are: pain, swelling, inability to move a joint, and contractures. There may be symptoms referrable to other systems (such as characteristic rash, pleuritic pain, Raynaud phenomenon) pointing to a specific diagnosis. Therefore a review of systems should be done carefully.

Pain in the joint is a common symptom for bringing the child to medical attention. Children fall and get hurt so often that history of trauma may not help in the diagnosis. However, this is an important piece of history and should be sought in all cases of joint pain.

Pain in a joint is not synonymous with arthritis. It is arthralgia. If there is joint swelling in addition to pain, it is more likely to be arthritis. Acute onset of pain suggests trauma or inflammatory disease. Pain that comes on slowly is more suggestive of collagen vascular disorder. Pain in one joint is likely to be due to trauma or inflammation, whereas polyarticular pain suggests a generalized disorder. Pain in a joint for 1 or 2 days is most often due to trauma, but may also indicate infection. Pain in a joint for a few days or months may be due to one of the collagen diseases.

Intense, acute pain is seen in acute rheumatic fever or septic arthritis. Extreme grades of pain are associated with vasomotor disease. Moderate pain is seen in juvenile rheumatoid arthritis. Arthritis with no pain suggests a neuropathic joint.

True migrating pain is characterized by pain in one joint in the morning, moving away to another joint by evening. This is called flitting, fleeting pain. Such pain is seen in acute rheumatic fever and in gonococcemia. Nonmigrating polyarticular pain is seen in other collagen vascular disorders.

Relief of joint pain with aspirin is another important point in history; it may indicate acute rheumatic fever or juvenile rheumatoid arthritis.

The relationship of pain to activity and sleep is another important point. Pain worse on activity is indicative of destructive joint disease, such as acute cartilaginous necrosis; whereas pain and stiffness early in the morning are indicative of juvenile rheumatoid arthritis.

Pain so severe that it interferes with sleep is often seen in vasomotor problems and bleeding into the joint. A child who goes to sleep but wakes up in the middle of the night complaining of pain probably has "growing pains" but such a history should also make one think of septic arthritis, osteomyelitis, or osteoid osteoma. Pain that does not interfere with sleep but gets worse in the morning is seen in juvenile rheumatoid arthritis.

Pain in one location may indicate a problem elsewhere (referred pain). For example, pain due to hip disease may be referred to other sites, such as the outer aspect of the ilium over the gluteus medius, to the inguinal triangle, or to an area over the anterior aspect of the thigh just above the patella. Pain in the sacroiliac joint is referred to deep in the buttocks. Cervical spine involvement in caries of the spine gives rise to pain over the occiput. Pain arising from intervertebral disc inflammation may be felt around the chest wall.

Inspection. Look for the presence or absence of swelling and its relation to the joint. Periarticular swelling and cellulitis can be easily mistaken for arthritis. Periarticular swelling usually involves only one side of the joint. Cellulitis usually extends well above and below the joint. True swelling of a joint with ill-defined edges merging into the surrounding area usually suggests effusion into the joint, whereas swelling of the joint with clearly defined edges suggests synovial thickening.

Sternoclavicular swelling is easily recognized, if present (consider juvenile rheumatoid arthritis if chronic, and gonococcemia if acute). Swelling of the elbow is characterized by obliteration of the dimples on either side of the olecranon. Swelling of the carpal joints of the wrist is seen more often dorsally, is diffuse without a clear edge, and is associated with limitation of wrist extension. Swelling of the extensor tendon sheath of the wrist is characterized by a clear, distal, oblique transverse edge. Diffuse swelling of the entire dorsum of the hand should suggest sickle cell disease, tenosynovitis of flexor tendons with lymphedema, or serum sickness. Flexor tenosynovitis is characterized by flexed clawlike fingers and edema of the dorsum of the hand.

Swelling of the knee joint is appreciated easily. If the fluid is very minimal, the "bulge sign" should elicit a fluid wave. To elicit a bulge sign, keep the knee in extension and push the fluid away by rubbing vertically along the medial border of the patella. This gets the fluid into the suprapatellar pouch laterally. Now, one gentle stroke with one or two fingers along the lateral edge of the patella should produce a bulge just medial to the medial border of the patella. Make sure it is not the patella that is moving. While examining the knee, look also for a popliteal cyst in the popliteal space.

Swelling of the ankle joint is characterized by swelling on either side of the tendoachilles posteriorly. If it is only on one side of the tendoachilles, it is probably a tenosynovitis. Swelling of the anterior aspect of the ankle is seen in edema.

Swelling of the plantar aspect of the foot *with tenderness* is seen in ankylosing spondylitis. Swelling of sole and dorsum of feet *without tenderness* is seen in serum sickness.

Palpation. Mild *temperature* differences between joints can be appreciated easily. Heat over a joint is one of the primary requirements for the diagnosis of inflammatory arthritis.

Tenderness over joints is another important point in the diagnosis of inflammatory arthritis. In the long term follow-up of juvenile rheumatoid arthritis, persistent tenderness over a joint is a good indicator of persistent inflammation. To elicit tenderness over the temperomandibular joint, place one finger into the external auditory meatus and feel forward (anteriorly). The cartilage will be palpable directly under the finger, and tenderness can be easily elicited.

Tenderness of the small joints of the fingers should be tested by squeezing each small joint individually. Percussion along the flexor tendon produces exquisite tenderness in flexor tenosynovitis, whereas tingling sensation along the outer three fingers when tapping the flexor aspect of the wrist suggests carpal tunnel syndrome.

There is no direct way of testing for tenderness of the hip. However, it is good to remember that pain so severe that the hip cannot be moved even 5° in any direction signifies septic arthritis, unless proven otherwise.

Tenderness along the femoral-tibial edges of the knee is not a feature of arthritis involving the knee. However, if the knee is kept straight (extended) and the patella pressed down against the femoral condyle while moving the patella laterally, exquisite tenderness is elicited in chondromalacia of the patella. (In an athletic girl, pain in the knee with frequent buckling of the knee should suggest this diagnosis.)

Subtalar tenderness is elicited by gripping the ankle firmly and moving the foot into inversion and eversion. Small joints of the foot should be tested individually as described earlier for the fingers.

The other most important point in testing for tenderness is to *exclude* tenderness of periarticular structures. Bony tenderness close to a joint may appear as if it is joint pain or tenderness. For example, during examination of a child with pain in the knee, remember to feel for tenderness over the tibial tubercle, since the child may have osteochondritis dissecans (Osgood-Schlatter). Always feel for tenderness of the bone proximal and distal to the joint, since pain at the metaphysis due to osteomyelitis may mimic joint pain. Bone pain of leukemia may mimic the joint pain of arthritis. Careful examination will differentiate bony tenderness from joint tenderness. Tenderness along the tendon attachment may mimic arthritis. This is important to recognize, since tenosynovitis of tendoachilles is seen in ankylosing spondylitis and polytendonitis in hyperlipidemia.

To elicit tenderness of the sacroiliac joint, one of the best tests is what we call the "Pretzel Test." Hold and cross one *lower limb* over the other lower limb (Fig. 7E-1) while crossing the *opposite upper limb* across the trunk. In this semitwisted position, hold the shoulder (of the upper limb being crossed over) and knee (of the lower limb being crossed over) and give a quick springlike stretching. This may elicit pain and wincing in the presence of sacroiliac joint disease, though no one clinical test is good enough to define and localize sacroiliac disease.

During palpation, also feel for nodules along the flexor tendons and periarticular tissues. Minimal synovial thickening can be appreciated after a few years of practice. Always compare the feeling over a joint with the corresponding joint on the opposite side and with a normal joint. Feel for the amount of tissue between your finger and the underlying bone. Feel also for its texture. Gentle palpation is necessary to appreciate synovial thickening, since on firm pressure the synovium collapses. A "cashmere velvet" feeling is the best description of hypertrophic synovium.

Percussion along the flexor tendon produces severe pain in ten-

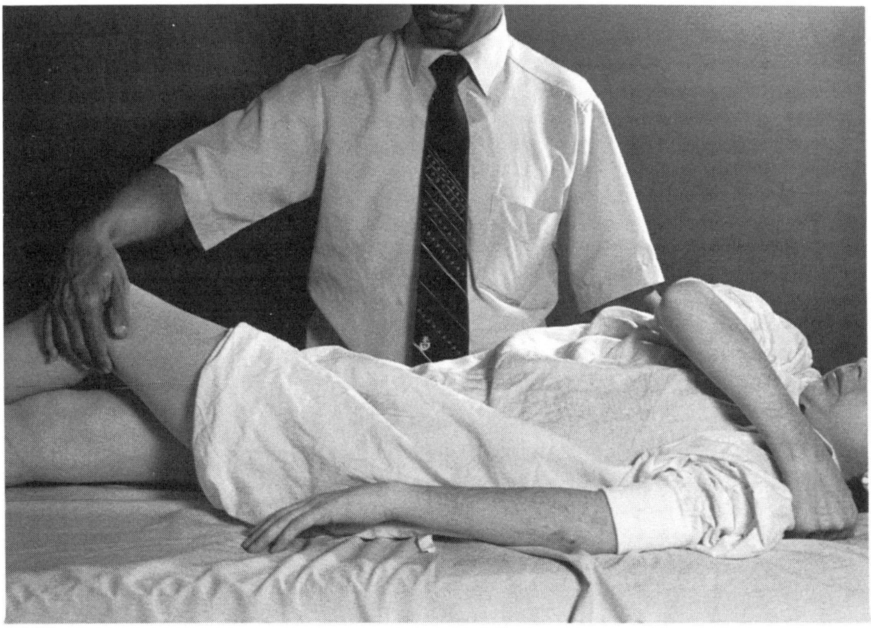

Figure 7E-1. "Pretzel Test" to elicit tenderness of sacroiliac joints. Note that the shoulder on one side and the thigh on the opposite side are pushed to cross over the midline. This stretches the sacroiliac joint on the side of the thigh that is being moved.

osynovitis. Percussion on the flexor aspect of the forearm at the lower end causes pain along the outer three fingers in carpal tunnel syndrome.

One can appreciate crepitus along the flexor tendons on auscultation in tenosynovitis of scleroderma and over the temperomandibular joint in juvenile rheumatoid arthritis.

Range of Movement. Precise testing of range of movement is essential in the long-term follow-up and rehabilitation of children with arthritis. This can be left to the specialists and therapists. A pediatrician should know how to test the range of major joints in a quick way.

Have the child look down, touching the chin on the chest (inferior cervical spine), look up (atlanto-axial joint), side-to-side (atlanto-axial joint), and bend laterally by touching the shoulder with the ear (lower cervical spine). Ask the child to raise the arms above the shoulder and touch the palms (abduction and internal rotation of shoulder). Ask the child to fold the hands in the Indian greetings positions and press hard (wrist extension, elbow flexion) (Fig. 7E-2). Ask the child to bend the fingers "as if you are going to scratch someone," (distal and proximal interphalangeal joints) and to close the fist (metacarpophalangeal joints). Have the child squat down

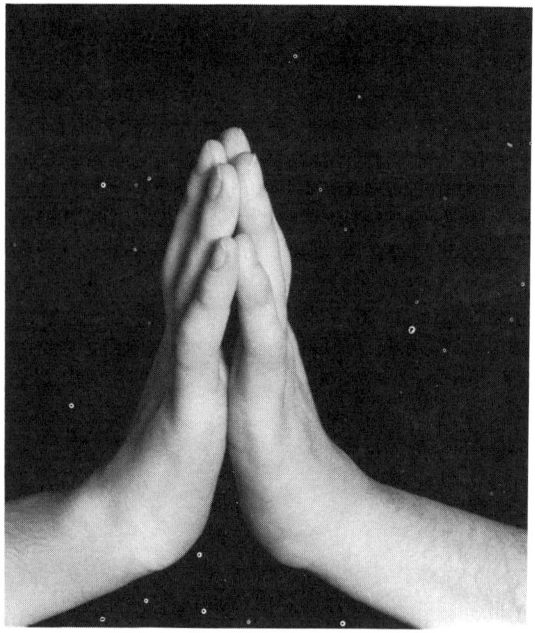

Figure 7E-2. Indian greeting position to test extension at the wrist joints. (Also note flexion deformities of the PIP joints.)

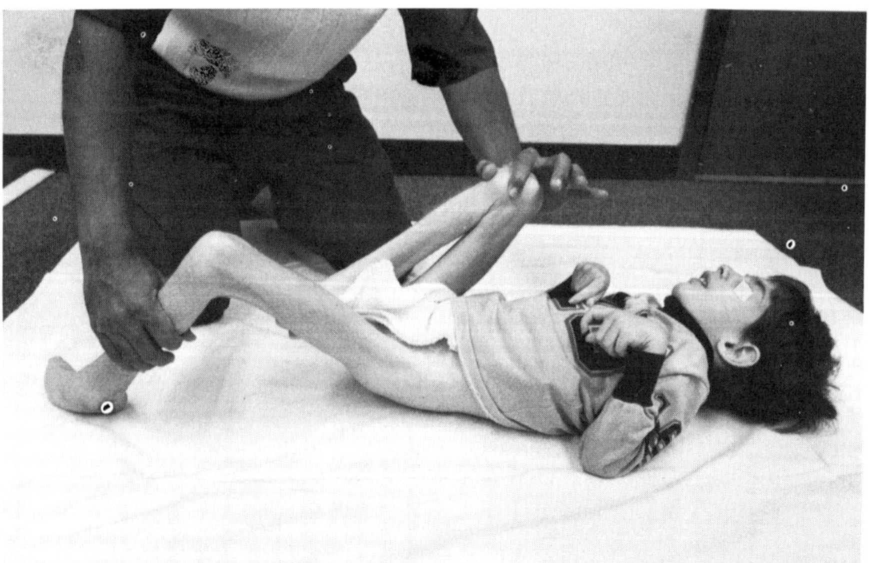

Figure 7E-3. Test for hip flexion contracture. The right hip is flexed fully to fix the spine, and the left hip is extended as far as possible. Normally, the posterior aspect of the thigh should touch the examining table.

(hip and knee flexion) and get up without support. If the child has trouble sitting down, suspect some joint problem. If there is trouble in getting up, suspect muscle weakness.

While testing the *hip*, look at its position at rest. If at rest it is in flexion and external rotation, it signifies an effusion into the hip joint. Hip flexion contracture is tested for as follows (Fig. 7E-3): Have the patient lie supine. Flex both hips as far as they can go. Now hold one hip at the maximum flexed position to fix the pelvis against the table and obliterate the lumbar lordosis. Now ask the patient to put the other hip down as far as it will go. (During this process, if the pelvis were not fixed, lumbar lordosis may occur and make it look as if the hips were extending.) If the back of the thigh does not touch the examining table, this signifies hip flexion contracture. Now repeat the same procedure on the opposite side.

Abduction and adduction are easy to test. But, remember to keep your fingers on the pelvis so that you can recognize if the whole pelvis is rocking.

To test for *rotation at the hip*, the best position is with the patient lying prone. Actually, four different things can be accomplished in this prone position (Fig. 7E-4).

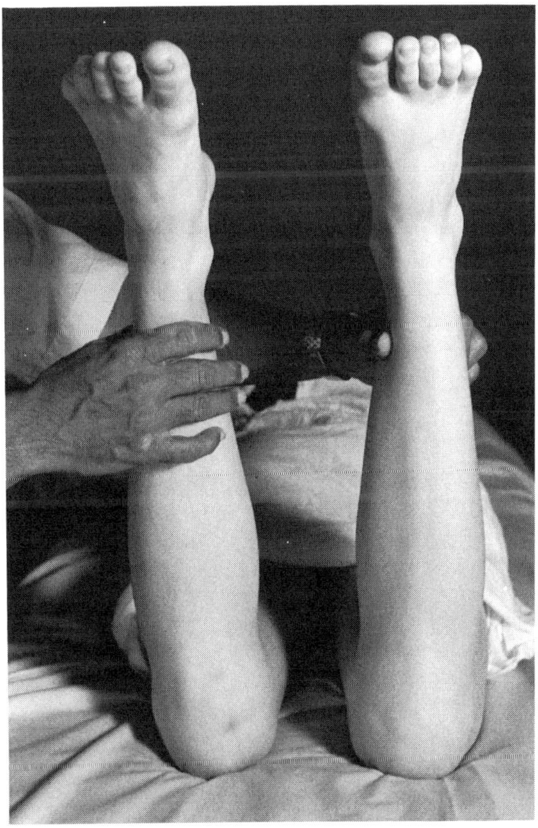

Figure 7E-4. Patient prone with knee joints in flexion. This is an ideal position to test the ankle, knee, and hip joints.

1. Have the patient lie prone and flex the knees as far as they will go. Normally, both heels should touch the buttocks. Also, both knees should be capable of the same range of movement. Thus, limitation of range of movement of the knee is demonstrated.
2. When the knee joints are flexed fully, if the hip raises off the table, that signifies hip flexion contracture.
3. With the knees in 90° flexion, rotate the femurs. When the heels cross over, you are testing external rotation at the hip and when the heels go apart, you are testing internal rotation at the hip (Fig. 7E-5 and Fig. 7E-6).
4. With the knee flexed, lift the thigh off the table. Ask the patient to hold the flexed limb in the air. This tests gluteus maximus.

Limitation of internal rotation is an early sign of many of the hip diseases—particularly slipped epiphysis and Legg-Perthes disease. Up to 18 months of age, excessive external rotation is a common normal finding.

The *knee* should extend to a straight line. In girls, it may even be 5 to

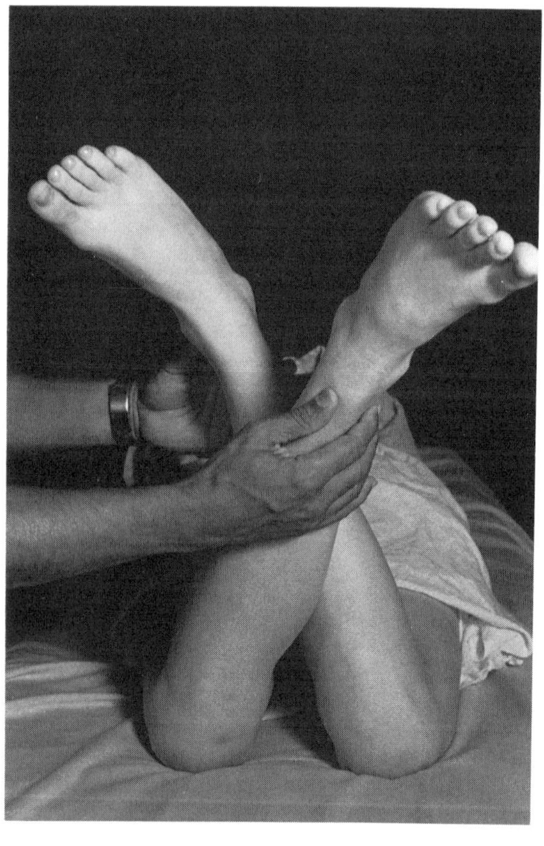

Figure 7E-5. Patient prone and the knee joints in flexion; external rotation of the hip is being tested.

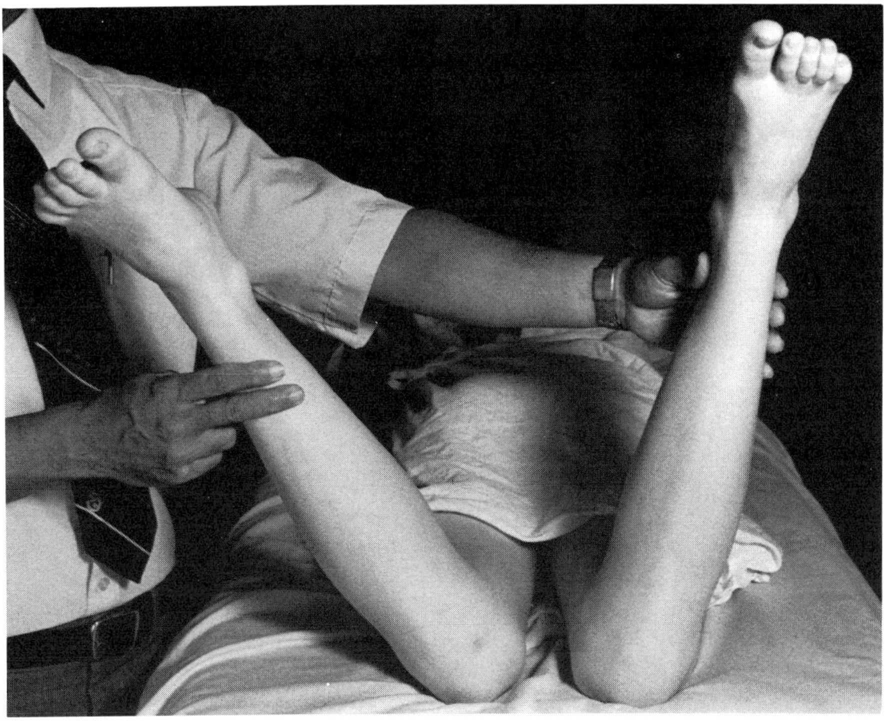

Figure 7E-6. Patient prone and the knee joints in flexion; internal rotation of the hip is being tested (note asymmetry).

10° of hyperextension. Loss of full extension is seen in various arthritides. Pain below the knee causing limitation of full flexion is seen in Osgood-Schlatter disease.

The *ankle* should have normal dorsiflexion and plantar flexion of about 30°. Have the patient sit at the edge of a table with the hip hanging loose to test for the ankle motion. Subtalar motion is usually 10 to 15° and is tested by fixing the ankle, holding the foot by the calcaneum and inverting and everting the foot.

Intoeing and *outtoeing* are common complaints during the developing age periods. These problems are related etiologically to various diagnoses, such as metatarsus adductus, internal tibial torsion, femoral anteversion and everted foot, and external rotation contacture of the hip (see Table 7E-2).

During evaluation of a child with these complaints one should obtain a history on the following points: (1) When was it noticed? Pronounced metatarsus adductus will be visible even at birth, whereas a flatfoot is appreciated only when the child starts walking; (2) What is the rate of progression? Most of these problems correct themselves by the age of 7 or 8 years. If,

TABLE 7E-2. TORSIONAL DEFORMITIES OF THE LOWER LIMB

	Intoeing	Outtoeing
Hip	Femoral anteversion	Physiologic (infancy)
Tibia	Internal torsion	External torsion
Foot	Metatarsus adductus	Flat foot or curved foot

(Modified from Staheli LT: Torsional Deformity. Pediatr Clin North Am 24(4):801, 1977. With permission from WB Saunders, Philadelphia.)

however, there is rapid progression, it may be necessary to treat the condition; (3) Family history of similar problems in other members of the family and the continuing observation may help decide on the management.

During the examination, look at the foot, the leg, and the hips with the child in a sitting position, prone, and with the child walking.

Foot: Look at the sole of the foot. The lateral border of the foot is normally straight. Convexity of this border should suggest metatarsus adductus (Fig. 7E-7).

Leg: Observe the child sitting at the edge of the examining table with the legs dangling freely. Normally, the tibial tubercle and patella face directly anterior, and a line drawn vertically from the tibial tubercle should run through the second metatarsal. In the presence of deformities of the forefoot this will not be true.

Tibial torsion is best looked for with the child prone on the examining table and the thigh flexed to 90° (Fig. 7E-8). Now, draw an imaginary line through the axis of the femur and another line from the heel through the axis of the foot. This angle, called the "thigh-foot" angle is between 10 and 30°. In internal tibial torsion it is less than 10°. In the first 2 years of life, internal rotation of the tibia is normally present.

The *hip* is also examined for internal and external rotation as described on page 187. In the first 18 months of life, it is common to see excessive external rotation and limitation of internal rotation. The external rotation may remain excessively greater, with limitation of internal rotation, particularly in hypotonic infants who lie supine all the time.

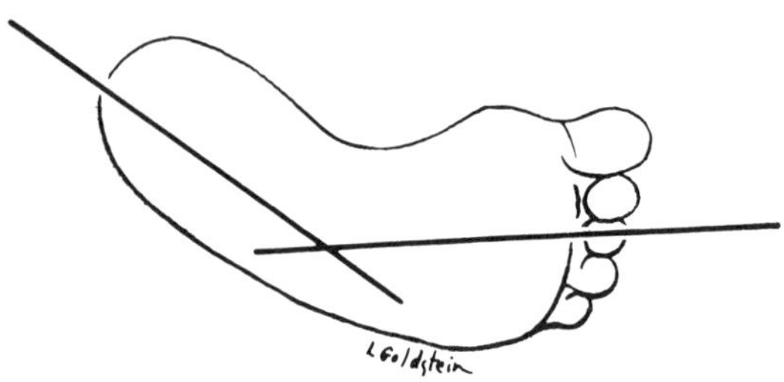

Figure 7E-7. Metatarsus adductus.

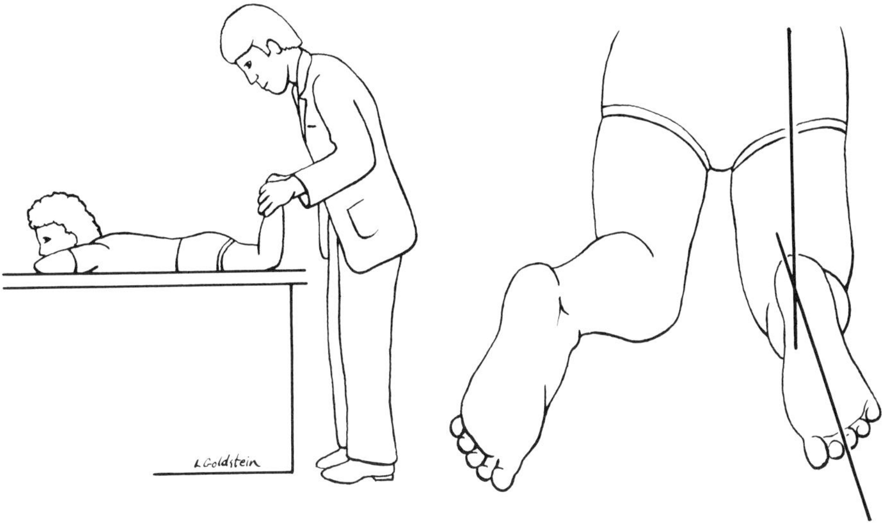

Figure 7E-8. Method to look for tibial torsion. (See text for description of the "thigh-foot" angle.)

Internal rotation is normally less than 70°. When it is greater than 70° it is likely to be due to femoral anteversion (Fig. 7E-9). This may also be exaggerated by children sitting in a "W" position. Significant limitation of internal rotation is seen in many intraarticular diseases of the hip.

Toddler gait: Normally, when a child walks along a straight line the feet make an angle of about 10° in external rotation (Fig. 7E-10). Intoeing and outtoeing are defined in relation to this observation. When the child's foot makes an angle of less than 10° to the straight line it is intoeing. If it is over 30°, it is outtoeing.

Intoeing gets worse when the child is tired or when the child is carrying the weight of a shoe. Intoeing due to femoral anteversion will be char-

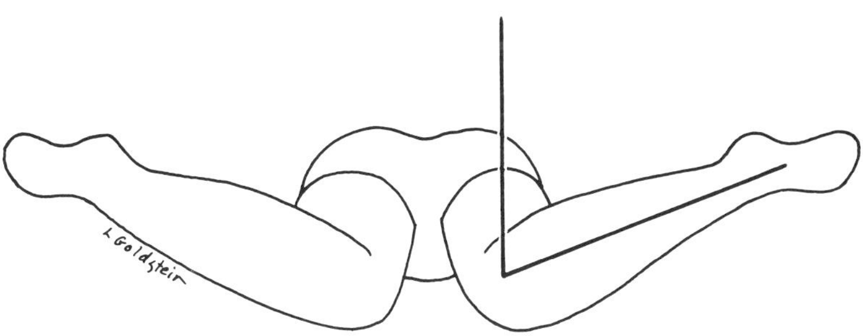

Figure 7E-9. Exaggerated internal rotation of the hip.

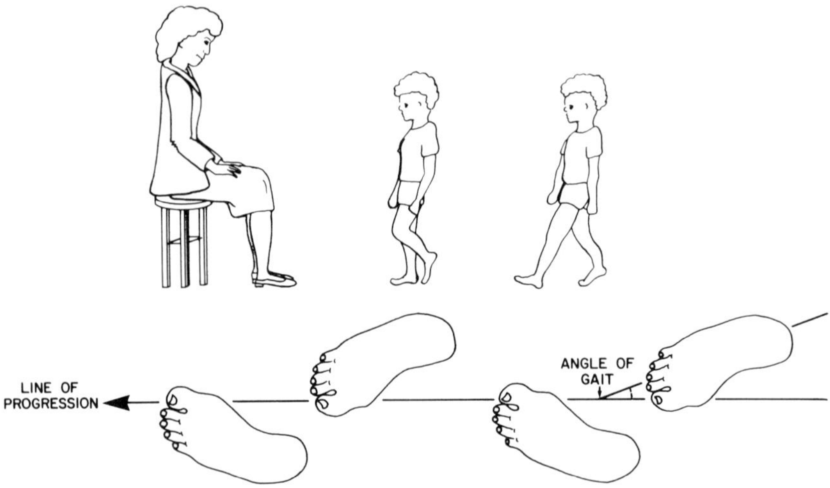

Figure 7E-10. Method for examining child's gait. This footprint suggests intoeing.

acterized by the observation that the patella faces medially during the child's walk. The entire foot will land in a medially rotated position and the patellae face medially. In forefoot problems and tibial torsion, the foot will land normally and then rotate inwardly during the weight-bearing phase.

To examine for *genu varum, genu valgum, flat foot,* and *pronated foot,* have the patient stand up erect without clothes. With the medial malleoli touching, there must be normally less than 2 inches (5 cm) space between the medial condyles. In genu varum (bow leg) the space is wider than 2 inches (5 cm). However, it is physiologic to see some bowing until 2½ years of age (Fig. 7E-11).

With the medial condyles touching, the space between the malleoli should be less than 2 inches (5 cm). Intermalleolar distance of over 2 inches (5 cm) is abnormal at any age, though knock-knee is "physiologic" between 2 and 5 years of age (Fig. 7E-12).

With the child standing erect look from behind. Normally, the tendoachilles makes a vertical line or has a very minimal medial curve. If it makes a "C" curve, it denotes a pronated foot (Fig. 7E-13). When the child is standing without shoes, look also for flatfoot. If there is flatfoot, the medial border of the foot touches the floor. This is normal in the first 18 to 30 months of life. (Plain and simple flatfoot does not need correction.)

Functional Tests for Joint Problems

1. Duration of morning stiffness
2. Grip strength
3. Gait

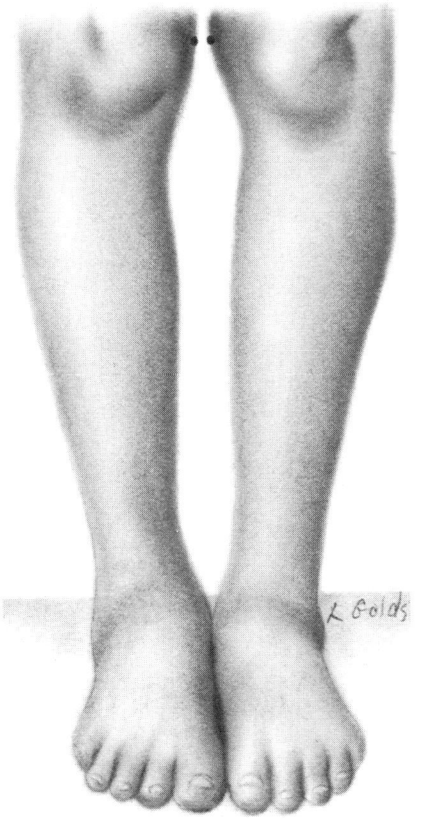

Figure 7E-11. To look for genu varum (bowleg), measure the distance between the medial condyles of the femur (*dots*) with the medial malleoli touching each other.

Duration of *morning stiffness* obtained by history is a reliable indicator of disease activity in rheumatic diseases.

Grip Strength: A blood pressure cuff is rolled and given to the child to hold in the hands. The cuff should be small enough that the fingers go around it. The bulb is squeezed by the examiner to reach a measurement of 20 mm Hg on the manometer. Now the child is asked to squeeze the bag as strongly as possible with one hand. After the child lets go and rests, this is repeated two more times and the best of three measurements is taken as the value. This is now repeated on the other side. Normally, children 6 to 10 years old can squeeze up to 120 mm Hg, and adolescents can squeeze the mercury out of the unit. The grip strength measures a composite of pain, tenderness, limitation of range of movement, and weakness of muscles of the hand. In long-term follow-up of children with arthritis, it is a good indicator of improvement or worsening.

Gait: Abnormalities of gait due to bone and muscle problems were described on page 62, Chapter 6. In a child with arthritis, certain special types of gait are seen. A child who bears weight for longer duration on one

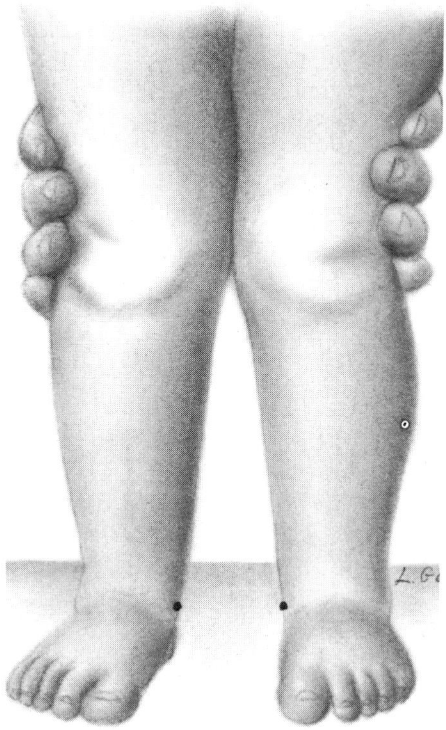

Figure 7E-12. To look for genu valgum (knock-knee), measure the distance between the medial malleoli (*dots*) with the child standing.

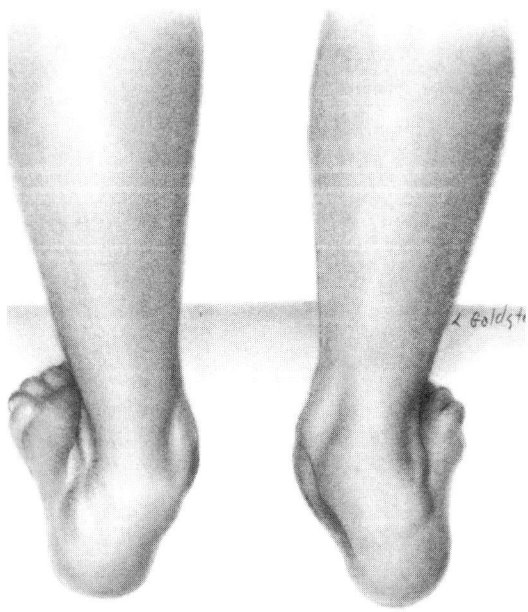

Figure 7E-13. Pronated feet; look for the outward curvature of the tendoachilles.

side than on the other side during walking has a painful limp. If he walks with the hip markedly flexed, holds his thigh while walking, and bears weight at the tip of the toes for as brief a time as possible, he probably has pain in the hip. If a child walks on the outer side of the foot, suspect a painful condition of the metatarsophalangeal joints of the great toe. If a child lifts the whole foot at once without a smooth heel-off-toe cycle, this signifies a stiff knee which cannot bend or a painful foot.

Other functional methods to test the mobility of the joints:

1. Give the child a piece of paper to see whether the child can pinch it.
2. Give a key and see whether the child can hold it between the opposing aspects of the thumb and index finger.
3. Give a pen and spoon to see whether patient can use them without difficulty and pain.
4. Have the patient sit down and get up from the chair.
5. Have the patient climb up and down the stairs.

Clues in other systems: Look into symptoms and signs in other systems that may give clues to the diagnosis of the musculoskeletal problem. Skin rashes give the best help in the differential diagnosis of arthritis. A list of rashes characteristic of various arthritides are given in Table 7E-3.

Spine

Inspection. Presence of a short neck or elevated shoulder and scoliosis in a young child should indicate the possibility of hemivertebrae. If you see a child walking extremely carefully to avoid pain, it should suggest the possibility of intervertebral disc inflammation or caries of the spine. A bunch of hair over the lower end of the spine should suggest the presence of lipomeningocele, particularly if associated with paraparesis, tight heel cord or urinary problems. A dimple at the lower end of the spine may be a sacrococcygeal dimple or pilonidal sinus. The points in favor of pilonidal sinus are its location (higher), color (tan, blue), and hair around it.

Normally, when the child is looked at from a lateral view, there is a C-curve over the cervical spine, convex curve of the thorax, and C-curve of

TABLE 7E-3. SKIN RASH AS A CLUE TO DIAGNOSIS OF ARTHRITIS

Type of Rash	Diagnosis
1. Erythema marginatum	Acute rheumatic fever
2. Evanescent macular rash	Juvenile rheumatoid arthritis
3. Malar rash	Systemic lupus erythematosus
4. Vesicles over extensor aspects of joints	Gonococcal arthritis-dermatitis
5. Purpuric spots over distal portion of extremities	Henoch-Schönlein purpura
6. Erythema chronicum migrans	Lyme arthritis

the lumbar spine. Loss of C-curve in the cervical spine suggests either juvenile rheumatoid arthritis or tuberculosis of the spine. Prominent thoracic curvature may indicate kyphosis, as in Morquio disease.

If there is a distinct angle at the apex of the kyphosis it is called gibbus and indicates the possibility of fracture or collapse of a vertebrae. Loss of lumbar lordosis is seen in ankylosing spondylitis. Prominent lordosis may be either familial, developmental (up to 7 or 8 years), or due to hip flexion contracture.

Points that suggest a child may have *scoliosis* (even before removing the clothing) are: elevated shoulder on one side, complaint about unequal bra cup-size in girls, family history of scoliosis, prominent scapula, and apparent leg-length discrepancy.

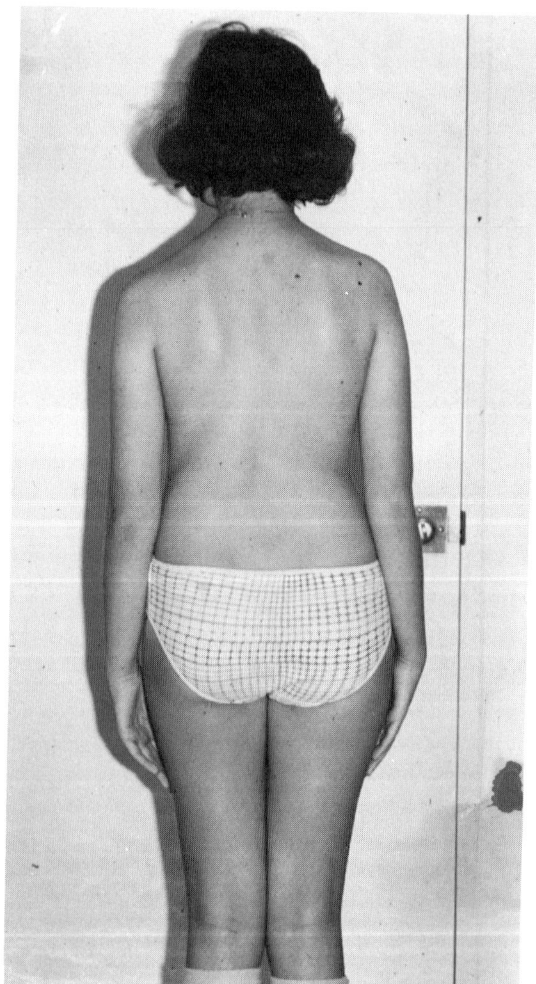

Figure 7E-14. Method to examine for scoliosis. Note that the right shoulder is at a slightly higher level, the right interscapular area is fuller, the right scapula more prominent, and the loin groove is more prominent on the left. *(Photograph courtesy of Dr. M Ecker.)*

Scoliosis is easily visible on examining the spine from the back (Fig. 7E-14). It is usually described as "Scoliosis with convexity to the right (or left)." Since scoliosis can be primary or secondary, one should make sure that there is no neuromuscular disease or leg length discrepancy. To measure for leg-length discrepancy, lay the patient down flat in the supine position. With the lower limbs in equal degrees of abduction from midline, measure the distance from the anterior superior iliac spine to the medial malleolus. The measuring tape should run across the thigh, over the medial surface of the knee, and along the medial aspect of the tibia.

Since the scoliosis may be a fixed lesion, test for this by asking the patient to lean forward as if to touch the feet with the hands (Fig. 7E-15). A curve that corrects during the procedure is obviously not fixed. In a small

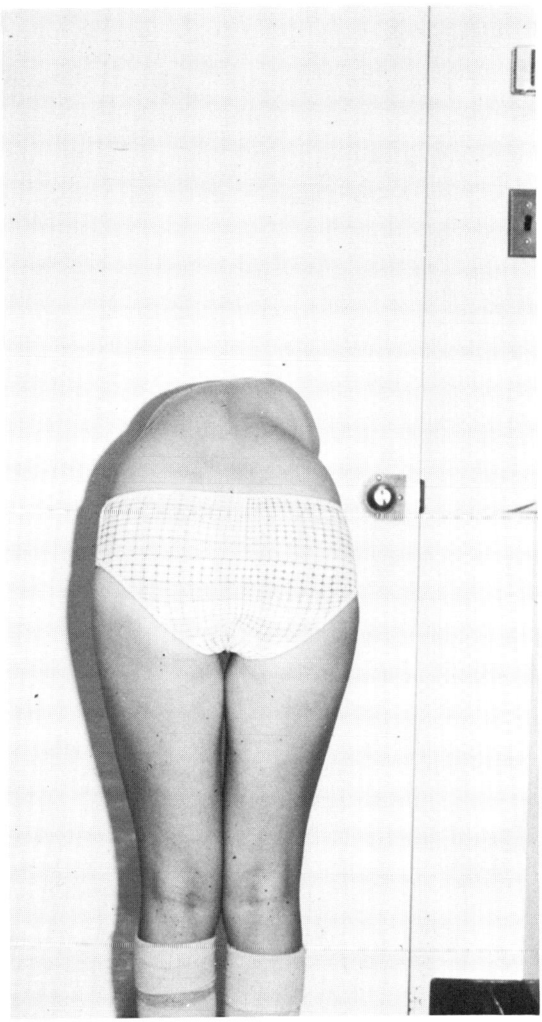

Figure 7E-15. Test for scoliosis. Ask the patient to bend forward. The hump is visualized without any difficulty. *(Photograph courtesy of Dr. M Ecker.)*

child, lift the child by the arms and hands vertically. A nonfixed curve will disappear.

Test for *mobility of the lumbar spine* using a modified Schober's method. Place a line across the back at the lumbosacral junction with the patient standing erect. Place a mark on the skin in the midline over the spine at a point 10 cm above the first point. Place another mark 5 cm below the first point. Now ask the patient to bend over to touch the feet. Measure the distance between the upper and lower marks. Normally, the back should stretch to at least 7 cm between the two points during this maneuver. A simpler clinical method is to place two fingers on adjacent spinous processes and estimate the separation of fingers when the patient bends forward.

Palpation. Palpate the spine for local tenderness, particularly if osteomyelitis or a vertebral tumor is suspected. Tenderness between the vertebrae may be elicited in disc inflammation.

HAND

In addition to its contributions to everything man has been able to do such as art, music, and everything else man creates, the hand gives clues to the diagnosis of many systemic diseases. The subheadings under which hands should be observed are:

- General clues: handedness, involuntary movements, neurologic
- Size of the hand and of the phalanges
- Shape
- Hand position
- Trophic changes
- Color of the palm and of the fingers
- Rash (palm, fingers, and nail)
- Nodules (palm, tendons, and fingers)
- Fingers: size, numbers, alignment, thumb
- Dermatoglyphics

General Clues

The general examination starts with observing which hand the child uses to receive a toy or object. Since definite handedness may not be established till 2½ to 3 years of age, a consistent approach with one hand at a very early age should arouse suspicion of hemiplegia. A child with no dominant handedness at 7 to 8 years of age also should arouse suspicion.

One can recognize the *handedness* of the child by looking for certain clues. Clinical clues are significant only in relation to a cluster of other findings. One cannot, therefore, swear by any of the following findings: (1) the dominant hand will have a wider thumb nail base than the nondominant one. The corner is also more squared rather than rounded on the dominant side; (2) If you spread the web-space between the thumb and the index finger, the angle is more obtuse on the dominant side; (3) If you ask the child to put his hands behind his back and raise the hands as far as possible between the shoulder blades, the dominant hand will reach higher.

Tremors may be observed on even a casual scrutiny of the hands. Tremor at rest is seen in essential tremor and Wilson disease. Tremor seen in sustained posture should suggest anxiety and fatigue and, rarely, disease states such as thyrotoxicosis and cerebellar disease. Intention tremor (tremor which comes on with an activity such as in the finger-nose test) is seen in cerebellar disease or in stress. Athetosis is characterized by writhing movements of the distal parts of the body and is observed most commonly in the hands. Carpopedal spasm also may resemble athetosis but is elicited by occlusion of vessels with a sphygmomanometer cuff. Asterixis (liver flap) is a flopping movement of the outstretched hand and is seen in hepatic failure (Reye syndrome).

One can feel the *power of grasp* during a handshake. Though a weak grasp by itself may not indicate disease, one should look for neurologic and joint diseases (juvenile rheumatoid arthritis) which interfere with grasp. On sustained grasp, alternate squeezing and relaxing by the patient (inability to sustain the grasp is seen in chorea). During the hand grasp, one may also recognize how anxious the child is if the palm is sweating. Nail biting and thumb sucking are also easily recognized by looking at the fingers and the thumb.

The easiest way to test for the motor components of the *three major nerves* of the upper extremity is to test the mobility of the thumb. Abduction and extension of the thumb are lost in radial nerve paralysis, adduction of the thumb is lost in ulnar nerve paralysis, and apposition of the thumb is lost in median nerve paralysis. The sensory portions of these three nerves are evaluated by testing sensation over the ulnar aspect of the little finger (ulnar nerve), the radial aspect of the index finger (median nerve), and the dorsal aspect of the web between the thumb and index finger (radial nerve).

Size

The size of the hand may be small (feet also small) in achondroplasia, Down syndrome, and deLange syndrome. The fingers are also small. Large hands are seen in gigantism, and long hands with spidery fingers are seen in arachnodactyly and homocystinuria. Hypoplasia of the radial aspect of hand is seen in Holt-Oram syndrome and Fanconi syndrome.

Shape

The shape of the hand in athetosis has been described above. "Mitten hand" with fused fingers is seen in Apert syndrome. Bifid clawlike hand is seen in Thalidomide syndrome.

Hand Position

The characteristic *position* of the hand in brachial plexus paralysis is one of "policeman receiving tip." In radial nerve paralysis there is weakness of extension of the wrist, with wrist drop. Ulnar nerve paralysis produces claw hand deformity in which the fourth and fifth fingers are extended at the metacarpophalangeal joints and flexed at the proximal interphalangeal joint. Ulnar deviation of the hand and volar subluxation at the wrist are seen in juvenile rheumatoid arthritis.

Trophic Changes

Observe for trophic changes in reflex sympathetic dystrophy, the thinning of the pulp of the fingers in scleroderma, and vasculitic ulcers at the tip of the finger in scleroderma.

Color

The color of the hands and fingers is flushed in high output cardiac failure, is pale, cold, and clammy in shock, and is blue in cyanosis. The yellow color of jaundice is seen in the creases of the palm. Raynaud phenomenon is characterized by periodic attacks of color changes of the fingers particularly on exposure to cold. Characteristically, the fingers first get pale, then get blue, and finally red. During the stage of pallor there may be associated pain and a feeling of heat during the stage of red color.

Rashes and Nodules

Various kinds of rash occur characteristically in the hands. Raynaud phenomenon was already mentioned. *Macular* lesions of the palm may be seen in systemic lupus erythematosus and secondary syphilis and erythema multiforme. Red, dry, and scaly lesions over the dorsum of interphalangeal joints are seen in dermatomyositis. Similar lesions on the dorsum of the hand between the interphalangeal joints are seen in lupus erythematosus. Telangiectasia and periungual erythema is seen in dermatomyositis. Common *papular* lesions of the palm are those of eczematous dermatitis and scabies. Lesions of scabies are seen in between the fingers, in the creases at the wrist, and in the palmar creases (Fig. 7D-4, page 172). These lesions may be papules or vesicles. *Vesicular* lesions are seen in scabies, herpes simplex, chicken pox, epidermolysis bullosa, and congenital syphilis. They are seen on the dorsum of joints in gonococcemia. The classical vesicular lesions of smallpox will never be seen again! *Pustules* are seen in impetigo and infected scabies. *Nodular* lesions are seen in rheumatoid arthritis on the dorsal aspect of joints and in granuloma annulare usually along the fingers. Nodules may be felt along flexor tendons in juvenile rheumatoid arthritis. *Purpuric* lesions of Rocky Mountain spotted fever and meningococcemia may be seen around the wrist and hands. In Rocky Mountain spotted fever, the lesions characteristically start around the wrist. *Vasculitic* lesions at the tips of the fingers are seen in scleroderma. Such lesions around the edge of the nail are seen in systemic lupus erythematosus. *Splinter hemorrhages* under the nails are seen in subacute bacterial endocarditis.

Fingers

One of the abnormalities associated with the *size and shape* of fingers is short fingers of equal length as seen in hypothyroidism and achondroplasia ("banana-bunch" fingers). However, in achondroplasia, there is a divergence between third and fourth finger giving the "trident sign." Polydactyly is common in Ellis-Van Creveld syndrome and Trisomy-13. Syndactyly is seen often in Apert syndrome, deLange syndrome, and Prader-Willi syndrome. (See page 71 for a description of clubbing.)

In acute tenosynovitis, the fingers are uniformly swollen, held in slight flexion, and are tender along the tendon sheaths. "Triggering" or locking of the finger suggests nodules along the flexor tendons.

Flexion deformity of the little finger is called camptodactyly (Fig. 7E-16). It is inherited through a simple dominant gene and is seen in 1.9 percent of the normal population. This is also part of various syndromes, however, such as Down, Carpenter, and Aarskog. Clinodactyly is the shortening of the radial aspect of the middle phalanx, resulting in radial deflection of the terminal phalanx. It is common in females and is seen in 0.3 percent of the normal population (Fig. 7E-17).

Hypoplasia of the metacarpal bones of all fingers is seen in syndromes such as Coffin-Siris and *cri-du-chat.* Hypoplasia of the fourth metacarpal causes a dimple at a location where a bump should be seen. This is seen characteristically in pseudohypoparathyroidism.

The appearance of the *thumb* can give clues to many diagnoses. Table 7E-4 lists various abnormalities of the thumb and associated syndromes. The thumb sign of Marfan syndrome is elicited by asking the patient to

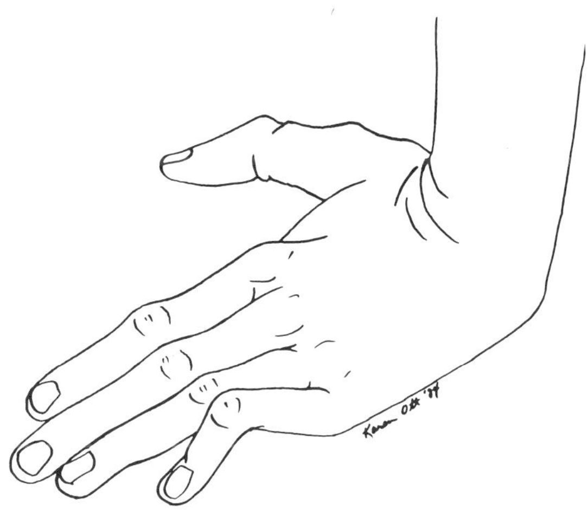

Figure 7E-16. Camptodactyly (flexion deformity of the little finger).

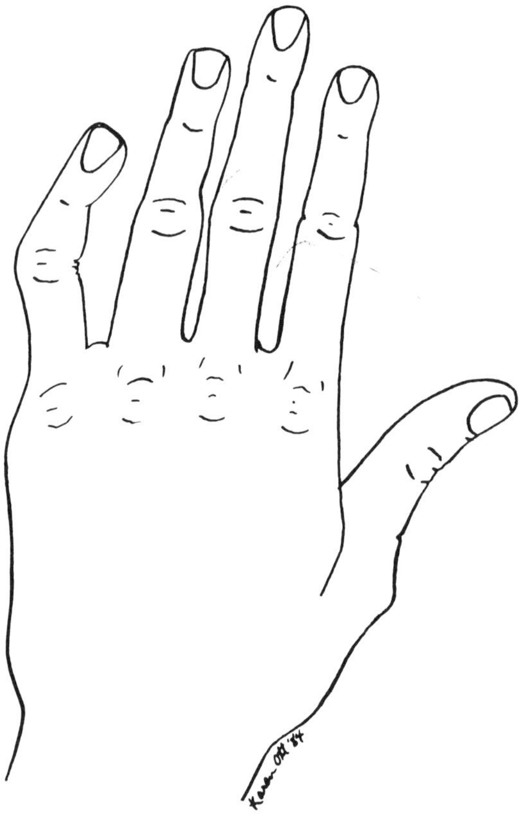

Figure 7E-17. Clinodactyly (radial deviation at the proximal interphalangeal joint of the little finger).

clench the fist with the thumb held inside the palm. The tip of the thumb protrudes past the ulnar border of the palm in Marfan syndrome and this is the "thumb sign." The sign is absent in homocystinuria, a condition in which other morphologic features are very similar to those of Marfan syndrome.

TABLE 7E-4. CLINICAL SIGNIFICANCE OF ABNORMALITIES OF THE THUMB

Abnormality	Syndrome
1. Triphalangeal thumb	Holt-Oram syndrome
2. Thumb aplasia	13 q syndrome
3. Broad thumb	Rubinstein-Taybi syndrome
4. Proximal placement of thumb	18 q syndrome
5. Flexed thumb	Arthrogryposis
6. Bifid thumb	Translocation 3/13

Dermatoglyphics

The epidermal ridges and creases of the palms of the hand are unique for each individual. Even identical twins will not have identical ridge characteristics. The thumbprint has been used as equivalent to a signature in India and China for many centuries. It was Sir Francis Galton who established the study of fingerprints (derma-skin; glyphic-curve) on a scientific basis, though Purkinje recognized the characteristics of finger patterns.

The three components of the dermatoglyphic patterns are:

1. Flexion creases
2. Ridge arrangement of palms
3. Finger patterns

Flexion creases. They are not strictly part of the dermatoglyphics, but are closely related. Usually there are three palmar creases. When the two distal creases are fused and run as a single crease across the entire palm reaching the ulnar border of the palm, it is called the simian crease (Fig. 7E-18). This

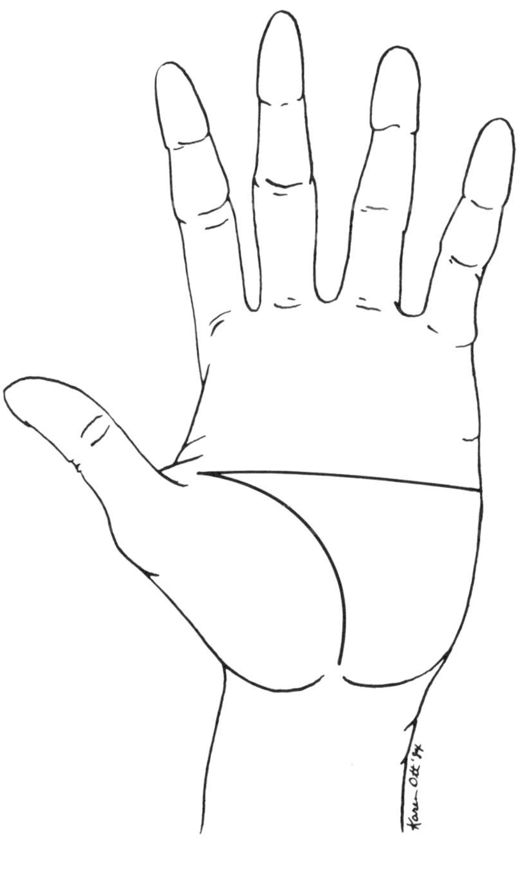

Figure 7E-18. Simian crease of Down syndrome.

is seen classically in Down syndrome. When there are two transverse creases and the proximal one runs across the entire palm, it is called Sydney line, seen in congenital rubella syndrome.

Look for a crease on the palmar surface of the fingers corresponding to the interphalangeal joints. Normally, there are two or three creases over the proximal interphalangeal joints but only one over the distal interphalangeal joints. Two creases over the palmar aspect of the distal interphalangeal joints are seen in patients with sickle cell disease. Usually the second crease is located just beyond the distal interphalangeal flexion crease.

Ridge Arrangement of Palms. The ridges of the palm run in different directions. In areas where three ridge systems meet, there are triradiate structures, aptly called triradii (Fig. 7E-19). There is one proximal (axial) triradius on the palm close to the wrist. This is designated as *t.* There are four other triradii (digital) situated one each under the index, middle, ring, and little fingers. They are designated *A, B, C, D.* The angle between the triradii located on *A, t,* and *D* is called the *AtD* angle and usually measures 40°. If, however, the axial triradius is located distally in the center of the palm, the *AtD* angle becomes obtuse (75 to 80°). Such a situation occurs in Down syndrome, Turner syndrome, and congenital rubella syndrome.

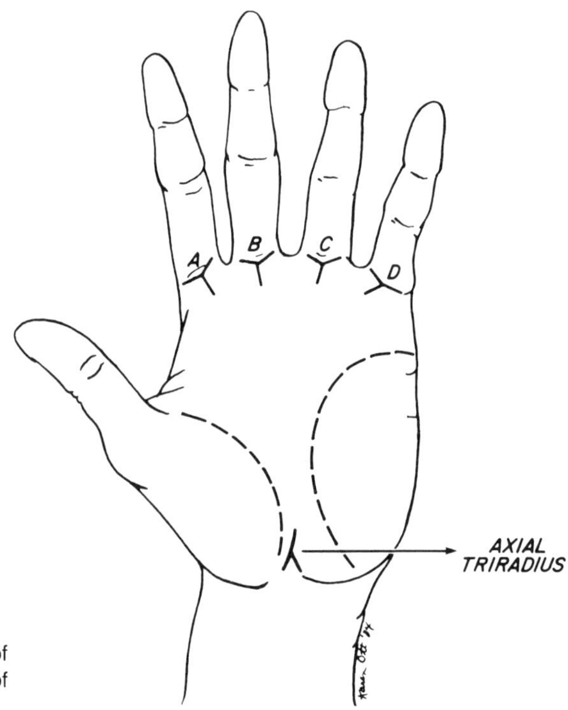

Figure 7E-19. Arrangement of ridges on the palm and location of triradii.

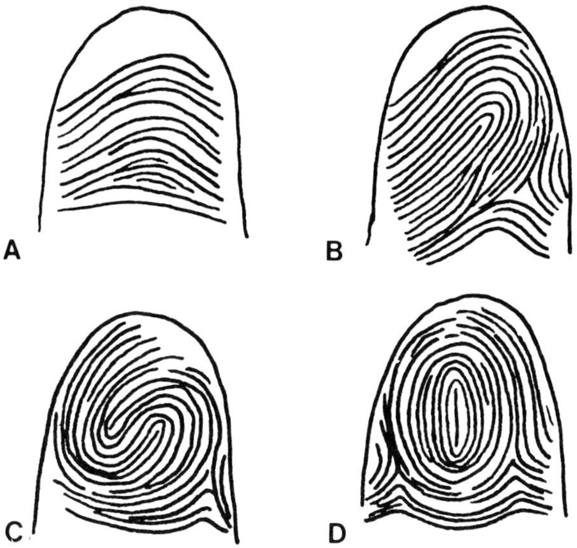

Figure 7E-20. Dermatoglyphic patterns of fingers: **A.** arch; **B.** loop; **C.** double loop; **D.** whorl.

Finger Patterns. There are three characteristic patterns on the finger tips: loop, whorl, and arch (Fig. 7E-20). The loop has only one triradius whereas the whorl has two. The loops may be ulnar loops (opening toward the ulnar side) or radial loops (opening toward the radial side). The usual pattern is ulnar loop of the little finger, radial loop of the index finger, and whorl or arch of the middle finger. One may occasionally have the same pattern in all fingers. This is rare in normals and is more often seen in congenital rubella syndrome (more whorls), Trisomy-18 (more arches), and Down syndrome (ulnar loop in all fingers). In Trisomy-18, there may be no patterns at all on the fingertips.

The number of ridges cutting across a line joining the center of a loop or whorl to the nearest triradius may be counted in each of the ten fingers (Fig. 7E-21) and added together to get the ridge count. The average value is 145 for males and 127 for females. The ridge count is increased in Turner syndrome and congenital rubella syndrome, since they have more whorls (average is 169) and decreased in Klinefelter syndrome (average is 27).

SPORTS INJURIES OF KNEES AND ANKLES

Trauma to soft tissues is common as part of sports-related injuries. It could be a s*t*rain (injury to muscle-tendon unit) or a s*p*rain (injury to ligaments).

In children, when there is a stress on a joint, fracture is more common than ligamental tears. Such ligamental injury can occur, however, particu-

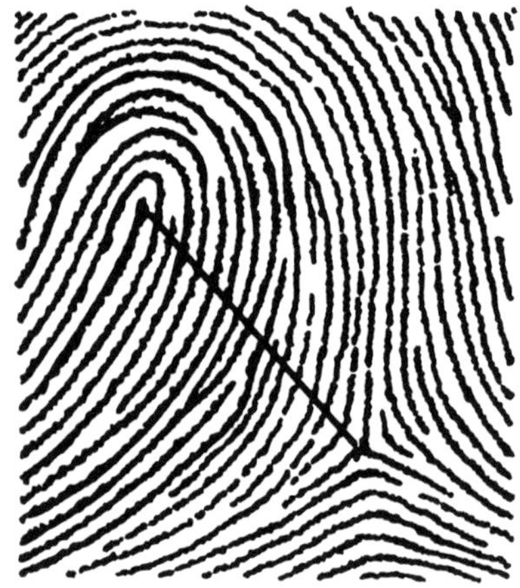

Figure 7E-21. Ridge count. (See text for description.)

larly in the sports injuries of adolescents. The knee and ankle joints are the commonest areas for these injuries.

The patella may be completely displaced from the intercondylar notch due to an acute violent force pushing the patella laterally. This can occur particularly in those with hyperextendible joints. There is usually pain and swelling on the medial aspect of the patella. Any attempt by the examiner to move the patella laterally produces great anxiety in the child.

The lateral collateral ligament of the knee is tested as follows. Holding the lower end of the leg with one hand place the palm of the other hand just below the knee on the medial aspect of the upper part of the leg. Give a gentle outward pressure on the upper part of the tibia and inward pressure on the lower part of the leg. This should stretch the lateral collateral ligament.

To test the medial collateral ligament, use the same procedure but apply inward pressure over the upper part of the tibia with the palm held on the outer aspect and apply outward pressure on the lower leg. There should be less than 5° motion and there should be no pain. Greater than 5° motion signifies instability. Pain inside the joint suggests damaged articular cartilage.

To test for the cruciate ligament of the knee, have the patient supine with the knee in flexion and the sole of the foot touching the examining table. Gently sit on the dorsum of the foot (if possible without imposing pressure) and grasp the upper end of the tibia with both hands. Now rock the tibia gently forward and backward. There should normally be no movement. Presence of gliding movement of the tibia on the femur suggests loss of integrity of the cruciate ligaments.

The severity of sprains of the ligaments around the ankle joints may be graded as I (minimal swelling and pain—no disability), II (moderate swelling, severe pain and some disability), or III (complete rupture of the ligament resulting in a snapping noise, severe pain, and disability). Type III sprain is associated with instability of the joint which may be tested as follows: (1) stabilize the lower leg with one hand; grasp the heel firmly with the other hand and try to push anteriorly to look for excess anterior movement of the talus in the ankle mortise as compared to the opposite side. This tests the talofibular ligament; (2) to test for the calcaneo-fibular ligament, grasp the heel as described in (1) and look for excess inversion of the foot (as compared to the opposite side).

BIBLIOGRAPHY

Block JE: Thumbs down on left-handedness. (Correspondence.) N Engl J Med 291:307, 1972.

DeJong R, Platou RV: Sickle cell hemoglobinopathy: An anatomic sign. Am J Dis Child 113:271–272, 1967.

Garrick JG: Knee problems in adolescents. Pediatrics in Review 4:235–243, 1983.

Harvey J: Ankle injuries in children and adolescents. Pediatrics in Review 2:217–222, 1981.

Holt, SB: The significance of dermatoglyphics in medicine: A short survey and summary. Clin Pediatr 12:471–484, 1973.

Lawrence JS: Rheumatism in Populations. London, Heinemann Med Bks, 1977.

Moll JMH, Wright V: Measurement of joint motion. Clin Rheum Dis 2(1):3–26, 1976.

Rang M: The Easter Seal Guide to Children's Orthopedics. Ontario, Canada, Easter Seal Society, 1982.

Shiono H, Kadowaki J: Dermatoglyphics of congenital abnormalities without chromosomal aberrations: A review of the clinical applications. Clin Ped 14:1003–1013, 1975.

Spiro AJ: Approach to diagnosis in the child with muscle weakness. Pediatr Ann 16:149–161, 1977.

Sports Medicine: Health Care for Young Athletes. Committee on Sports Medicine. American Academy of Pediatrics, 1983.

Staheli LT: Common orthopedic problems. Pediatr Clin North Am 24(4):663–919, 1977.

7F. Central Nervous System

Some common complaints associated with diseases of the central nervous system are: loss of consciousness, seizures, developmental delay, developmental regression, weakness of parts of the body, unsteady gait, limping, clumsiness, involuntary movements, floppiness, and headaches. Loss of vision, loss of hearing, and vertigo as presenting symptoms are less common.

EXAMPLES OF HISTORY TAKING

Before describing the methods of physical examination, two of the common manifestations, viz., loss of consciousness and seizure, will be discussed as examples for history taking and classification.

Loss of consciousness (coma): When dealing with a child in coma, the following points in history are relevant. Was the onset sudden or gradual? Is there a history of trauma (intracranial bleeding)? If there was trauma, did the patient lose consciousness at once (severe intracranial bleeding, cerebral contusion) or after a period of lucid interval (middle meningeal bleeding)? Is there a history of headache and vomiting preceding the onset of coma (encephalitis, tumor)? Did the patient have fever before onset of coma (encephalitis, meningitis)? Is there a history of ingestion of drugs or toxins? Are there any members of the family taking medications (possibility of ingestion of drugs)? Is there a history of preceding illness such as diabetes, systemic lupus erythematosus, or sickle cell disease? If so, has the patient been taking any drugs for this illness?

Seizures: Some of the important points in history to be obtained in any patient with seizures are as follows: What is the nature of involuntary movement? Are they tonic-clonic (grand mal)? Are they sudden, single, or repetitive muscular contractions (myoclonic)? Are they complex, seemingly purposeful acts (psychomotor attacks)? Are they confined to one extremity or to one side of the body? Does the attack start in one area of the body and march in a definite sequence (focal motor seizure with march) or does it come all at once (grand mal)? How long does the attack last? (grand mal usually lasts less than 5 minutes; petit mal lasts for less than 10 to 20 seconds; myoclonic and akinetic seizures are very brief and momentary in nature; psychomotor attacks last less than 2 minutes). Does the patient lose consciousness? (in grand mal he loses consciousness first, immediately followed by the convulsions; in petit mal there is brief loss of consciousness; in psychomotor seizure, the patient performs coordinated acts but is amnesic). Does the patient fall down? (in grand mal, the patient loses balance and falls; in petit mal, he or she does not; in myoclonic jerks, the movement may be so violent that the patient is thrown off the chair or bed; in akinetic seizure, there is sudden loss of tone and the patient collapses to the floor). Does the patient lose control of the bladder and bowel? (this occurs in grand mal and rarely in petit mal; loss of control of bladder and bowel at night may be suggestive of a seizure which no one saw). What happens after the attack? (in grand mal, the patient may sleep for a few hours and appear dazed; in petit mal, the patient may appear momentarily confused or have lip-smacking and chewing movements; in psychmotor seizures, the patient may also have lip-smacking or chewing movements and be amnesic to events that happened during the seizure). How many attacks are there per day? (this establishes the severity and seriousness of the problem). Are there any precipitating events? (examples are light stimulation starting a grand mal and startle response initiating myoclonic jerks).

PHYSICAL EXAMINATION OF THE SENSORIUM*

Appearance

Normal components of appearance include:

- Awareness
- Position and spontaneous movements of the body
- Responsiveness to touch and handling
- Activity
- Orientation

Awareness. A normal child is alert and responsive. A comatose child is unresponsive but may be aware of his surroundings. The vacant looks of a retarded child or a blind child are easy to recognize after some experience. Certain children after head injury and meningitis, may be aware of the surroundings but not able to verbalize.

During the management of a patient with coma, a standardized examination which can be administered quickly with high consistency and can be duplicated easily by observers is needed to assess the integrity of important neurologic functions. Table 7F-1 is one such standardized format, listing all the items of importance in history and physical examination. Items of importance in the history were already referred to on page 208. Routine neurologic examination is discussed later in this chapter. The following comments refer to the neurologic profile.

The neurologic profile (Table 7F-1) includes items that evaluate arousal (verbal response and eye opening), pupillary responses, eye movements (both spontaneous and in response to stimuli), corneal responses, breathing pattern, motor responses, tendon reflexes, and muscle tone. For each category, enter the best level of function on admission and during each 24 hours. A flow sheet with these data will be of great help in the management of patients in coma. The best verbal response is oriented speech and gets the highest score, whereas no speech obviously indicates a deeper state of coma.

Patients with spontaneous eye opening and movements get the best score and are obviously not comatose, though many may not be aware of

*For a detailed description of neurologic examination of children see Baird, 1983.

TABLE 7F-1. EXAMINATION OF THE COMATOSE PATIENT

History (from parents and friends)
- Onset of coma (abrupt, gradual)
- Recent complaints (headache, depression, focal weakness, vertigo)
- Recent injury
- Previous medical illnesses (diabetes, uremia, heart disease)
- Previous psychiatric history
- Access to drugs (sedatives, psychotropic drugs)

General Physical Examination
- Vital signs
- Evidence of trauma
- Evidence of acute or chronic systemic illness
- Evidence of drug ingestion (needle marks, alcohol on breath)
- Nuchal rigidity (examine with care)

Neurologic Profile
- Verbal responses
  - Oriented speech
  - Confused conversation
  - Inappropriate speech
  - No speech
- Eye opening
  - Spontaneous
  - Response to verbal stimuli
  - Response to noxious stimuli
  - None
- Pupillary reactions
  - Present
  - Absent
- Spontaneous eye movements
  - Orienting
  - Roving conjugate
  - Roving dysconjugate
  - Miscellaneous abnormal movements
  - None
- Oculocephalic responses
  - Normal
  - Full
  - Minimal
  - None
- Oculovestibular responses
  - Normal
  - Tonic conjugate
  - Minimal or dysconjugate
  - None
- Corneal responses
  - Present
  - Absent
- Respiratory pattern
  - Regular
  - Periodic
  - Ataxic

(continued)

TABLE 7F-1. (Continued)

Motor responses
Obeying commands
Localizing
Withdrawal
Abnormal flexion
Abnormal extension
None
Deep tendon reflexes
Normal
Increased
Absent
Skeletal muscle tone
Normal
Paratonic
Flexor
Extensor
Flaccid

(From Plum F, and Posner JB: The Diagnosis of Stupor and Coma, 3rd ed. Philadelphia, FA Davis Co., 1980.)

their surroundings. Those with severe brain injury have no eye opening at all or open the eyes only in response to a painful stimulus. Reactions of the pupils to light (including the diameter), should be recorded, if possible during each examination. Look for spontaneous eye movements in which patients look toward a stimulus. Roving conjugate and dysconjugate eye movements signify deeper stages of coma. One should also record any unusual types of eye movements such as bobbing.

Oculocephalic response should *not* be looked for in patients suspected of having a severe neck injury. The methods to elicit oculocephalic response and oculovestibular responses are given elsewhere (pages 223 and 231). Corneal response to a stimulus is recorded as present or absent. Respiratory patterns are recorded in those not on a mechanical respiratory device.

Patients who can move a limb on verbal command, are obviously not comatose. If there is no response to verbal command, apply pressure (squeeze) over the nailbed, tendon, or the glabella. Presence of a higher degree of function allows the patient to locate or resist the noxious stimulus by using an extremity. Rapid withdrawal with hip or shoulder adduction is a more primitive response. Abnormal accentuation of flexor or extensor tone of the extremities denotes even deeper stages of coma. Tendon reflexes are often exaggerated in a comatose patient. Absent reflex may be an indication of a deeper stage of coma. The presence of flaccidity also denotes a deeper stage of coma.

Body Position. A child's normal position in bed is of varying styles. Some sleep on the side with both upper and lower limbs partially flexed. Some sleep on their abdomen with the face turned to one side. But a child with meningitis or subarachnoid hemorrhage does not like to be handled, is irritable, and lies down with eyes tightly closed, turning the head away from light. In the presence of severe meningeal irritation and in tetanus, the child is opisthotonic with the occiput burrowing into the pillow.

A child with decerebrate rigidity has lower limbs in full extension, upper limbs in extension at the shoulder and elbow, forearm pronated, and the thumb adducted (Fig. 6-1, page 60). In decorticate rigidity the lower limbs are in extension, the shoulders are in external rotation, but the elbows are flexed and thumb adducted into the palm (Fig. 6-2, page 61). The child with severe hypotonia is in a pithed frog position.

Responsiveness. A normal child is appropriately happy or reacts adversely to being handled by strangers. Babies with multiple caretakers (institutionalized babies) and those with mental retardation do not seem to appreciate these differences. On the other hand, battered children are afraid of all types of human contact. An autistic child does not even make eye contact with the examiner, but the child may handle the coat pocket or the stethoscope as if these items have no connection to the human being carrying them. A child with meningitis or painful conditions such as fractures does not like to be handled.

Activity. A normal child has equal spontaneous movements of all parts of the body. Unequal movements of the limbs suggest varying conditions like monoplegia, paraplegia, and hemiplegia, or painful conditions (e.g., fracture).

Orientation. Most normal children can identify right and left on their own body by 6 years and on another's body by 9 years. Orientation in time and space is altered in the presence of infections, and toxic and vasculitic diseases of the brain. Simple questions to determine whether the child knows where he or she is, where home is, what day of the week it is, what time of the day it is, and when he or she is next going to have a birthday will help assess this function of the brain.

Memory

To test short-term memory, the simplest method is to give a set of numbers and ask the child to repeat them forward and backward. For example, if the examiner says 5, 6, 7 the child has to say 5, 6, 7 and then 7, 6, 5. The backward repetition is affected more often in organic brain syndromes. (Normal: A normal 6 year old can repeat 5 digits forward and count 3 digits backward; a 10 year old can count 6 digits forward and 4 digits backward.)

Another test for immediate memory is to tell a story and have the child repeat it. This also tests attention span, comprehension, and confabulation.

To test intermediate recall, give the child the name of a flower, city, and food at the beginning of an examination. After varying intervals during the examination ask him to repeat the items from memory.

To test long-term memory ask the child about his home address, telephone number, birth date, and names and ages of siblings.

Intelligence will be discussed in Chapter 8 as part of the assessment of child development.

Speech

The components of speech to be tested are:

- Presence or absence of speech (spoken word and written word)
- Quantity of speech—age appropriateness
- Quality of speech—volume
phonation
articulation
content
rhythm
- Examination of the anatomic structures of mouth, pharynx, and larynx

Presence or Absence. A child may have normal speech but may never open his mouth in the presence of strangers or in the doctor's office. A complete and thorough speech examination may not be possible and is not totally necessary. One may have to rely on the history and careful observation of whatever communication is available. If there are sufficient reasons, we may have to refer the child to a speech pathologist for a thorough examination. Certain points, however, are within the reach of all interested clinicians and can be evaluated with most children. These normal milestones in speech and prespeech developments are given in Table 7F-2.

Failure to speak any word by 18 months and failure to make meaningful sentences by 3 years are abnormal. Complete absence of speech is mutism and may be an evidence of deafness, mental retardation, or autism.

Quality. In testing for quality of speech, see if the patient can produce an adequate *volume* of air and control it. Patients with intercostal muscle paralysis may not be able to speak long sentences without frequent pauses. They may have no voice or a breathy voice. A simple way to test for this is to make the child take a large breath and count as many numbers as possible in one breath. The other simple method is to have the child blow out a match held at a distance of 2 to 5 inches.

Vocal cords are essential for *phonation*. The patient may have normal respiration and strong respiratory muscles, but if vocal cords do not move normally, one may have aphonia (no voice). The vibration of air by vocal cords gives rise to pitch and intensity of the sound. Listen, therefore, to the

TABLE 7F-2. SEQUENCE OF 29 LINGUISTIC AND AUDITORY MILESTONES

Sequential Milestone Item	Months of Age
1. Alerting*	1
2. Social smile*	1–1½
3. Cooing	3
4. Orient to voice*	4
5. Orient to bell (1)*	5
6. "Ah-goo"	5
7. Razzing	5
8. Babbling	6½
9. Orient to bell (11)*	7
10. Gesture	7½
11. "Dada/mama" (inappropriate)	8
12. Orient to bell (111)*	9½
13. "Dada/mama" (appropriate)	10
14. One word	11
15. One-step command (w/ gesture)*	12
16. Two words	12
17. Three words	14
18. One-step command (w/o gesture)*	15
19. Four to six words	15
20. Immature jargoning	15
21. Seven to twenty words	18
22. Mature jargoning	18
23. One body part*	18
24. Three body parts*	21
25. Two-word combinations (N + N)	21
26. Five body parts*	23
27. Fifty words	24
28. Two-word sentences (S + P)	24
29. Pronouns (I, me, you; inappropriate)	24

*Age levels are approximate and still need to be standardized on different normal populations. The sequence of development for items at different age levels demonstrates much less variability, especially in delayed subjects. Attempts should be made to directly observe asterisked items; when a child is uncooperative during a particular evaluation, parental observation may be recorded.

(From Capute AJ, Accardo PJ: Linguistic and auditory milestones during the first two years of life: A language inventory for the practitioner. Clin Pediatr 17:847–853, 1978.)

pitch. Monotonous speech without inflections is seen in deafness. A deaf child also may have a very high-pitched voice if the deafness is central. Many normal children may have a high-pitched voice, particularly in the prepubertal period.

Coordinated movement of the tongue, palate, and lips are required for *articulation.* A simple test for articulation is to make a child say "ka, pa, ti, ka" repeatedly and quickly. Because the sound "ka" comes from the back of the throat, the word "pa" produced by the lips, and "ti" produced by the tongue and the palate, these three sounds test the major components of articulation effectively. Problems of coordination will also be evident when the child tries to say these words fast.

The components of articulation are intelligibility and coordination. There are a number of test words such as "Methodist, Episcopal," or "round the rugged rock the ragged rascal ran" to test for intelligibility and coordination. The *content* of the speech as to appropriateness and orientation and irregularity of *rhythm* (stuttering) are easily discerned just by listening to the child's conversation.

Nasal resonance during phonation is another point to look for—suggesting cleft palate, chronic adenoiditis, or palatal paralysis. If this is suspected, ask the child to say words ending with "ng" (e.g., coming, walking) which he or she may not be able to pronounce properly.

CRANIAL NERVES

Olfactory Nerve (First nerve)

Testing the sense of smell is very difficult, even in adults. In children it is more difficult. Present common items such as toothpaste, oranges, and chewing gum to each nostril with the other side closed. The child should have his eyes closed and should guess the item from the smell. In infants, change of facial expression may be the only clue.

Optic Nerve (Second nerve)(Fig. 7F-1)

Presence or absence of vision

- Acuity
- Fields
- Fundus

Presence of Vision. A simple test to show that a child has *intact cortical vision* is to make a menacing gesture, as if to poke the eye. A consistent blink response indicates cortical vision, However, this response is not present routinely before 10 months of age. Inconsistent response indicates that the vision is intact, but the interpretation of vision is impaired, as in parietal lobe lesions. If a child follows a moving light or object, intact cortical vision is confirmed.

Acuity. There are many tests for visual acuity. The simplest is the illiterate *E* chart which can be used for children as young as 3 years. There are many other tests and refinements, but the *E* test is as good as any other for

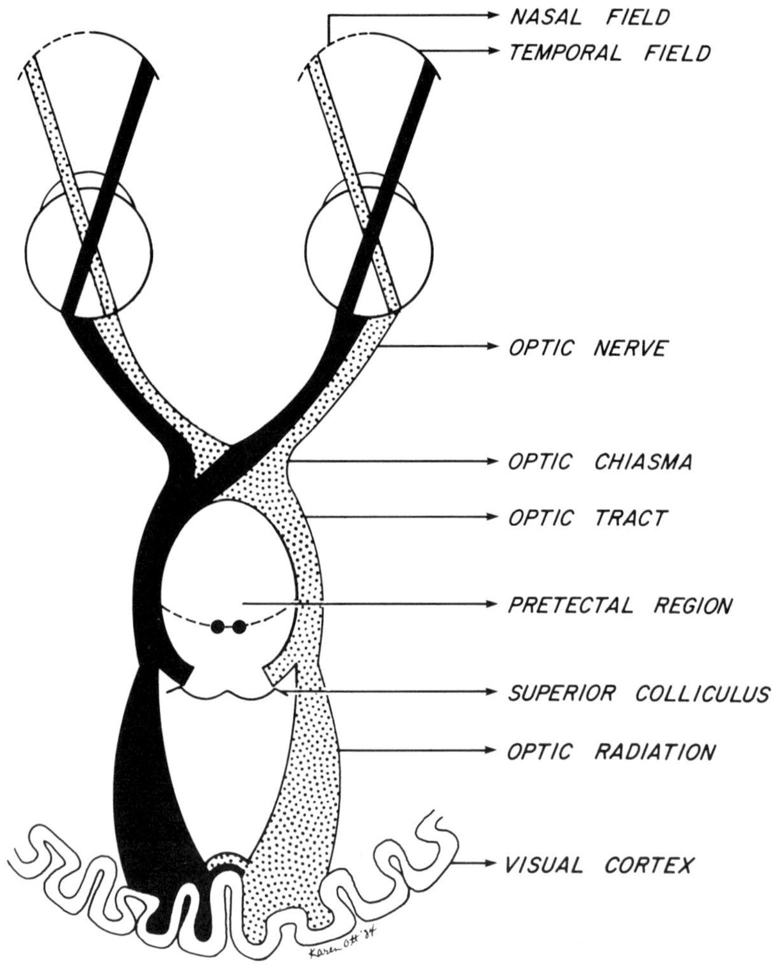

Figure 7F-1. Diagram of visual pathway.

screening. The *E*'s in the chart are in different directions so that the limbs are pointing up, down, right, and left. The chart is fixed at the child's eye level in a well-lit hallway at a distance of 20 feet from the child's seat. The child is asked to show with fingers the direction to which the limbs of the E are pointing. Test each eye separately and then both together. At least 50 percent or more of the letters in each line should be recognized correctly by the child to get a "pass" for that line. Physiologically, children are far-sighted till 6 to 7 years of age. Children in the first three grades of school should be able to read 20/20 or better with each eye. A compact eye testing machine which electrically projects the charts in front of the child's visual field is even more accurate and takes very little space in an office. One example is the Titmus Vision Tester (Titmus, P. O. Box 191, Petersburg, VA 23804).

Field of Vision. The field of vision is tested by a confrontation method till the child is old enough to cooperate with perimetry. Some simple methods are: (1) use a colorful toy and approach the eye from each side sequentially. If the child's response (as shown by turning to the object) is obvious when approached from one side but not the other, hemianopsia is suspected. (2) If the child tilts the head to read, hemianopsia or muscle imbalance is to be suspected. (3) Ask the child to look at a measuring tape when it is being pulled out of its container. Ask the child to fix the eye on the opening in the container from which the tape comes out. Do it first with the tape coming out from right to left and then from left to right. Normally, the eye will follow the tape for a short distance as it comes out and return back to the opening of the tape container. This is called opticokinetic nystagmus. If there is hemianopsia, this reflex will be absent in the direction opposite to the hemianopsia. (4) The child is asked to sit and look at the examiner's eyes which have to be level with the eyes of the child. Now two objects are dangled with threads behind the child's head and are slowly brought forward. As soon as the peripheral field of the eye catches the object, the child will move the eye. If this occurs consistently in one direction but not the other, it indicates a field defect. (5) Another method is for the child to look into the examiner's eyes, which are placed at the same level as those of the child's. Now the examiner takes his hands to the periphery of the visual field (Fig. 7F-2), with the index fingers extended and at diagonally op-

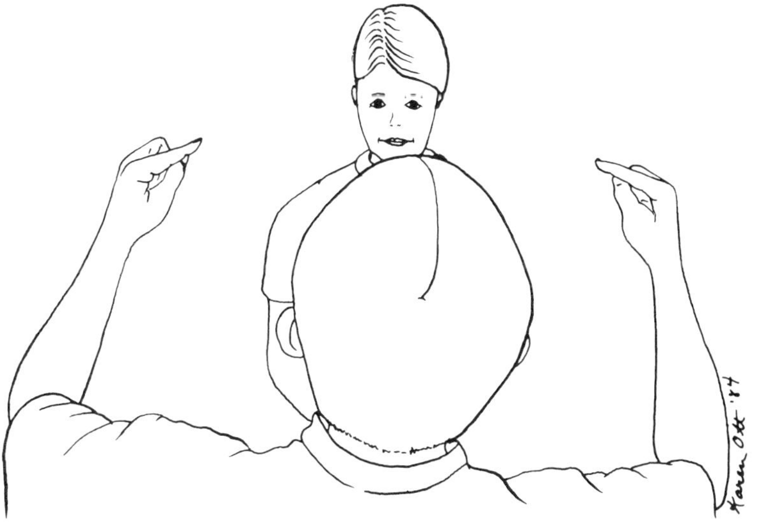

Figure 7F-2. Confrontation perimetry.

posite positions. He quickly flexes one of the fingers and the child is asked to show which finger moved. This is repeated at different points in the perimeter of the field.

Remember that false results can be obtained. Cooperation is needed for these tests, and staring at a child's eyes can frighten him or her.

Fundus. The optic fundus is examined with an ophthalmoscope. The following is a brief description of the parts of the ophthalmoscope and their use.

Ophthalmoscope: The ophthalmoscope consists of a handle, batteries, and the ophthalmoscope head. Most models operate on batteries (3 volts) and are easily carried. Some models (particularly those used by ophthalmologists) can be connected to electric outlets through a transformer (12 volts). Always use fresh batteries to obtain maximum light and good visualization.

The head has a rubber guard to prevent scratches to the examiner's glasses if he or she wishes to use the instrument with glasses on. The rotary disc on the head has numbers in red on the left side and numbers in black on the right side of the "0" mark. The red numbers indicate minus lenses in the viewing aperture, and black numbers indicate plus lenses. *Myopia* in the patient's lenses is neutralized by the minus lenses and *hyperopia* by the plus lenses in the ophthalmoscope. One can get 15 to 20 diopters of power through these discs. Plus 8 to 15 lenses also are used to focus on the iris margin and the lens.

Ophthalmoscopes also have devices to give different kinds of beams of light. The control is usually on top or behind the instrument head. Two round apertures (one large, one small), a slit, a grid, and a red-free filter are usually provided. The large round is for large pupils and the small round is for small pupils. The slit is used to recognize the convexity and concavity of the retinal lesions. In the presence of a raised or depressed retinal lesion, if the light from the vertical slit is focused on the lesion and the adjoining normal retina, there will be a steplike distortion of the beam at the junction of normal retina and the lesion. If the distortion is convex pointing towards the observer, the lesion is an elevation. If it bends away from the examiner, it is a defect in the surface of the retina. The grid is used to measure the size of the vessels. The green filter (red-free light) makes the blood vessels stand out as dark stripes and allows recognition of small aneurysms and hemorrhages. With fresh batteries, this filter may also help differentiate between melanin (not very black) and old hemorrhage (intense black).

Techniques in using the ophthalmoscope: Certain practical points to remember are: (1) Many children and infants are curious and eventually will look directly into the light if you leave them alone and wait, but if you touch the lid to open the eye, the fight will get tougher. (2) Younger children are best examined when they are lying down. Some older children cooperate better if they are sitting up. (3) Some children may require anesthesia. If the problem is significant enough to warrant such a risk, an ophthalmologist should be looking at the eye! (4) Dilation of the pupil is necessary for a thorough examination of the eye, though a satisfactory examination of the optic nerve head can be accomplished without mydriasis. For routine office use, 1 drop of 10 percent phenylephrine in each eye is adequate.

For better pupillary dilation, the following procedure is recommended:

- For children less than 1 year of age: either tropicamide (1 percent) applied 3 times at 10 minute intervals or Cyclomedrin (combination of 0.5 percent Cyclopentolate and 0.5 percent Tropicamide) used once. Examine after 30 to 40 minutes.
- For children over 1 year of age:
  If the child has seizures: 0.5 percent Tropicamide and 10 percent Neosynephrine applied 2 or 3 times over a 10 minute period.
  If the child has no seizures: Cyclopentolate 1 percent solution (once).
  If the child has dark eyes: add Tropicamide 1 percent solution (once). Examine after 20 to 30 minutes.

Start by using a +8 lens which will show any scars or large deposits in the *cornea* as black spots in the midst of the red reflex. By changing the lens to +10 or +12, the edge of the iris becomes easily visible. Determine if the edge is clear and round. In the presence of iridocyclitis, the iris edge will show fine serrations, instead of a smooth round contour.

Now look for the red reflex. Occasionally, the normal red reflex is replaced by a "white" or "yellow" reflex, also called the cat's eye reflex. A white reflex should indicate serious eye disease and requires immediate consultation with an ophthalmologist. Retinoblastoma, angiomatosis of the retina, Toxocara canis, and retrolental fibroplasia can cause a white reflex. Congenital cataract will also give a white reflex instead of the red reflex but one can judge the point of origin of the reflex by changing the power of the lens. A +10 or +12 lens will be needed to locate the white reflex of a cataract.

Now look at the *characteristics of the fundus*. Look at the periphery and move slowly toward the optic disc by following the vessels. Take note of the characteristics of the arteries and veins. Finally, look at the macula. The fovea is the center of the macula and is located approximately 2 disc diameters temporal to the disc. The major points to look for in the macula are: (1) pigmented deposits with exudates of toxoplasmosis, and (2) the cherry red spot of Tay-Sach's disease.

Important findings to look for in the fundus of children are related to the *retinitis* of congenital infections, degenerative diseases, phakomatosis, optic atrophy, and papilledema. Look for the "jet-black" deposits of retinitis pigmentosa which starts in the equatorial region, spreading later to the periphery, and for a yellow-white exudate of congenital syphilis which later turns into pigments all over the fundus. Also look for retinal exudates which appear as faint clusters or masses.

Next look at the *blood vessels*. The central retinal artery divides into superior and inferior segments. Each of these segments divides into a temporal and nasal branch. There are veins corresponding to these four arterial branches. Normally, veins are larger than arteries (3:2) and darker. The vessels have a central stripe which is more prominent in the arteries. The arteries and veins are graceful in their course without too many curvatures and acute bends. On locations where the arteries and veins cross each other, the veins pass underneath the arteries.

It is important to be familiar with these normal characteristics, because in hypertensive retinopathy one sees an increase in the reflex stripe along the arteriole, loss of reflex stripe of the veins on either side of A-V crossing, and narrowing of arterioles. Increased tortuosity of vessels in black patients may indicate sickle cell disease. Perivascular sheathing is seen in vasculitis of various kinds. Hemorrhages along blood vessels are seen in severe papilledema, hypertension, and systemic lupus erythematosus. (These may show better with a red-free light.) Vascular tumors may be recognized during this portion of the examination. Fullness of the veins and loss of venous pulsation of the optic cup are seen in papilledema.

Next, look at the *optic disc* and characterize the following features: shape, size, color, depth, the edge, and the vessels. Normally, the disc is round. The central portion of the disk is a shallow paler area and is called the physiological cup. The vessels fan out from the center of the cup. The physiological cup is symmetrical and occupies about 30 percent of the disc. In glaucoma, the cup extends almost to the periphery and is asymmetric. The vessels are pushed nasally. In primary optic atrophy the entire disc is white; the disc margins are clear and the vessel undisturbed. In secondary optic atrophy, the disc is pale—not white—with sheathing of vessels and indistinct margins.

The margins of the disc get indistinct and the color hyperemic in optic neuritis and in papilledema. There are fullness of veins, loss of pulsation of veins, and retinal hemorrhages in both conditions. The physiologic cup is filled out. It may be difficult to differentiate between these two conditions. In addition to history, two other useful points in differentiating these two conditions are: (1) decreased visual acuity in neuritis as opposed to usually normal vision in papilledema, and (2) presence of inflammatory cells in the vitreous seen in optic neuritis (Table 7F-3).

Oculomotor, Trochlear, and Abducent Nerves (Third, Fourth, and Sixth nerves)

These nerves supply the extraocular muscles and the pupil. Consequently, examination of these nerves involves movements of the eyeball spon-

TABLE 7F-3. APPEARANCE OF OPTIC FUNDUS IN THREE IMPORTANT CLINICAL CONDITIONS

	Papilledema	Papillitis	Optic Atrophy
Depth	Elevated disc Physiological cup obliterated	Elevated disc Physiological cup obliterated	Shallow
Edge	Blurred edge	Blurred edge	Very sharp
Vessels	Engorged	Engorged	Narrow/few
Color	No venous pulse Hyperemic Hemorrhages	No venous pulse Hyperemic Hemorrhages	Pale to white
Vision	Good; or enlarged blind spot	Poor vision; or loss of central vision	Reduced vision

taneously and on demand (Fig. 7F-3). It is obvious that during the examination one should systematically observe the following:

1. Position of the eyes at rest; squint
2. Movements of the eyes independently of each other
3. Movements of the eyes together (conjugate)
4. Movement of the eyes in relation to the head movements and body movement

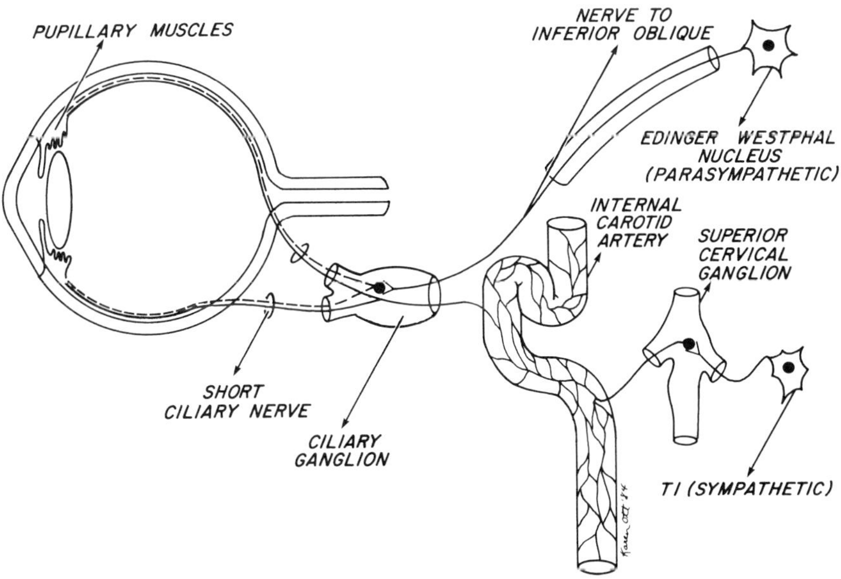

Figure 7F-3. Nerve supply to the pupil and to the extraocular muscles.

Also evaluate:

1. Nystagmus (discussed on page 230)
2. Double vision
3. Pupils

Some of the clinical clues to lesions of the third, fourth, and sixth nerves are: (1) ptosis—which is drooping of the eyelids; (2) an eye that is deviated down and out; (3) inability to look outwards, and (4) diplopia.

Position of Examination. Younger children are best examined when they are sitting on their mother's lap facing the examiner. The eyes of the examiner should be at the same level as the child's. Covering the eyes can scare the child. The child should therefore be examined with both eyes open before examining with the eyes closed. Also, the examiner should use his or her own hand to cover the eyes of the child rather than use any occlusive device. Use of a flashlight or a sparkler toy is bound to make the child follow with the eye.

Testing for Squint. With the child looking at the object directly in front of the eye, look for the reflection of the light from the surface of the pupils. Normally these should be at comparable points, but in the presence of squint, the reflections are at nonconjugate locations. Strabismus (squint) which is obvious with both eyes open is called heterotropia. Esotropia is convergent strabismus, and exotropia is divergent strabismus.

Tendency for deviation is called phoria. Esophoria is the tendency to converge and exophoria is the tendency to diverge. Testing for phoria uses the cover–uncover test. The child looks at an object or light. Cover one eye, then the other with a cardboard or with your thumb held in front of the eye. Do it slowly and rapidly. *Look at the uncovered eye always.* If there is definite movement of the uncovered eye on rapid, alternate covering, phoria is present. When one eye is covered, if the uncovered eye moves to fix on the finger, it was originally not looking at the object. Now if the covered eye is uncovered (and is found to be moving) to fix on the object, it was obviously deviating when the other eye was looking at the object. This indicates the presence of a tendency (phoria) for squint.

Independent Eyeball Movements. Next, test for movements of the eyeball in all directions by having the child follow a bright light or sparkler, first with both eyes moving and then one eye at a time (Table 7F-4). The third nerve innervates the medial rectus, superior and inferior recti, inferior oblique, levator palpebrae superioris, and the pupillary constrictors. Therefore, if the third nerve is paralyzed, one expects to see ptosis, pupillary dilatation, and loss of all movements except lateral deviations and downward movement with the eyes in abduction. Paralysis of the fourth nerve (superior oblique muscles) is tested by looking for slight upward deviation of the eye

TABLE 7F-4. CHART OF PARALYSES OF INDIVIDUAL EYE MUSCLES

Muscle	Nerve	Deviation of Eyeball	Diplopia Present When Looking*	Direction of Image
Internal rectus	III	Outward (external squint)	Toward nose	Vertical
Superior rectus	III	Downward and inward	Upward and outward	Oblique
Inferior rectus	III	Upward and inward	Downward and outward	Oblique
Inferior oblique	III	Downward and outward	Upward and inward	Oblique
Superior oblique	IV	Upward and outward	Downward and inward	Oblique
External rectus	VI	Inward (internal squint)	Toward temple	Vertical

*Dioplopia is noted only when the affected eye attempts these movements.
(From Chusid JG: Correlative Neuroanatomy and Functional Neurology, 17th ed. Los Altos, Calif., Lange Medical Publications, 1979. Reproduced with permission.)

in abducted position because the inferior oblique is dominating. In paralysis of the sixth nerve, there is paralysis of abduction (lateral movement) of the eye.

To test for recti and oblique muscles, one must test the eyes in either abduction or adduction. On abduction of the eye, the superior rectus acts as an elevator and the inferior rectus as a depressor. On adduction of the eye, the superior oblique is a depressor and the inferior oblique is an elevator of the eye. In midline position all these muscles have a rotatory component.

Conjugate Eyeball Movement. Conjugate deviation of the eyes (both eyes moving parallel) *at rest* with the gaze directed to one side indicates either a corticulo-bulbar irritative lesion on the opposite side or a destructive lesion on the same side. After observing for any conjugate deviation at rest, test for conjugate eye movement *on command.* If it is absent, it denotes injury to the frontomesencephalic pathway. In children with head injury, one may see conjugate deviation at rest and inability to produce conjugate movement on command. Inability to get superior conjugate movement is called Parinaud syndrome and denotes a lesion in the corpora quadrigemina.

Eyeball and Head Movements. The next step is to examine the movement of the eye as the position of the head is changed. With the eyelids held open, the head is rotated from side to side. A positive doll's eye reflex (oculocephalic reflex) is said to be present if there is conjugate deviation of the eyes in a direction opposite to the direction of movement of the head (head rotated toward right, eyes deviating to left). Such a reflex is absent in a normal, awake person but may be present in patients with coma.

Double Vision (Diplopia). Usually double vision is a definable complaint in older children, but younger children and infants may not be able to explain this. In the presence of diplopia (particularly of recent onset) the infant may refuse to open the eye and may lie down with the eyes buried. Or, he or she may rotate the head to one side (sixth nerve) or tilt the head (third, fourth nerve).

With both eyes open, have the child look at a finger or pencil held around the periphery of the field of vision, first to the patient's right. Find out whether two images are seen. A false image appears in the direction toward which the paralyzed muscle usually pulls. Repeat the test with the object to the left of the patient, up and down (Table 7F-4). A simpler method is to do the cover–uncover test (as in testing for squint) in right, left, up, down, and oblique positions. Any deviation of the uncovered eye in any of these positions is likely to be associated with diplopia. This test does not require the child's response.

Pupils. In evaluating the pupils the points to be looked for are: (1) size; (2) shape; (3) equality between both sides; (4) response to light on the same side; (5) response to light on the opposite side; (6) response to pain; and (7) response to accommodation.

Afferent fibers involved in the light reflex leave the other fibers along the optic tract before the fibers reach the lateral geniculate body and go to the pretectal region (Fig. 7F-1). The afferent fibers involved in accommodation reflex course toward the superior colliculi. The afferent fibers for pupillary control are through parasympathetic and sympathetic fibers. Pupillary constrictors arise in the Edinger-Westphal nucleus and medial nucleus of the third cranial nerve and course along the third nerve to the ciliary muscles. Pupillary dilators originate from the cervical sympathetic ganglion and course along the internal carotid artery. Both parasympathetic and sympathetic fibers course through the ciliary ganglion and short ciliary nerves (Fig. 7F-3).

Small pupils are common in black children—actually it is difficult to see the small dark pupil in the center of a dark iris. A trick which one of the authors has used is to cover the flashlight with yellow cellophane paper and shine the yellow light at an angle.

Very small pupils may be normal but may also indicate head injury, deep coma, or drug toxicity. In Horner syndrome, a small pupil is a feature together with ptosis, enophthalmos, and lack of sweating on the ipsilateral side of the face.

Large pupils are seen in third nerve paralysis, fear, anxiety (sympathetic overactivity), and in certain stages of coma. A fixed dilated pupil without reaction to light in a comatose child may be a sign of ipsilateral hippocampal herniation.

Unequal pupil size may be normal. It may be due to a small pupil on one side (local use of drugs, Horner syndrome, or irritative lesion of the third nerve), or a large pupil on one side (drugs applied locally, Byrne response of pain to one extremity, complete paralysis of the third nerve on one side), or aniridia on one side.

Reaction to light is tested by having the child looking away from the major source of light in the room and shining a flashlight on the pupil. Normally the pupil reacts quickly. At the same time, the opposite pupil also contracts (consensual light response).

To test the accommodation reflex, the child is asked to look at a distant object. Then a finger is held close to his or her nose and the child asked to focus on the finger. Normally the eyes should converge and the pupils constrict in attempting to look at a close object.

For the ciliospinal reflex, the skin of the neck is pinched. This should cause dilation of the pupils. In Byrne reflex, pinching one lower extremity causes dilation of the pupil on the opposite side.

The interpretation of the reflexes described above is as follows: (1) loss of direct pupillary response on one side with loss of consensual response on the other side and retention of accommodation reflex is seen in lesions of the optic nerve close to the eyeball. (2) Homonymous hemianopsia without loss of pupillary responses indicates lesions past the point where pupillary fibers leave the optic tract. (3) Loss of direct and consensual responses on the same side with retention of accommodation reflex suggests lesions close to the Edinger-Westphal nucleus or ciliary ganglion ("Argyll-Robertson pupils"). (4) Absolute paralysis of the pupil on one side suggests lesions of the oculomotor nerve (Figs. 7F-1 and 7F-3).

The presence of ptosis on one side may mean third nerve palsy, in which case the pupil will be dilated, or Horner syndrome, in which case the pupil will be small. The appearance of ptosis may be spurious because of widening of the palpebral fissure on the opposite side (seventh nerve palsy). Bilateral ptosis is seen in myasthenia.

Trigeminal Nerve (Fifth nerve)

The fifth cranial nerve has a motor and a sensory component. There are three divisions of the fifth nerve: ophthalmic, maxillary, and mandibular. The first two are sensory, the third has a sensory and a motor component (Table 7F-5).

To test for the *motor component,* ask the patient to clench the teeth. Palpate the masseters and the temporalis muscles. Ask the patient to open and close the mouth. If one side is paralyzed, the jaw will be deviated to the nonparalyzed side when the mouth is opened.

Somatic Sensory. Sensory innervation of the face is given in Figure 7F-4. Touch and temperature are tested in the usual manner (described on pages 239–241). A child in pain because of teething will frequently pull at the ear because of transmission along the mandibular portion of the trigeminal nerve.

Corneal Reflex. The easiest way to test for corneal reflex in young children is to blow air into the patient's eye, causing a blink. The more acceptable

TABLE 7F-5. MAJOR BRANCHES OF THE TRIGEMINAL NERVE AND THEIR FUNCTIONAL SIGNIFICANCE

Branch	Sensory Supply	Motor Supply	Disability If Cut
Ophthalmic	Conjunctiva (except lower lid) Lacrimal gland Medial part of skin of nose up to its tip Upper eyelids Forehead and scalp, to the vertex	None	Loss of corneal reflex Trophic changes in eye Loss of sensation in areas described under Sensory Supply
Maxillary	Cheek, front of temple, lower lids and conjunctiva, side of the nose, upper lip, upper teeth, mucous membrane of nose, upper pharynx, roof of mouth, soft palate	None	Loss of sensation in areas described under Sensory Supply Loss of palatal reflex
Mandibular	Lower part of face Lower lip Tongue, lower teeth and part of ear Salivary glands	Muscles of mastication	Paralysis of masticators Loss of sensation in areas described under Sensory Supply

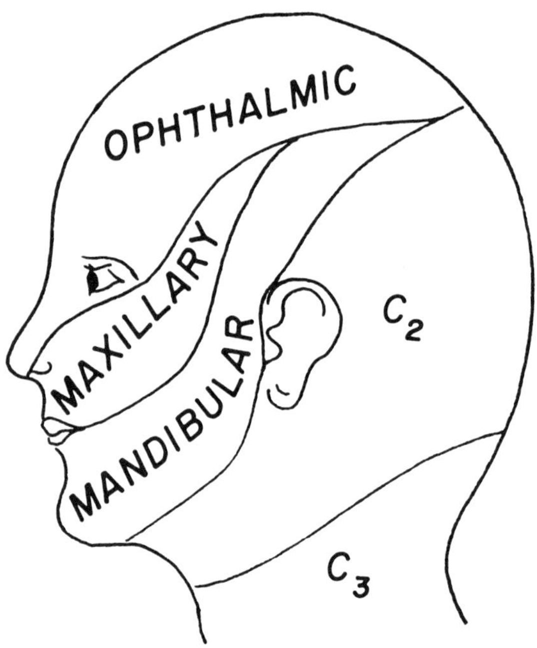

Figure 7F-4. Sensory supply of the face (fifth nerve).

method is to twist a small thread out of a cotton ball and touch the cornea with it. Have the child look in one direction and approach the cornea from the opposite direction (to avoid a visual blink reflex rather than a corneal blink). Test on both sides.

Jaw Reflex. Have the patient open the mouth gently. Place a finger at the tip of the mandible and tap it with a percussion hammer. Normally, one gets a mild contraction of the masseter muscle. An exaggerated reflex indicates upper motor lesion above the fifth nucleus. This reflex may be absent, even in normal individuals.

Facial Nerve (Seventh nerve)

The anatomy of the seventh nerve is described diagrammatically in Figure 7F-5. The seventh nerve is almost entirely a motor nerve. It supplies all the muscles of the face and scalp (except the levator palpebrae superioris) and also the platysma and the stapedius. The chorda tympani, which runs parts of its course with the facial nerve, supplies taste to the anterior two thirds of the tongue. Autonomic afferent fibers to the lacrimal gland and the submaxillary and submandibular glands also run with the facial nerve.

Motor Function. While talking to the parents, observe casually the patient's face and the facial expression. In the case of unilateral facial paralysis, the facial furrows are flattened and saliva may accumulate on the affected side. The palpebral fissure may be wider on that side, and the eyeball may roll

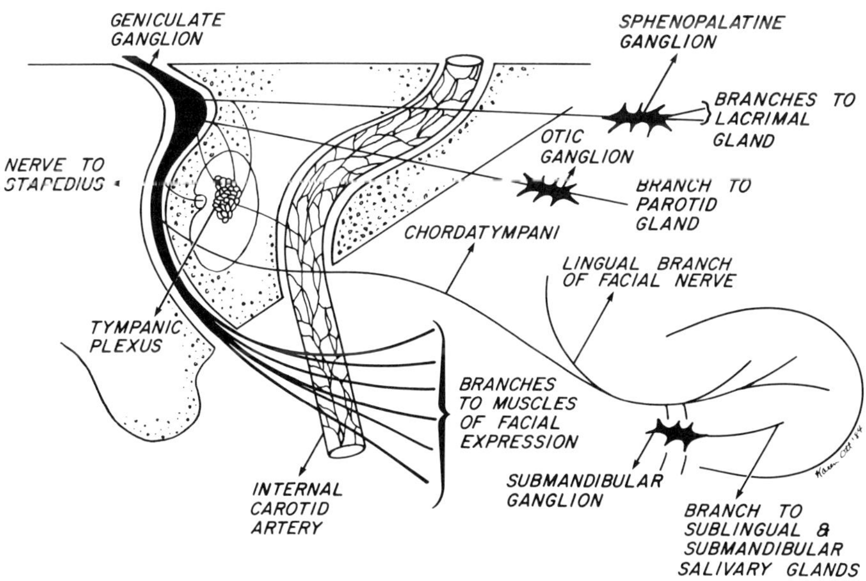

Figure 7F-5. Anatomy of the seventh cranial (facial) nerve.

up under the upper eyelid rather than the upper lid moving down on the eyeball. Blinking may be less forceful on the affected side.

Unilateral facial weakness has to be differentiated from weakness of the depressor anguli oris, which may be congenitally absent (Hufnagel palsy). If the latter is the case, only the lower part of one half of the face below the angle of the mouth is involved.

Look for bilateral facial weakness, which may be part of Guillain-Barré syndrome, various myopathies, and Moebius syndrome. If voluntary movements are lost but emotionally induced movements, such as smiling, are intact, it indicates supranuclear lesions. In nuclear or peripheral lesions voluntary and emotional movements are both lost.

Determine whether only the movements of the lower part of the face are lost (intranuclear lesion) or movements of both upper and lower halves are lost (lower motor).

The various simple tests to evaluate the motor function of the nerve are:

1. Have the child close the eyes as tightly as possible. Normally, the upper lid will descend with some movement of the eyeball upward. There will be closure of the lids, with lashes buried inward, and lifting of the corners of the mouth upward.
   In cases of facial paralysis, the upper lid does not close down, even though the eyeball moves upwards (Bell's phenomenon). The eyelashes are not buried in the closure. The angle of the mouth either does not move at all or moves much less than on the unaffected side.
2. Ask the child to whistle—if he or she can understand and try.
3. Ask the child to blow up one cheek and try to push out the air against closed lips. It is much easier to push air out of the paralyzed side.
4. Ask the child to show the teeth or smile. The face is flat on one side and the pull is toward the unaffected side.

Sensory Functions. Examination of *taste* over the anterior two thirds of the tongue should be a part of examination of the seventh nerve. This is hard to do. If one has to, the method is as follows. Have the child put the tongue out as far as possible. Hold the tip with a moist filter paper. Dry one half of the tongue with filter paper. Place over the anterior two thirds of the tongue with an applicator or a small dropper the following substances one at a time: 5 percent glucose solution (sweet), 3 percent sodium chloride (salt), 1 percent citric acid (sour), and 0.1 percent quinine hydrochloride (bitter). The drop should be placed carefully. The child should not draw the tongue in but should indicate the taste with finger clues or pointing to a set of cards with the names of the tastes written on them. After each drop the tongue is thoroughly washed, and the next taste is tested. Bitter should be the last tested, for obvious reasons. The taste is lost in lesions along the course of the seventh nerve from the internal auditory meatus to the place where the chorda tympani branches off.

Autonomic Functions. In recent lesions of the facial nerve, increased lacrimation and salivation are common.

Reflexes. Certain motor reflexes of the face are affected in the presence of facial nerve lesions, though most of these reflexes indicate a premature nervous system or regression to an infantile status or frontal lobe lesions. These are the glabellar reflex and snout reflex. Glabellar reflex is elicited by repeated tapping of the glabellar region. Normally there will be a blinking response of the lids for five to six times and then the response extinguishes. An abnormal response is the persistent blinking response as long as tapping over the glabella is continued. Snout reflex is characterized by pouting of the lips when the area of the philtrum of the upper lip is tapped. This reflex should be absent in normal children after the first 2 months of life.

Chvostek's sign is elicited by tapping the facial nerve in front of the ears. Marked contractions and spasm following such a tapping suggests hypocalcemia. (This response is not a reflex. This is a response caused by an increased irritability of nerve fibers to mechanical stimulation.)

Auditory Nerve (Eighth nerve)

The auditory nerve has two components: one supplying the cochlea and serving auditory functions and the other supplying the semicircular canals and serving functions of equilibrium of the body. The auditory fibers reach the cochlear nuclei in the pons and the vestibular fibers reach the nuclei in the pons and medulla. From these locations, the secondary tracts decussate partially and terminate in the inferior colliculi and medial geniculate bodies and at the cortical center for hearing, which lies in the temporal lobe.

Evaluation of the Auditory Component (Hearing). In young infants, in children up to 3 to 4 years of age, and in retarded children, hearing tests are complex to administer. Many clues in the patient's history may point to the nature of the problem. For example, failure to respond to normal sounds (except very loud sounds), excessive response to visual stimuli, delayed speech, and a monotonous voice with normal motor development make one suspicious of nerve deafness. *Inconsistent* response to sounds, delayed speech, avoiding eye contact, ignoring visual clues, and unusual body movements suggest psychogenic reasons for deafness. Finally, normal but *delayed* response to sounds, with normal reaction to visual stimuli and delayed development in all areas of development suggest retardation.

Have the child sit on the mother's lap facing the examiner. Use the rustling of a piece of paper, the flicking of the examiner's nails, a rattle, a small bell, or a tuning fork (256–512 cps) to make noise. Observe the child's face as the noise is made. Hold the object used to make the noise slightly behind the child's ear, first on one side and then on the other. Evidence of intact hearing is a change in the expression of the face, reaction of the pupil, and the child turning to the source of sound.

In older children, one can use a tuning fork or a watch or whisper (with the mouth hidden) to make sounds. Ask them whether they hear and, if they do hear, whether there is any difference between one ear and the other.

If there are any abnormalities and suspicion about hearing, one should obtain both a tympanometry and audiogram or, in the younger infant, an evoked response audiometry. The old tests with a tuning fork, such as Rinne test and Weber test, are of historical interest only. These two tests are based on the comparison of air conduction to bone conduction. If the middle ear is affected, bone conduction is better than air conduction. If the nerve is affected, both air and bone conduction are decreased, but air conduction remains better than bone conduction.

Rinne's test: tap a tuning fork (256–512 cps) and hold it next to the ear. If it can be heard, place it on the mastoid. If it can be heard again, compare to see which is heard louder and longer. Normally, air conduction is louder and is heard longer. In middle ear disease, bone conduction is louder and is heard for longer periods.

In Weber's test, a tuning fork is tapped and held over the forehead in midline. In middle ear disease on one side, the sound is heard louder on the affected side. If there is loss of nerve conduction on one side, the sound is louder on the unaffected side.

Abnormal Sounds. Ringing in the ears (tinnitus) may be due to salicylate toxicity. Hyperacusis is common in facial nerve paralysis. Auditory hallucination may be seen in systemic lupus erythematosus and in psychosis.

Vestibular Functions. Children cannot explain vertigo. The only clues, therefore, may be unexplained crying, the child trying to bury the face and not wanting to open the eyes, and vomiting with a change of posture. Other clinical clues for vestibular dysfunction are imbalance and nystagmus.

Nystagmus. A nystagmus is the involuntary movement of the eyeball which may be either rhythmic or nonrhythmic. Usually nystagmus has a fast and a slow component; less frequently it is symmetrical, with rhythmic to-and-fro oscillations called "pendular nystagmus."

Nystagmus may be physiologic or pathologic. It may occur at rest or only on movement of the eyes. Nystagmus may be horizontal or vertical or rotary or mixed. Nystagmus may be fine (less than 1 mm movement) or coarse (over 3 mm movement). Nystagmus that occurs when the eye is looking toward the direction of the fast component is mild (first degree).

Moderate nystagmus is seen when the eye is in median position (second degree). The nystagmus is severe when it occurs with the eye deviated toward the direction of the slow component (third degree).

To test for nystagmus, ask the child to look at the flashlight or a toy held in front of the eye. Move the object rather fast, first to one side and then to the other, and ask the child to follow. Also move it up and down. Keep the flashlight or toy in extreme positions for a few seconds to see if the nystagmus disappears after five or six beats. This is the characteristic of end-point fatigue nystagmus.

Coarse, slow, searching movements and pendular movements are seen in blind children (if vision was bad early in life). The slow component of nystagmus to the affected side is seen in vestibular lesions, whereas the quick component to the affected side is seen in cerebellar lesions. When the direction of fast component reverses from right gaze to left gaze, it is a cerebellar lesion.

A *Caloric Stimulation Test* to elicit nystagmus helps identify eighth nerve function. Before the test is done, exclude perforation of the ear drum and blocking of the external meatus with wax. Clean the canal if needed. Place the child in a semireclining position (30°) with pillows. Hold the child with assistance, since proper positioning of the semicircular canals is essential. Cold water is drawn into a 10-ml syringe with polyethylene tubing. The tubing is placed into the external meatus so that the water when injected will be directed at the tympanic membrane. Inject the water very slowly over a period of 30 seconds and observe the eyes carefully. Normally this should produce slow deviation of the eyes toward the side of injection with the rapid phase of nystagmus away from the side of injection. In other words, if the right vestibular tract is intact and if the right ear is being stimulated, the eyes will slowly deviate to the right with a sudden jump toward the left to bring the eye back to neutral. This response is repetitive, with the eyes again deviating to the right and jumping back to the left. This response is lost if the vestibular nerve is damaged and may be hard to elicit if there is brain stem damage.

Glossopharyngeal, Vagus, and Accessory Nerves (Ninth, Tenth, and Eleventh nerves)

The glossopharyngeal nerve carries sensory fibers for the posterior third of the tongue, and motor fibers for the stylopharyngeus and middle constrictors of the pharynx. The only clue to unilateral paralysis of the ninth nerve may be a slight flattening of the arch of the palate on the affected side at rest.

The vagus nerve is motor for the soft palate, pharynx, and larynx. Its parasympathetic portion supplies the respiratory, cardiovascular, and gastrointestinal systems.

The accessory nerve carries motor fibers only to the sternocleidomastoid and to the trapezius muscles.

The following findings suggest lesions of the ninth and tenth nerves:

1. Presence of stridor in the absence of mechanical obstruction is suggestive of denervation of the larynx and vocal cords (recurrent laryngeal nerve paralysis).
2. Hoarse voice suggests recurrent laryngeal nerve paralysis.
3. Aphonia.
4. Loss of swallowing reflex with drooling and choking.
5. Nasal regurgitation when swallowing liquids suggests palatal weakness.
6. Ineffective cough reflex.
7. Inability to pronounce words such as *egg* (which sounds as "eng") and words ending with a *k* sound.
8. Palatal reflex—in unilateral paralysis, palate may droop on the affected side and not move on phonation. Palatal reflex is tested by touching the soft palate with a tongue blade. This produces elevation of the soft palate and retraction of the uvula. (The sensory nerve is the ninth and the motor nerve is the tenth for this reflex.)
9. Gag reflex (afferent nerve is the ninth nerve and motor is the tenth nerve for this reflex). The stimulus is produced by touching the base of the tongue or the pharyngeal wall with a tongue blade. The normal response is elevation of the pharynx and tongue retraction.
10. Loss of sensation of taste in the posterior one third of the tongue.

The eleventh nerve supplies the sternocleidomastoid and the trapezius muscles. Ask the patient to shrug the shoulder against resistance (elevate shoulder). This tests the upper part of trapezius. To test the lower fibers of the trapezius, have the patient lie prone with the arms abducted 90° and rotated laterally. Ask the patient to adduct the scapula against resistance. The movement should take place between the scapula and the thorax. The sternomastoid is tested by asking the patient to rotate the head to one side when resistance is applied against this movement at the chin.

If one sees torticollis, which implies rotation of the chin to a direction opposite to that of direction of rotation of the occiput, one should also make sure that there is no head tilting or spasmodic involuntary movement of the head. Torticollis and head tilting are seen in athetoid cerebral palsy, hiatus hernia, rheumatoid arthritis with cervical spine involvement, enlarged cervical lymph nodes, retropharyngeal abscess, mastoid disease, vocal cord tumors, paralytic torticollis, and as compensation for visual field cuts and diplopia.

Hypoglossal Nerve (Twelfth nerve)

The twelfth nerve is a purely motor nerve supplying muscles of the tongue and depressor muscles attached to the hyoid bone.

Look at the normal position of the tongue at rest when the mouth is slightly open. If the tongue is in midline, ask the patient to put the tongue out. In the presence of unilateral paralysis, the tongue may be deviated toward the unaffected side. This may be difficult to interpret if there is facial weakness. Hold a pencil vertically from the midline of the nose and compare the position of the tongue in relation to this midline. Also ask the child to push against a tongue blade, first on one side and then on the other, to look for inequality in power. Finally, look for fasciculations (seen best on the under surface of the tongue) and for wasting.

After completion of examination of the cranial nerves, examine the rest of the central nervous system: motor system, sensory system, reflexes, and neurodevelopmental reflexes.

MOTOR SYSTEM

The five areas to be examined in evaluating the motor portion of the nervous system are:

- Strength
- Tone
- Coordination
- Involuntary movements
- Bulk (muscle mass)

Strength

There are two kinds of strength: *kinetic,* in which the muscle is used to move a joint through a range against resistance, and *static,* in which the muscle is used to keep a joint in one position against the pressure used by the examiner to move the joint in the opposite direction. The strengths are about equal, though in extrapyramidal conditions one may see loss of kinetic strength but retention of static strength.

Muscle testing can be a quick screening or an elaborate one, such as those done by experienced physical therapists. All pediatricians must be aware of some simple items that can be tested easily. In the case of young children, one may have to rely on the parents' history and simple observations such as unequal moro reflex, poor swinging of one arm while walking, too much wear of the front of the shoe, and resistance to examination.

Some of the simple tests for important large muscles are as follows:*

1. Anterior neck flexors: Ask the patient to lift the neck off the pillow from a lying down position.

*For detailed descriptions of testing of muscles, refer to Daniels L, Worthingham C: Muscle Testing Techniques of Manual Examination, 3rd ed. Philadelphia, Saunders, 1972.

2. Deltoid: Ask the patient to abduct the shoulders to 90°.
3. Elbow flexors (biceps and brachialis): Have the patient flex the elbow against resistance.
4. Hip flexors: Have the child lie supine with the knee flexed. The child is asked to flex the thigh against resistance.
5. Hip extensors: Ask the child to climb stairs; ask the child to stand up from a sitting position in a chair.
6. Quadriceps: Test the child's ability to extend the knee with the patient sitting at the edge of a table.
7. Hamstring: With the patient lying prone, test the ability to flex the knee.
8. Gastrocnemius: Ask the child to walk on tiptoes.

In certain situations, it may be hard to decide whether muscle weakness is true or due to malingering. The presence of spontaneous reflex movements such as contractions of the latissimus muscle during cough, offer a simple way for ruling out malingering. A test specifically applicable to differentiation between hemiplegia and hysterical paralysis is performed as follows. The patient is lying on the back and the palms of the examiner's hands are placed under the heels of the patient. Now, the patient is asked to lift one leg off the table and then the other. In the presence of true hemiplegia, when the patient lifts the paralyzed leg off the table, the examiner can feel the counterpressure of the nonparalyzed side on the examiner's palm kept under the heel. If a patient with hysterical paralysis is asked to lift the so-called paralyzed side, the examiner will not feel any counterpressure of the normal leg because the patient is making no effort to lift the leg. This is called Hoover sign.

One other clue is obtained when the patient is asked to contract a muscle and the examiner applies resistance to this movement. If the muscle is not truly paralyzed (malingering) when the resistance is withdrawn, there will be no movement. In true paralysis there will be follow-through movement.

Tone

Though there are many neurophysiologic discussions on the stretch reflex, a clinician is really testing resistance to passive movement when describing tone. The tone is either normal, poor-reduced (hypotonia), or increased (hypertonia, spasticity, rigidity).

The examiner puts the major joints through their full range and notes the range of motion possible and the resistance offered to this passive motion. (Of course one should exclude bone deformity or tendon contracture as the cause of the resistance, if resistance is present.)

Resistance to passive movement may be very little or none, allowing the limbs to be placed in various grotesque positions, as in various myopathies or myelomeningocele. This is called *hypotonia*. One should exclude hyperextensible joints as the cause of excessive movements of the joints. Hypotonia may be found in a primary muscle disorder in peripheral nerve lesions, in disease of anterior horn cells (polio), and in cerebellar lesions. Sudden and episodic hypotonia may signify akinetic seizure or syncope due to whatever cause.

Spasticity

Spasticity is characterized by increased tone of the muscles with exaggerated tendon reflexes. In spasticity, limitation of range of movement is only mild to moderate, and contracture is possible. Spasticity is marked by resistancc occurring as soon as the passive range is started, with intermittent, jerky yielding ("clasp-knife" type). *Rigidity* is characterized by resistance to passive stretching and normal tendon reflexes. There is marked limitation of range of movement but no persistent contracture. Rigidity is marked by uniform resistance throughout the range but allows a full or nearly full range (similar to the experience of bending a metallic flexible pipe and aptly called "lead-pipe" type).

In addition, one should note whether, in trying to move, children demonstrate any unusual patterns. In cerebral palsy and following brain injury the child may have some coarse voluntary movements, but these follow a set pattern. For example, when the child is asked to extend the great toe against resistance, the lower limb may adduct at the hip, and extend at the knee and at the ankle—this is an "extensor synergy" pattern. Similarly, when the child is asked to open the fingers, the shoulder adducts, the elbow flexes, and the wrist flexes and pronates. This is the "flexor synergy" pattern.

In cerebral palsy, one has to differentiate between the spastic type and the athetotic-extrapyramidal type (dyskinetic). Table 7F-6 summarizes Dr. Gillette's suggestions for differentiating between these two types of cerebral palsy.

Increased muscle tone (hypertonicity) may also be due to reflex spasm of muscles secondary to pain (for example, spasms of hip flexors in synovitis of the hip and in iliopsoas abscess, and spasm of cervical muscles in

TABLE 7F-6. DIFFERENCES BETWEEN SPASTIC AND DYSKINETIC TYPES OF CEREBRAL PALSY

Spasticity	Athetoid-Extrapyramidal (Dyskinetic)
Exaggerated stretch reflex; clonus	No clonus; more of continuous resistance to passive stretch
Tone greatest in arm flexors and leg extensors	Tone greatest in extensors throughout
Contractures common and appear early	Contractures occur later

(From Gillette H: Systems of Therapy in Cerebral Palsy. Springfield, Ill., Chas. C Thomas, 1974.)

meningeal irritation). Increased tone due to disease of the muscle itself must also be ruled out.

Coordination

A child steadying the upper arm against the chest while trying to carry out hand activity probably has unsteadiness of hands and lack of coordination. Other clues for poor coordination in children are: frequent falls, dropping objects, bumping into furniture, poor penmanship, and clumsiness. For proper coordination of muscle movement, the muscle must be strong, agonists and antagonists should act together, proprioceptive impulses from the muscles and joints should be received by the cerebellum and cortex, and body orientation should be intact. Obviously, lesions involving any of these areas will affect coordination.

Tests for Coordination.

1. *Finger-nose test:* The patient touches the nose with the finger, then touches the tip of the finger of the examiner held in space and then touches the nose again. *Intention tremor* appears when the patient is attempting the finger-nose test but subsides at rest. Presence of intention tremor may signify a cerebellar lesion. In addition, one may see *dysmetria* (inability to coordinate for distance) and *past pointing* (consistently missing the examiner's finger on the same side), both indications of cerebellar lesion. *In chorea, the coordination is normal,* but is periodically *interrupted* by the involuntary movements.
2. *Rapid alternating movement:* The patient is asked to repeatedly pronate and supinate the forearm by slapping the thigh with the palm and back of the hand alternately. The other method is to ask the child to repeatedly touch the tip of the index finger with the tip of the thumb as fast as possible. The same test is done on the foot by asking the child to repeatedly do tapping movements of the forefoot of the child against the examiner's palm held close to the foot. Inability to perform rapid alternate movement is called *dysdiadochokinesis* and is present in cerebellar lesions and in spasticity. Normally children above 5 years of age should be able to do these rapid alternate movements.
3. *Rebound test of Holmes:* The patient flexes the elbow against resistance by the examiner. Now the examiner suddenly withdraws the resistance. In the presence of problems in controlling and checking muscle contraction, the arm flexes uncontrollably and even may hit the face. Positive rebound test implies a cerebellar lesion.
4. *Maintenance of posture* is tested by asking the patient to extend the arms in front, with the fingers slightly separated to see if the patient

can maintain this posture. Tremor, chorea, and athetosis are recognized during this maneuver.

5. Other methods of testing for coordination include asking the child to run, to climb stairs fast, to ride a cycle, to tie the shoes, to write, and to draw a person.

Involuntary Movements

There are many types of abnormal movements that are involuntary.

1. *Tic:* Tics are purposeless but *repetitive* movements. They do not interfere with normal activities of a child and disappear during sleep. They get worse when others are watching. The areas usually affected are the eye muscles, facial muscles, and upper limb muscles.
2. *Fasciculation:* What is commonly referred to as "fibrillation" is actually "fasciculation." True fibrillation is an event occurring in the individual muscle fiber and cannot be seen clinically by the naked eye. The rapid twitching movements of bundles of fibers which leave a furrow on the skin over the muscle are fasciculation. It occurs in conditions associated with dysfunction of anterior horn cells; for example, poliomyelitis and Werdnig-Hoffmann disease. In the latter disease, the tongue is a good place to look for fasciculation.
3. *Chorea:* Chorea is purposeless but *nonrepetitive* movement. These are aggravated by activity and emotional stress. There is usually hypotonia and poor coordination in various activities such as eating and writing. The children may run into objects and hurt themselves.
4. *Myoclonus:* Intermittent contractions of a single muscle or groups of muscles resulting in quick jerky motion of a limb is myoclonus. It is made worse by voluntary activity and emotional stress. This usually occurs in association with lesions of the brain stem nuclei and reticular formation.
5. *Athetosis:* Slow, rhythmic movements of the extremities and the face are brought on by voluntary activity and emotional stimuli. The limbs take characteristic postures. The movements involve the distal muscles more than the proximal muscles.
6. *Dystonia:* This is characterized by fluctuations in tone and involvement of proximal muscles of the extremities resulting in strange postures and torsion spasms. If resistance is applied to a movement the spasm gets even worse. It disappears in sleep.
7. *Tremor:* These are rapid oscillatory movements present at rest or elicited by asking the child to extend his arms in front (see page 199, Chapter 7E).

Muscle Mass

Wasting and atrophy of muscles implies lower motor-neuron disease or disuse from whatever cause. Wasting is obvious in certain diseases, such as poliomyelitis, but it may be difficult to assess if it is only minimal.

One should observe for symmetry or asymmetry of wasting. Also note if it is proximal wasting only (myopathies) or wasting of distal muscles (peripheral neuritis). In conditions associated with wasting of muscles from early childhood, the affected limb may be smaller or shorter.

Hypertrophy may occur with excess use (such as in the upper arms of paraplegics who walk with crutches or adolescent boys and girls who perform weight lifting) or in diseases, such as myotonia congenita or congenital hemihypertrophy. Pseudohypertrophy is seen in Duchenne muscular dystrophy and is localized usually to the gastrocnemius.

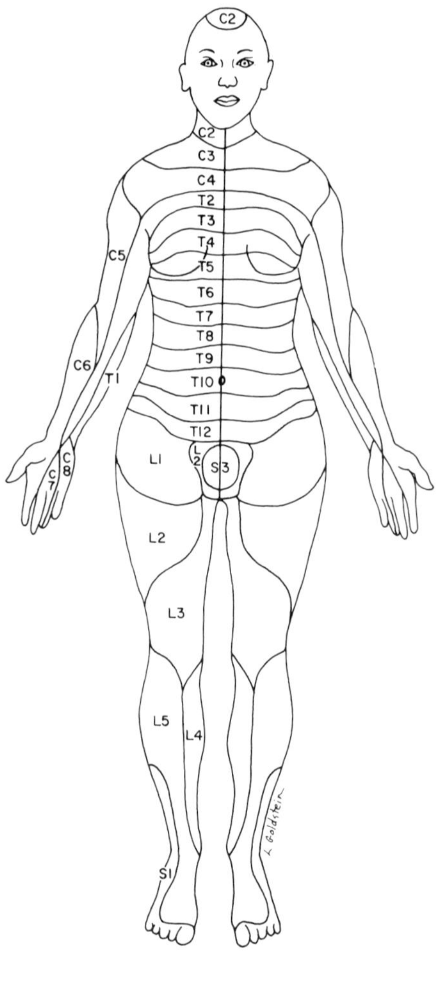

Figure 7F-6. Sensory innervation of the skin—anterior aspect.

SENSORY SYSTEM

The sensory system (Figs. 7F-6 and 7F-7) is very difficult to examine in children. Many children and infants obviously cannot cooperate and respond. They get frightened, distracted, and fatigued easily. Therefore, patience and ingeniuty are needed. Besides, even if the child cooperates he or she may be correct 50 percent of the time by chance. If the findings are essential, one may have to examine on more than one occasion to get reasonable cooperation from the child. On each occasion one may have to confine oneself to testing a single sensory modality.

The modalities to be tested may be classified under four headings:

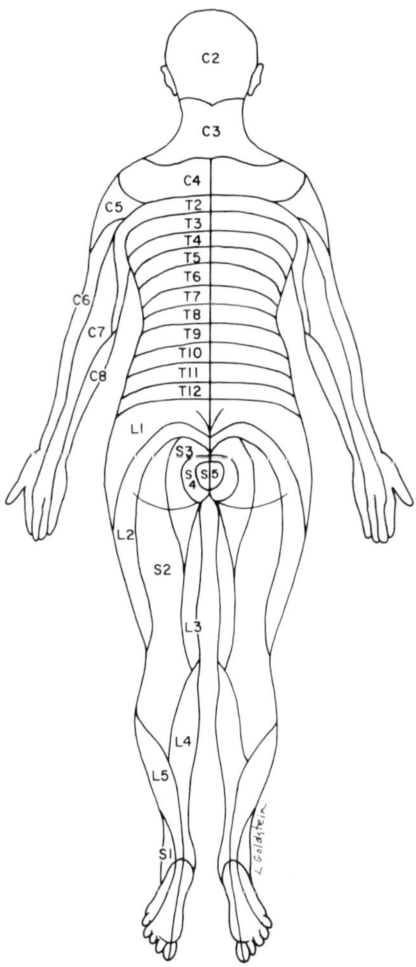

Figure 7F-7. Sensory innvervation of the skin—posterior aspect.

- Superficial Sensory: Touch
Pain
Temperature: cold, hot
- Deep Sensory: Pressure
Joint position
Vibration sense
- Cortical Sensory: (discriminatory) Stereognosis
Discrimination
Extinction
- Special Sensory: Smell
Taste
Hearing
Vision

Superficial Sensory

Equipment needed for testing is a cotton ball or soft tissue paper, a safety pin or ball head pin, and a metal tube for hot and cold water.

Method: Ideally, the child's eyes should be closed (another frightening experience for small children) as the examiner touches the skin gently, going from one area of the body to the other in an organized fashion. For example, go from the neck to the shoulder, outer aspect of the upper arm, outer aspect of the forearm, outer aspect of the palm, inner aspect of the palm, inner aspect of the forearm. First complete this on one side and then go to the opposite side. Such an organized approach will ensure covering all the areas (don't forget the perianal area supplied by S2–S4). Obviously this is time consuming and may have to be done at more than one examination. The child has to indicate whether he felt the touch by saying "now." During this procedure the examiner should not give any clues as to whether he is touching or not. In other words, he should not ask, "Do you feel?" every time he touches.

To test for pain, a similar approach is used with the stimulus being the tip of a pin. The child should be instructed to respond by saying "sharp" or "dull," not just saying "now" every time he feels the sensation. This is done to avoid having the child respond to the pressure aspect of the pin prick. If the child cannot respond verbally, his facial expression and withdrawal of the limb is used as an indication of intact pain sensation.

To test for temperature sensation, use two tubes, one filled with cold water and the other with hot water. The water should not be excessively hot or cold. The test should be done as described above. The skin is touched first with one tube, then the other, randomly alternating the sequence, and asking the child to respond by saying "hot" or "cold" depending on the stimulus. Again, the response should be spontaneous each time the child feels something touch the skin—not on questioning by the examiner.

Interpretation: Loss of sensation on one side of the body (hemianesthesia) is rare and may be seen following a head injury. The cutoff point exactly at the midline suggests hysteria, since in true hemianesthesia the cutoff point is just lateral to the midline. In spinal cord injury, the level of anesthesia has to be remembered in relation to the injured vertebrae since the number of the vertebra does not correspond to the spinal cord segment. The levels to be remembered are:

Vertebra	*Spinal Segment*
C1	C1
C7	C8
T10	T11
T12	L3
L1	End of cord

During the examination for cord injury, test for anesthesia, first going from above downward, then from below upward. If the point at which sensations are not felt is higher when you test from below upward than from above downward, incomplete cord lesion is indicated. In myelomeningocele, the level is never strictly defined. It is patchy and uneven between the halves of the body. Loss of sensation for pain and temperature with retention of sensation of touch and position sense and vibration sense in the upper limb is seen in syringomyelia. Hyperesthesia is seen in transverse myelitis, peripheral neuritis, reflex sympathetic dystrophy, herpes zoster, and in children with hemiplegia and hemianesthesia during the recovery phase of head injury.

Deep Sensory

Deep sensations originate from deeper structures, such as muscles, tendons, and joints. Vibration sense is usually included with these proprioceptive sensations. The impulses originate from muscle spindles and other endings in muscles and tendons. Some travel along the spinocerebellar tracts to the cerebellum. Others constitute the afferent arc of the stretch reflex and still others travel through posterior columns and the medial lemniscus to the thalamus and thence to the parietal lobe. Parts of these nerve fibers and connections are thus involved in other functions, such as tendon reflexes and sense of position. Tendon reflex tests the peripheral arc of this system. Sense of position tests the spinocerebellar tract, whereas the special tests of proprioception to be described in the following paragraphs test the entire system.

Deep sensory tests have to be explained adequately to children. The child should be old enough to understand and follow directions. Generally they are hard to do in children less than 3 years old.

To test for proprioception, the toes should be moved up and down passively by the examiner with the child's eyes closed and suddenly stopped in an up or down position. The child should be able to say whether the toe is up or down. Before the test is done the child should have a good explanation with the eyes open. Also, when testing up or down, the toes should be held on the lateral aspects, not held by the nail and the pulp, since the sense of touch may give clues. Finally remember children can say "up" and "down" and be correct 50 percent at each testing purely by statistical chance.

Other tests for proprioception are: (1) have the child touch the tips of corresponding fingers of both hands in space with eyes closed, and (2) arrange the finger of one hand in space in varying positions (eyes closed) and ask the child to put the finger of the opposite hand in the same position.

Vibration sense is tested by using a tuning fork of 128 vibrations per second. The fork is placed over various bony prominences, sometimes with vibrations and sometimes without, and the child is asked to say if he feels the vibrations or not.

Interpretation: Loss of proprioception and of vibration sense indicates posterior column lesions, such as in spinocerebellar ataxia. Loss of proprioception is seen also in parietal lobe lesions.

Cortical Sensory

Subjects for testing include:

- Stereognosis
- Two-point discrimination
- Texture
- Weight discrimination

Stereognosis is tested at the bedside by asking the child to close his eyes and placing in his hands common objects, such as a coin, a key, or blocks, (from the Denver kit), and asking him to name the object. For more precise testing, one has to use standard geometric shapes, such as cubes and spheres, and these methods are well described in texts listed in the references.

Discrimination of two points is tested by using a paper clip or hairpin. The patient must first understand with the eyes open what "one" and "two" mean. Now the test is done with the eyes closed. Touching the patient with one or two points should be done at random. Both points should touch simultaneously when testing is done for two points. The distance between the two points should be narrow in certain areas such as fingertips (2 mm) and wider (20 mm) in areas such as the forehead.

Textures can be tested using silk, wool, and plastic. The test for extinction is performed as follows: the child is asked to close the eyes and the examiner touches two parts of the body: both cheeks, both hands, one hand and one cheek, one hand and one foot—simultaneously and with equal pressure. The child is asked to name or point to the areas that were touched. When the cheek and the hand are touched, if the child recognizes that the cheek was touched but does not recognize the hand was touched, extinction of distal stimulus is to be suspected.

Interpretation: Loss of stereognosis and of two-point discrimination suggests parietal lobe syndromes. Extinction of distal stimulus (when face and hand are touched) is also seen in parietal lobe deficits.

REFLEXES

Reflexes can be grouped under four headings:

- Superficial
- Deep
- Developmental (infantile automatisms)
- Autonomic

Superficial Reflexes:

- Plantar
- Cremasteric
- Abdominal
- Anocutaneous
- Palmar

Plantar Reflex (Babinski). The reflex arc runs through the tibial nerve to the spinal cord (L4-S1).

How to elicit? The sole of the foot is stimulated by pressing along the plantar surface of the foot with a blunt instrument, such as the handle of the reflex hammer or a key, or the end of a ball-point pen. Start near the heel and carry the stimulus over to the base of the metatarsals, ending near the ball of the great toe.

Normal response: Plantar flexion of great toe is the normal response. Other toes also flex and adduct. In children, particularly the ticklish ones, the entire leg may be withdrawn.

Abnormal Response: Dorsiflexion of the great toe with fanning of other toes is an indication of a pyramidal lesion. In some cases, there may be dorsiflexion of the ankle and withdrawal of the entire extremity. In these cases, Babinski response may be elicited by stimulating other areas. In other words, the afferent area has enlarged. The following are some of the other stimuli which may elicit a Babinski response:

1. Method of Oppenheim: pressing firmly with thumb and stroking along the anterior border of the tibia.
2. Method of Gordon: Squeezing the calf.
3. Method of Gonda: Flexing and twisting any toe.
4. Method of Bing: Stroking the big toe along the lateral side.

Babinski is considered positive, if the great toe dorsiflexes with or without fanning of the other toes.

Cremasteric Reflex. A reflex tested, obviously, only in males by scratching the upper medial aspect of the thigh with a blunt instrument.

Normal Response: Contraction of the cremasteric muscle with elevation of the scrotum on the same side.

Abnormal Response. This reflex is lost in lesions above L-2.

Abdominal Reflex. This is elicited by stroking the four quadrants of the abdominal wall with a blunt instrument, such as a key or ball-point pen.

Normal response: Contraction of the abdominal wall at the stimulated quadrant, as shown by the movement of the umbilicus toward the quadrant stimulated.

Abnormal Response: Loss of abdominal reflex, which indicates pyramidal lesion above T-8.

Anocutaneous Reflex. Stimulation of the perianal skin by a pinprick.

Normal Response: Contraction of the external anal sphincter, with resultant indrawing of anal opening.

Abnormal Response: Loss of this reflex is seen in lesions involving S-2, S-3, and S-4.

Palmomental Reflex. This is elicited by scratching or tapping the thenar eminence of the hand.

Normal Response: No movements in the face.

Abnormal Response: Contraction of the mentalis and orbicularis oris muscles on the ipsilateral side. Abnormal response indicates bilateral frontal lobe lesion.

Hoffman's Sign. The patient's hand is held at the wrist, palm facing down and hanging loosely. The tip of the middle finger is grasped with the examiner's thumb and index finger. The nail of the middle finger is given a snap with the examiner's thumb.

Normal Response: No movement of the patient's thumb.

Abnormal Response: If the reflex is present, the thumb on the same side flexes and adducts into the palm. All the other fingers also flex. Presence of abnormal response indicates a pyramidal lesion above C-7.

Deep Reflexes

Biceps Reflex (C5,C6). To test for the biceps reflex, the patient's arm is held with the elbow in flexion and supported by one hand of the examiner. The thumb of the supporting hand is held over the insertion of the biceps tendon and the thumb is tapped with a reflex hammer. A normal response is flexion of the biceps, with or without flexion at the elbow.

Triceps (C6–C8). With the arm flexed 90° at the elbow, the forearm is supported by the examiner. A sharp tap over the triceps tendon causes contraction of the triceps, with or without elbow extension.

Brachioradialis (C5–C6). With the patient's arm between pronation and supination and the forearm supported by the examiner, the styloid of radius is tapped. Normal response is flexion of forearm and supination.

Knee Jerk (L2–L4). There are various positions in which to test knee jerks: (1) Patient may sit at the edge of the table with the knees hanging free and loose; (2) Patient lying supine, the knees are supported by the examiner's hand, relaxed and flexed to 30° or 40°; (3) In newborns, flexing the knee and placing the foot flat over the examiner's abdomen.

Tapping the patellar tendon with a reflex hammer produces visible contractions of the quadriceps. Response is extension at the knee. This reflex is sometimes hard to elicit. One may either divert the child's attention by talking about some subject of interest to the child. One may also augment this reflex by asking the child to hook the fingers and then to pull the fingers apart (Fig. 7F-8) (Jendrassik's maneuver) or by closing the eyes tightly.

Ankle Jerk (S1–S2). There are various positions to test the ankle jerk. The best position is for the patient to be prone with the knee flexed 90°. Now

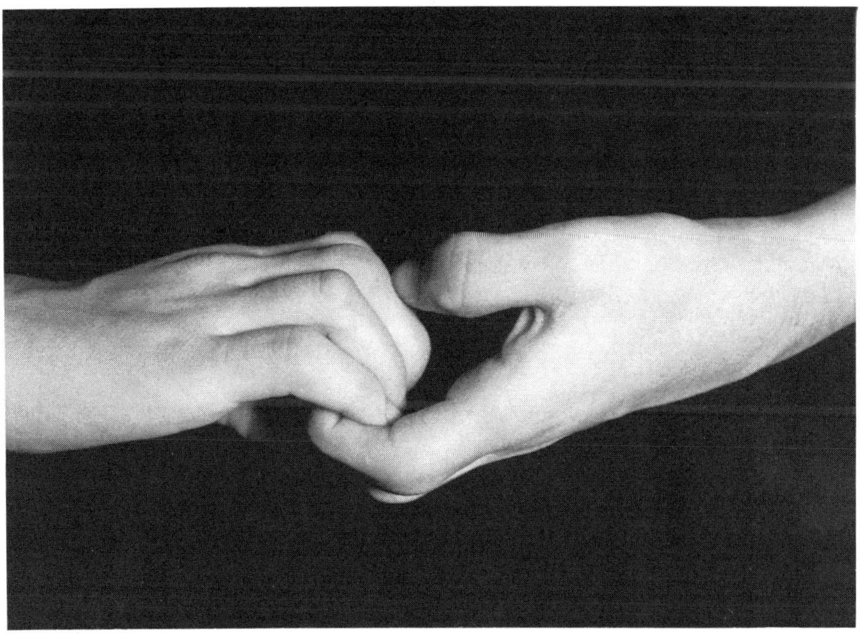

Figure 7F-8. Jendrassik's maneuver to augment knee jerk.

hold the toes down firmly and tap the tendoachilles (Fig. 7F-9). Another position is with the patient lying supine, hip flexed and externally rotated, and the knee flexed with the foot lying over the anterior aspect of the other leg (Fig. 7F-10). Now press firmly against the sole of the foot to dorsiflex the ankle and tap the tendoachilles.

Normal response is plantar flexion.

Interpretation of all tendon reflexes:

Exaggerated responses are seen with spasticity (pyramidal lesions).

Decreased deep tendon reflexes are seen in myopathies; and absent reflexes are more characteristic of peripheral nerve lesions.

Clonus. Clonus is characterized by rapid movements of a particular joint due to alternating contractions of agonists and antagonists. This is brought about, if present, by sudden stretching of a tendon (such as tendoachilles) and maintaining the stretch.

Ankle clonus is elicited as follows:

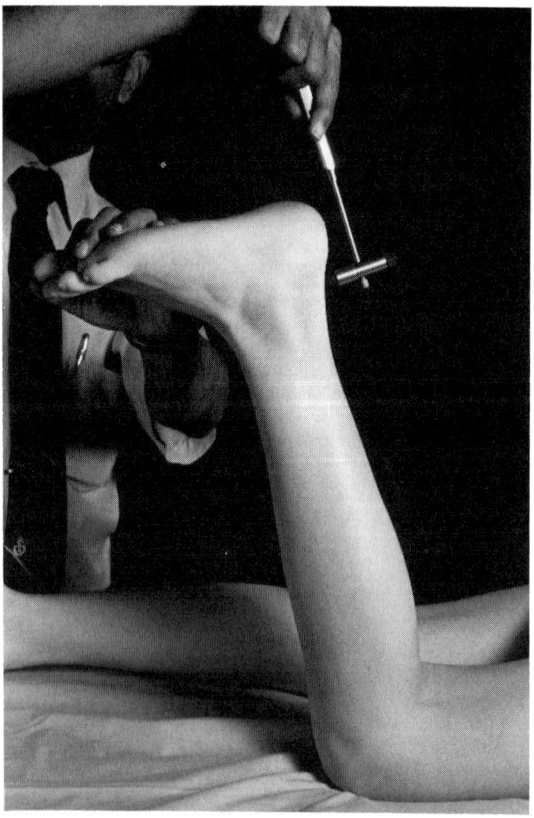

Figure 7F-9. Testing ankle jerk with patient in prone position and knee flexed.

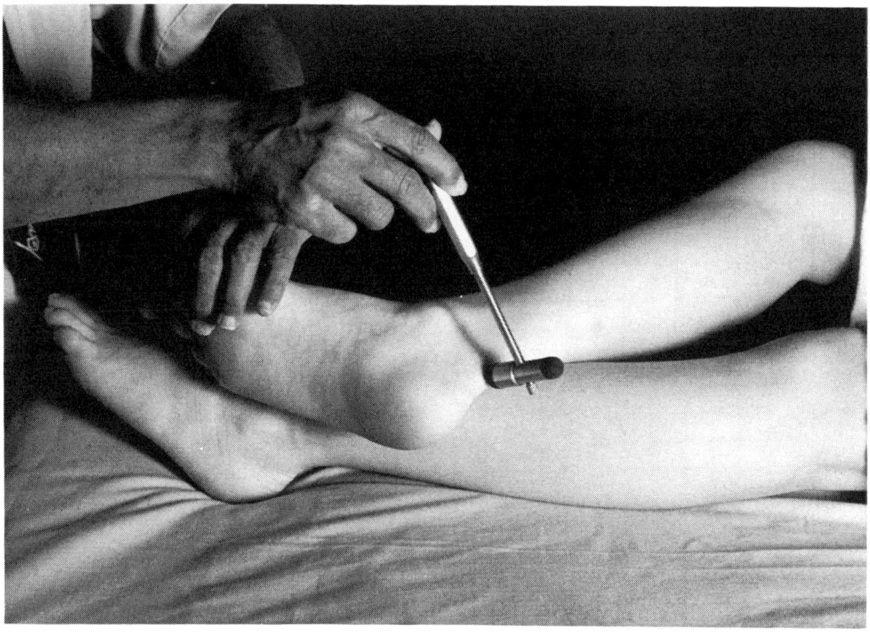

Figure 7F-10. Testing ankle jerk with patient in supine position and partial knee flexion.

With the patient in the supine position, the knee is flexed by the examiner. The forefoot is held by the other hand and dorsiflexed with a quick movement and the position maintained. If clonus is present, the foot will go through plantar flexion-dorsiflexion movements repeatedly. In certain children (cerebral palsy), such a clonus may be elicited just by the ball of the foot touching the floor, thus making it impossible for them to walk.

Patellar clonus is elicited using the following method: The patient is in the supine position with the knee in extension. The superior border of the patella is held by the examiner and quickly pushed toward the foot (caudal) and held. If clonus is present, the patella will move up and down repeatedly (caudal-cephalic movement).

The significance of clonus is the same as marked hyperreflexia, indicating impairment of higher control, and is seen in pyramidal lesions. Also, fewer than three or four beats of the ankle and knee may be elicited in any normal child, particularly if they are tense and hold their muscles tight.

Signs of Meningeal Irritation. With the patient supine and flat, if passive flexing of the neck causes the knees to flex and rise from the table, it is due to meningeal irritation (Brudzinski sign). Kernig sign has the same connotation and is also tested with the patient supine; the hips are flexed to about 90° and the knees then passively extended. The sign is positive if the *knees* cannot be fully extended.

NEURODEVELOPMENTAL REFLEXES

All children go through neurodevelopmental reflexes before they take the characteristic human form of bipedal walking. There are various kinds of body righting and balancing (automatic) reflexes which help to keep the balance while walking. Some of these reflexes are mediated at the spinal cord level, some at the brain stem level, some at the midbrain level, and some at the cortical level (Table 7F-7). They evolve from the caudal toward the cephalic level of control. (For more detailed descriptions see Fiorentino, 1979. Also, see Chapter 9, pages 299–302.)

Timing of Developmental Reflexes

In the natural course of development, *spinal cord reflexes* are present immediately after birth and disappear within 1 to 2 months. *Brain-stem reflexes* start appearing at about the 2nd week of life and should disappear by the 6th month.

In other words, spinal cord and brain stem reflexes are primitive reflexes and should disappear by 6 months of age. Persistence of these reflexes after this time indicates brain damage *in utero* or in early life. One may also find that these reflexes reappear in children who, after normal progression, had a cerebral insult such as a head injury or meningitis or anoxia (drowning). These children have obviously regressed. As long as spinal cord reflexes and brain stem reflexes are dominant, children cannot walk and cannot even crawl. (In essence they will be lying supine in various positions.)

TABLE 7F-7. DEVELOPMENTAL REFLEXES

	Reflex	Mediated at
Group A	Flexor withdrawal Extensor thrust Crossed extensor	Spinal cord level
Group B	Asymmetric tonic neck Symmetric tonic neck Positive supporting Tonic labyrinthine	Brain stem level
Group C	Neck correcting body Labyrinthine right reflex Optical righting reflex	Midbrain
Group D	Various balancing reflexes	Cortical/cerebellar
Group E	Automatic movement reactions Moro reflex	Stretch receptors of the neck
Group F	Parachute reflex Landau reflex	Semicircular canals

Most *midbrain reflexes* start appearing at about the 4th month but become suppressed by cortical influences after 2 years of age. Persistence of midbrain reflexes after 2½ years of age is abnormal. One sees these abnormalities in children with cerebral palsy and after cerebral insult. Children with dominant midbrain reflexes after 2½ years of age, can crawl easily but walking may be difficult without protective devices. Children who do not develop the midbrain reflexes may not be able to walk at all, except on all fours.

Absence of *cortical reflexes* beyond 2½ years is abnormal, though it is not incompatible with walking. These are balancing reflexes and contribute to safety in walking.

Spinal Cord Reflexes

Flexor Withdrawal. *How to elicit?* Pinch the sole of the foot (without tickling) with the child supine, head in neutral position, and *legs in extension.*

Response to look for? Dorsiflexion of the foot with uncontrolled flexion at the knee is positive response. The avoidance response of older normal children is considered a negative reaction.

What is normal? Flexion response described above till 2 months of age and avoidance response in older children.

What is abnormal? Persistence or reappearance of slow uncontrolled flexion response after 2 months of age.

Extensor Thrust. *How to elicit?* With the patient supine, stimulate sole of foot of *flexed leg* by pinching the sole.

Response to look for? A nondeliberate extension with adduction is considered a positive reaction.

What is normal? The above response is normal up to 2 months of age.

What is abnormal? The above response persisting or recurring after 2 months of age.

Crossed Extensor. *How to elicit?* With the patient supine and both lower limbs in extension, stroke the plantar aspect of the foot.

Response to look for? Flexion followed by extension and adduction of the opposite lower limb.

What is normal? The above described response is normal till 2 months of age.

What is abnormal? Persistence of the above described response after 2 months of age.

Brain Stem Reflexes

Asymmetric Tonic Neck Reflex. *How to elicit?* With the child in the supine position and arms and legs extended turn the head to one side.

Response to look for? Extension and stiffening of arms and legs on the side toward which the face is turned, together with flexion of the arms and legs of the opposite side (occiput side), is considered a positive response (Fig. 7F-11).

What is normal? This reflex is seen normally up to 4 to 6 months of age.

What is abnormal? Persistence of this reflex after 6 months of age.

Symmetric Tonic Neck Reflex. *How to elicit?* Support the child prone on the thighs of the examiner who is seated on a chair. Passively flex the neck; after observing the response of the arms and legs to passive flexion, extend the neck.

Response to look for? When the neck is flexed, arms flex and legs extend. When the neck is extended, arms extend and legs flex.

What is normal? Positive response as described above is normal until 4 to 6 months of age.

What is abnormal? Response as described after 6 months of age.

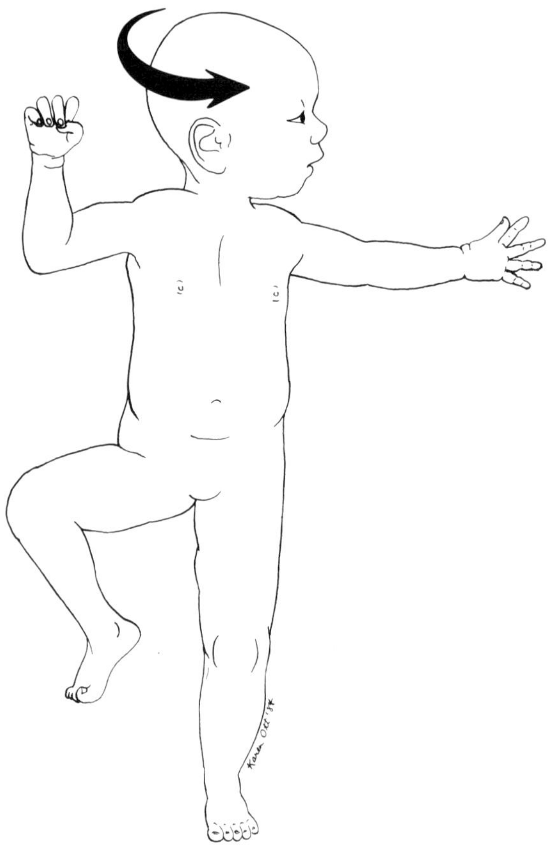

Figure 7F-11. Asymmetric tonic neck reflex ("fencing posture").

Positive Supporting Reaction. *How to elicit?* Pick up the child by the axilla and bounce several times so that the feet touch the floor.

Response to look for? When the feet are in contact with the floor, hold the child in a vertical position. Look for increase of adductor and extensor tone in the legs and ability of the child to bear weight. Look for sustained position in plantar flexion *with adduction.*

What is normal? Positive supporting reaction to bear weight is present at birth and disappears by 2 or 3 months.

What is abnormal? Sustained plantar flexion with increased tone of adductors after 4 months of age. Positive supportive reaction reappears at 6 months of age in preparation for walking but not with significant adduction or plantar flexion.

Tonic Labyrinthine Reflex. *How to elicit?* Examine the tone of flexors and extensors of arms and legs with the child in prone and supine position and the head in midline.

Response to look for? Flexor tone dominates when the patient is prone and extensor tone dominates when the patient is supine.

What is normal? Response as described above till 4 months of age.

What is abnormal: Response as described above after 4 months of age.

Midbrain Reflexes

Neck on Body Correcting Reflex. *How to elicit?* With the patient lying supine, turn the head toward one side.

Response to look for? Positive neck righting reaction is rotation of the body non-segmentally in the same direction.

What is normal? This non-segmental reflex is present at birth and disappears by 2 months of age. The mature segmental rotation of the thorax followed by the pelvis appears after 2 months.

What is abnormal? Presence of non-segmental response after 6 months or the absence of segmental response after 6 months of age.

Labyrinthine Righting Reflexes. *How to elicit?* With the child blindfolded, support the child in space in a prone position. Repeat the same test by suspending the child in space in a supine position. Next, hold the child by the pelvis in the vertical position and tilt the body to one side and then the other.

Response to look for? Positive responses for the four positions are as follows: With the child prone or supine, the head rises to normal position with the face vertical and the mouth horizontal. With the child in vertical position, the head tilts back to neutral position with the face vertical and the mouth horizontal.

What is normal? Positive response to prone position is normal after 2 months of age throughout life. Positive responses to other positions come on normally at about 6 to 9 months of age. They are suppressed by cortical influences after 2½ years of age.

What is abnormal? Absence of the positive response after 2 months in prone position and absence of the response to other positions between 6 months and 2½ years of age are abnormal.

Optical Righting Reflex. The test is performed the same way as described for the labyrinthine righting reflex and is interpreted the same way, but the labyrinthine righting reflex is tested with the eyes *closed* and the optical righting reflex with the eyes *open.*

Cerebral Cortical and Cerebellar Reflexes

These reflexes test the balancing ability of the child and are influenced by the cerebral cortex and cerebellum.

How to elicit? With the child sitting or standing, first push the child to one side (taking care the child does not fall to the opposite side in case these reflexes are not developed); then, to the other side.

Response to look for? If the child is sitting, the arm on the side toward which he is falling extends, fingers open, and the neck corrects so that the head is brought to neutral position. If the child is standing, the same response is seen. In addition, the knee on the side toward which the child is falling flexes, the opposite knee extends and tries to cross over toward the direction of the momentum.

Now, with the child standing and held by the axilla, gently push the child forward and then backward. If the child is pushed forward, the neck extends to bring the head to neutral and the child takes forward steps to catch up with gravity; if the child is pushed back, the neck flexes and the child takes backward steps.

What is normal? Positive responses as described above for balance in sitting position should appear by 6 to 8 months of age. Reflexes for balance in standing position should appear by 12 to 15 months of age.

What is abnormal? Absence of balancing reflexes for sitting after 8 months of age and absence of balancing reflexes for standing after 15 months of age are abnormal; asymmetric responses are also abnormal.

Automatic Movement Reactions

Moro Reflex. *How to elicit?* Produce a sudden noise away from the visual field of the infant. Another method is to support the child in the semisitting position and suddenly drop the upper part of the body. The upper part of the body is caught by the examiner's hand before hitting the table (without of course hurting or dropping the child hard on to the examining table).

Response to look for? Sudden extension and abduction at the shoulders quickly followed by flexion at the shoulder and the elbow in a movement like an embrace. The fingers open during this reflex.

What is normal? Presence of this response is normal in newborns and infants up to 4 months of age.

What is abnormal? Persistence of this response after 4 months of age.

Parachute Response. *How to elicit?* Hold the child by the waist and tilt the child forward as if to be dropped on the face.

Response to look for? Extension and abduction of the upper limbs with extension of the fingers as if to break a fall.

What is normal? This response should be present in most normal infants after 6 to 8 months of age.

What is abnormal? The absence of this response after 8 months is abnormal; unilateral response is abnormal.

Landau Reflex. *How to elicit?* Suspend the child in space (carefully) in a prone position by supporting the thorax.

Response to look for? Neck spontaneously extends with some stiffening of the back and lower extremities.

What is normal? Presence of this reflex between the age of 6 months and 2½ years.

What is abnormal? Failure of this reflex to develop by 10 to 12 months is abnormal.

Significance and Uses of the Neurodevelopmental Reflexes in Pediatric Practice

1. Abnormal responses in these categories suggest brain damage (e.g., cerebral palsy, post-head injury, and post-meningitis).
2. Persistence of reflexes mediated by the brain stem and spinal cord after 4 to 6 months of age signifies brain damage.
3. Delay in the appearance of reflexes mediated at the midbrain and cortical level after the appropriate age signifies brain damage.
4. Asymmetric responses (such as lack of parachute response on one side and unilateral Moro) signify hemiplegia.
5. These reflexes may mature at a slower pace in children with cerebral palsy (e.g., Landau reflex may not appear until age 2).
6. Older children with head injury and infectious brain insult lose their advanced reflexes and regress to spinal cord and brain stem level soon after the cerebral insult. They then redevelop through the various stages during the recovery period.
7. These reflexes are useful as indicators of prognosis in walking for children with cerebral palsy. For example, strong asymmetric tonic reflex, crossed-extensor reflex and Moro together with absence of parachute response give poor prognosis for walking.

8. These reflexes can be useful in physical therapy. For example, rolling an infant over a large beach ball will elicit a parachute response, if present. This will help open a spastic adducted thumb, since opening of the palm and extension of fingers is part of this response. The child with severe persistent tonic labyrinthine reflex may get equinus deformity if he is allowed to remain in the supine position most of the day, because extensor tone is increased in a supine position in the presence of active tonic labyrinthine reflex. If this child is treated in a prone position most of the day, flexor tone is accentuated as part of the same reflex.

ASSOCIATED MOVEMENTS

A normal child has freely swinging arms during walking. In the presence of pyramidal or extrapyramidal disease, this movement is lost. A paralyzed upper arm also does not move and swing normally during walking.

The other major associated movement is the mirror movement that occurs when the child attempts rapid, repetitive activity with one hand or foot. This may elicit a spontaneous movement of the corresponding part of the opposite limb until 5 to 6 years of age. After this age, mirror movements indicate cerebral disease, such as cerebral palsy.

AUTONOMIC REFLEXES

The two areas of importance, other than the vital signs, are skin and sphincters.

The two most important points to observe in the *skin* are: (1) vasomotor instability and color changes associated with severe pain, as in reflex sympathetic dystrophy, and (2) lack of sweating, as in Horner syndrome.

Anal sphincter is first observed to see whether the opening is normal and contracted or patulous. A rectal examination will tell us about sphincter tone. Anocutaneous reflex is tested by pricking the perianal skin by a pin: normal response is a brisk contraction of the external sphincter.

Since the *bladder* cannot be adequately examined clinically one relies on the history. History of dribbling, lack of awareness of full bladder, lack of desire to void, and inability to hold urine should make one suspicious of neurogenic bladder.

In the presence of bowel and bladder sphincter problems, the motor and sensory systems should be examined carefully to rule out lesions of the spinal cord (such as myelomeningocele or lipomeningocele).

BIBLIOGRAPHY

Baird HW, Gordon EC, Oppe TE: Neurological Evaluation of Infants and Children. In Clinics in Developmental Medicine. London, Heinemann Med Bks, 1983, Vol 84/85.

Capute AJ, Accardo PJ: Linguistic and auditory milestones during the first two years of life: A language inventory for the practitioner. Clin Pediatr 17:847–853, 1978.

Chusid JG: Correlative Neuroanatomy and Functional Neurology, 17th ed. Los Angeles, Lange Medical Publications, 1979.

Fiorentino MR: Reflex Testing Methods for Evaluating CNS Development, 2nd ed. Springfield, Ill., Chas. C Thomas, 1979.

Plum F, Posner JB: The Diagnosis of Stupor and Coma, 3rd ed. Philadelphia, F. A. Davis Co., 1980.

Teasdale G, Jennett B: Assessment of coma and impaired consciousness. Lancet 2:81–84, 1974.

SECTION IV

Specialized Examinations

CHAPTER 8

Developmental and Behavioral Assessment

The burgeoning field of developmental and behavioral evaluation is not strictly within the scope of this book. The complexities and the often contradictory findings of workers in developmental pediatrics are detailed comprehensively in Levine et al., 1983. Nevertheless an informal or formal developmental assessment must be a part of all pediatric examinations. In this brief chapter, therefore, we will describe evaluations that can be performed readily in the pediatric office as part of the well-child examination and on those children referred with the following problems: (1) developmental delay or distortion; (2) behavioral problems; (3) speech and language problems; and (4) handicapping conditions.

Developmental examinations differ in two major respects from system examinations: (1) they involve assessment of functions rather than of a disease process; (2) the physician needs the help of other professionals to complete the evaluation.

DENVER DEVELOPMENTAL SCREENING TEST (See Fig. 8-1)

Many of the tests of child development in use today are derived from Gesell's work. The most popular of these is the Denver Developmental Screening Test (DDST). This is not a diagnostic test and not an intelligence test. DDST is a screening test which a pediatrician or a trained nonphysician can use to assess whether an individual child is in the normal range for developmental milestones. If the DDST leads to doubts as to whether the child is developing appropriately, detailed testing has to be performed by someone trained in administering and interpreting the proper tests.

Since it requires about 20 minutes to administer DDST, two other tools have been introduced. One is a questionnaire (Denver Prescreening Developmental Questionnaire) and the other is a shortened version of DDST. It is recommended that all children get a screening with one of these two tools at the following ages: 3 to 6 months, 9 to 12 months, 18 to 26 months, and at 3, 4, and 5 years of age. Those who show abnormalities in either of these prescreening procedures should be screened utilizing the standard DDST.

"The DDST, which was standardized on a cross-sectional sample of Denver children, can be accurately applied to all racial groups. It provides not only a valid, concrete method for measuring a child's performance against a standardization sample, but also a one-page profile of the child's progress during the preschool years.

On the DDST form, there are 105 tasks that most children perform before the age of 6 years. These tasks were selected from existing infant and preschool scales on the basis of their validity, ease of administration, and clarity of scoring. For example, one task on the form is "walks well." This task, like all others on the test, represents skills that are acquired by different children at different ages. One child might begin walking at 10 months; another perfectly normal child may not walk until 14 months. This range could be represented on a cumulative frequency curve.

Because this type of graph would be cumbersome on a test form, the information on the graph was condensed into a bar. This bar graph is placed on the DDST form in relation to the age lines at the top and bottom of the form. The left end of the bar corresponds to the age when 25 percent of the children normally perform this item. The hatchmark indicates when 50 percent perform the task; the left end of the colored shading marks when 75 percent perform it; and the right end of the bar indicates when 90 percent of the children normally perform the task.

On the DDST (see Fig. 8-1), the tasks are arranged in developmental sequence. For example, the majority of children perform the task "walks backwards" at a later age than "walks well." Therefore, the bar is placed on the age line slightly to the right of the "walks well" tasks, as can be seen in the gross motor sector.

The 105 tasks on the DDST are arranged under four major headings. Those tasks measuring self-help skills and ability to get along with people are in the personal-social section. The second section, fine motor-adaptive, measures the child's ability to perceive, use his or her hands, pick up objects, and draw. Those tasks which measure language—the child's ability to respond to sound, follow instructions, and speak—are presented in the language section. And finally, tasks relating to locomotion and body posture are presented in the gross-motor section.

In administering the DDST, it is not necessary to ask the child to perform all of the test items. Instead, a vertical line is drawn on the form at the exact age of the child (calculated according to instructions in the reference manual). This line, cutting through all four sections of the test, helps determine which tasks the child should be asked to perform. It is usually only necessary to administer about 25 or 30 items for each child.

DIRECTIONS

This Denver Developmental Reference Chart has been developed as a parent counseling aid to parallel a smaller version of the Denver Developmental Screening Test, which helps to determine whether or not a given child's developmental status falls within established norms. Health professionals need to administer and interpret each item on the Screening Test according to standardized procedures and then plot the development of each child in their practice on a separate form. They then may use this Reference Chart, which has been designed in size and format for this purpose, as an office aid to discuss a child's development with the parents.

1. Try to get child to smile by smiling, talking or waving to him or her. Do not touch him or her.
2. When child is playing with toy, gently pull it away from him or her. Pass if he or she resists.
3. Child does not have to be able to tie shoes or button in the back.
4. Move yarn slowly in an arc from one side to the other, about 6″ above child's face. Pass if eyes follow 90° to midline. (Past midline; 180°)
5. Pass if child grasps rattle when it is touched to the backs or tips of fingers.
6. Pass if child continues to look where yarn disappeared or tries to see where it went. Yarn should be dropped quickly from sight from tester's hand without arm movement.
7. Pass if child picks up raisin with any part of thumb and a finger.
8. Pass if child picks up raisin with the ends of thumb and index finger using an overhand approach.
9. , 10., 11., 12. (See directions on face of chart. When giving items 9., 11., and 12., do not name the forms. Do not demonstrate 9. and 11.)
13. When scoring, each pair (2 arms, 2 legs, etc.) counts as one part.
14. (See directions on face of chart.)
15. Tell child to: Give block to Mommie; put block on table; put block on floor. Pass 2 of 3. (Do not help child by pointing, moving head or eyes.)
16. Ask child: What do you do when you are cold? . . . hungry? . . . tired? Pass 2 of 3.
17. Tell child to: Put block *on* table; *under* table; *in front of* chair; *behind* chair. Pass 3 of 4. (Do not help child by pointing, moving head or eyes.)
18. Ask child: If fire is hot, ice is ____? Mother is a woman, Dad is a ____(man)? A horse is big, a mouse is ____? Pass 2 of 3.
19. Ask child: What is a ball? . . . lake? . . . desk? . . . house? . . . banana? . . . curtain? . . . ceiling? . . . hedge? . . . pavement? Pass if defined in terms of use, shape, what it is made of, or general category (such as banana is fruit, not just yellow). Pass 6 of 9.
20. Ask child: What is a spoon made of? . . . a shoe made of? . . . a door made of? . . . (No other objects may be substituted.) Pass 3 of 3.
21. When placed on stomach, child lifts chest off table with support of forearms and/or hands.
22. When child is on back, grasp his or her hands and gently pull him or her to sitting. Pass if head does not hang back.
23. Child may use wall or rail only, not person. May not crawl.
24. Child must throw ball overhand 3 feet to within arm's reach of tester.
25. Child must perform standing broad jump over width of test sheet (8½ inches).
26. Tell child to walk forward, heel within 1 inch of toe. Tester may demonstrate. Child must walk 4 consecutive steps, 2 out of 3 trials.
27. Bounce ball to child who should stand 3 feet away from tester. Child must catch ball with hands, not arms, 2 out of 3 trials.
28. Tell child to walk backward, toe within 1 inch of heel. Tester may demonstrate. Child must walk 4 consecutive steps, 2 out of 3 trials.

Figure 8-1. Denver Developmental Screening Test (revised).

DENVER DEVELOPMENTAL REFERENCE CHART

Ross Growth & Development Program

Based on developmental data provided by
William K. Frankenburg, MD,
John F. Kennedy Child Development Center,
University of Colorado Health Sciences Center, Denver

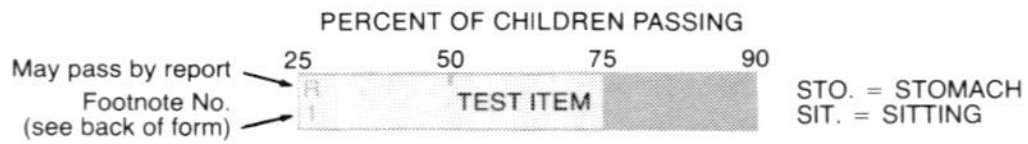

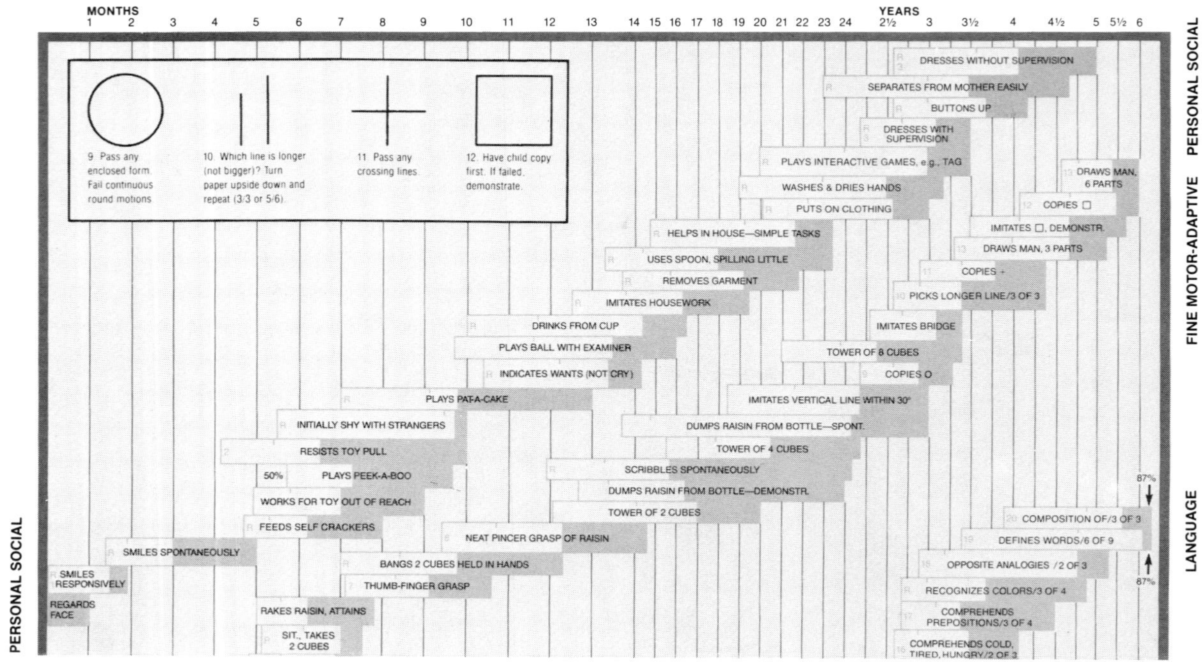

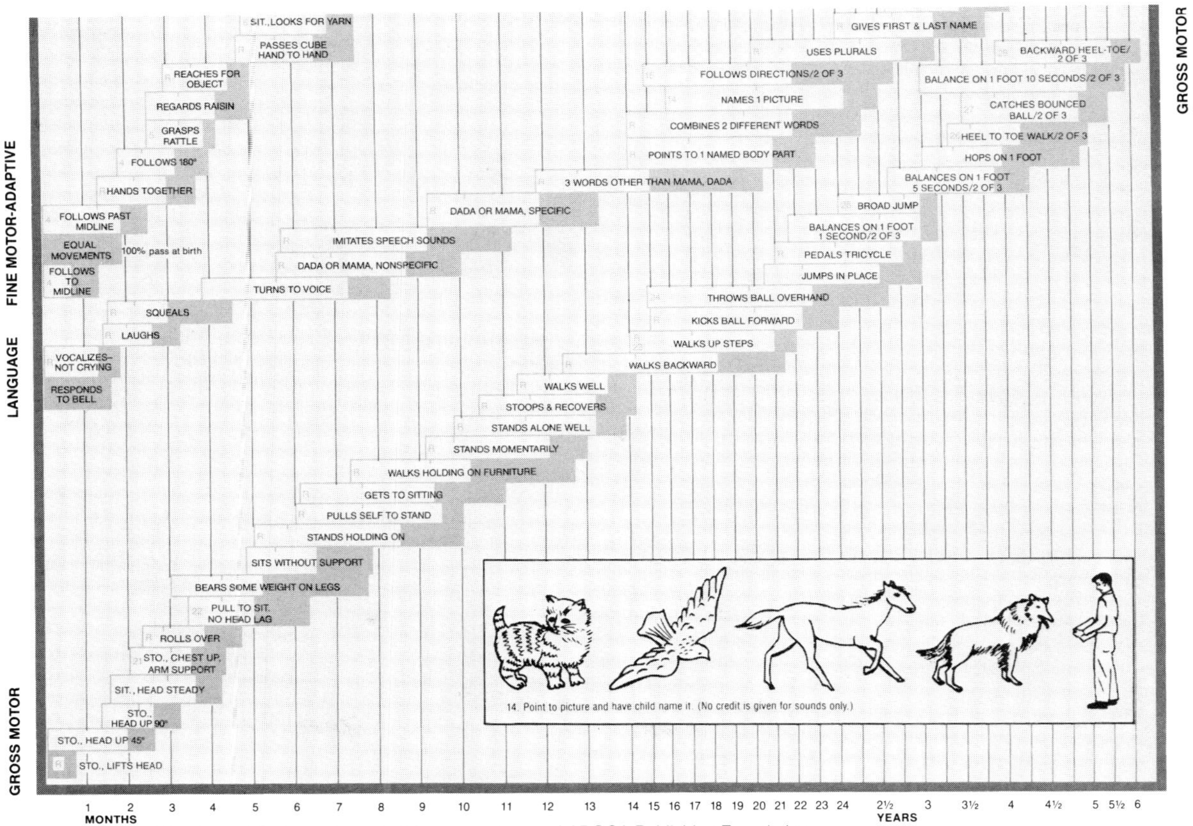

The Denver Developmental Screening Test (DDST) Reference Manual, test kits, and instructional films, as well as 8½″ x 11″ revised DDST forms for individual patient use, may be ordered from a sheltered workshop for mentally retarded persons:

LADOCA Publishing Foundation
East 51st Avenue at Lincoln Street
Denver, Colorado 80216
(303) 629-6379

In administering the test, the examiner seeks to determine whether the child can perform tasks that a normal child of that age can perform. Responses must be interpreted in strict accordance with guidelines given in the reference manual so that the child's performance can be correctly evaluated and compared with that of the standardization sample.

Some items are passed by observing the child perform the tasks. Others, such as whether or not the child can dress himself or herself, may be scored upon the report of the parent. As the child passes or fails an item, a "P" or "F" is placed on the bar.

After each item has been scored, the next step is to identify delays. Inability to perform any item that falls completely to the left of the age line should be considered a delay. In other words, 90 percent of normal children can pass that item at a younger age than the age of the child being tested. Failure to perform an item that touches the vertical age line is not considered to be a delay.

The number of delays and their location within the sectors are important in determining a total test result of normal, abnormal, questionable, or untestable. A formula given in the reference manual is used to determine the child's overall score. Abnormal, questionable, or untestable scores are considered to be positive test results. Approximately 10 percent of the children between birth and 6 years of age will receive positive test results. Determining why the result is positive and what should be done about it are two of the major responsibilities of the physician and other professionals serving the child.

In order to use the DDST properly, a potential examiner should study the test manual, view the demonstration film, and complete the proficiency evaluation. Without carefully studying these training materials, professionals and paraprofessionals alike will not be able to administer a valid test. If the items are not administered and interpreted in the standardized manner, the test may only represent a subjective interpretation by an individual examiner."*

HIGHER CORTICAL FUNCTIONS

Higher cortical functions include: (1) integrative functions (e.g., visual-motor); (2) speech and language; (3) intelligence; and (4) behavior. Failure of development of these functions at the appropriate time or loss of these functions may be due to organic brain damage. This damage may be the result of genetic or acquired reasons, but these functions are affected also by environmental and socioeconomic factors. Proper assessment of these functions and interpretation of the test results are therefore, very difficult,

*Information on DDST reproduced with kind permission of the author and the publisher from WK Frankenburg (ed): Pediatric Developmental Diagnosis. Thieme Stratton, N.Y., 1981, pp. 18–19.

and the pediatrician can properly interpret only a few simple screening tests.

Integrative Functions

The brain has to receive information through various sensory channels before responses can be initiated. Once the stimulus is received, the brain has to process the information. This includes identifying, distinguishing, and selecting the appropriate signal from a mass of information received, followed by suppression of irrelevant stimuli. After this processing of the stimuli, the brain has to integrate the stimulus received through one sensory system with stimuli received through other sensory systems and finally integrate the sensory system with the motor system to respond through one of the modalities (vocalization or movements). Integration is only one of the central processes.

Integration may be between one sensory system and another (auditory-visual, visual-tactile) or between one sensory system and one expressive or motor system (auditory-vocal, auditory-motor, visual-motor, visual-vocal, tactile-vocal, tactile-motor). These links develop mostly during the second half of the first year of life. Visual-motor integration is the most important of these and some of the well-known tests such as those of Frostig, Berry, and Bender are used to evaluate visual-motor integrative functions.

Though Bender's visual-motor Gestalt test is well known and has been widely used for many years, other better-standardized instruments are available now. Berry's test for visual-motor integration is a relatively simple test to administer and score. Familiar figures such as vertical stroke, horizontal stroke, square, circle, and triangle are used in this test, and the child is asked to duplicate them. This test is *not* a diagnostic tool but is a measure of visual-motor integration designed for educational assessment of children between 2 and 5 years of age. Poor performance in this test may be due to difficulty in visual perception, motor coordination, intellectual capacity, or motivation, and therefore should be followed by further testing in these specific areas.

Another test that is included in this area is Goodonough's Draw-a-Man Test. Though ability to draw (manipulation, fine motor skill) is the prime requisite to complete this test, many other areas of child development are also tested simultaneously. They are: perceptual awareness, visual-motor coordination, awareness of body parts, and concepts of self-image. The child is asked to draw a person on a sheet of paper, and the drawing is scored to arrive at an approximate mental age for the child.

Speech and Language

The earliest relationship of an infant with the mother is based on nonverbal communication. The child soon learns to communicate with cooing, gurgling, smiling, and crying. Later, a child may be able to use nonverbal self-expression, such as facial expressions. Speech as an expression of needs usually starts in the second year of life but language as a vehicle of thought comes considerably later.

For language development to progress, the child must be able to hear and, before speaking, must have verbal recognition and considerable comprehension. The central processing includes sensory integration (stimuli received through the ears, eyes, and skin), concept formation, symbolization (inner language), and sensory-motor links. This is a complicated process, and it is not possible for most pediatricians to test these areas without the help of specialists.

There is no simple screening test for assessment of language development. The pediatrician, however, can do simple tests in his or her office. The room has to be quiet (a difficult task to accomplish in a pediatrician's office). The pediatrician should speak softly and look for the child's response. He or she should ask the child to point out two or three familiar objects. (This tests the child's ability to hear, understand, and carry out an instruction.) Next, the physician can give some commands, starting with simple single items and proceeding to commands involving two or three steps. During the process of examination and when the child is playing, listen to the speech, the clarity of the speech, the word context and sentence structure. Finally, the child may be shown some pictures and asked to tell a story based on the picture. Table 7F-2 on page 214 summarizes the normal stages of development of speech.

The Peabody pictorial vocabulary test (for receptive language) and the Slossan oral reading test (reading readiness) also can be administered by pediatricians in office practice. More detailed language tests have to be administered by psychologists or speech therapists trained in administering and interpreting them. These include: (1) auditory discrimination test (Wepman); (2) test for verbal conprehension-receptive language (Reynell Developmental Language Scale); (3) test for central language processing (Illinois Test of Psycholinguistic Abilities); (4) test for expressive language (Reynell Developmental Language Scales); and (5) tests for articulation (Renfrew Articulation Test).

Intelligence Testing

Aristotle classified mental characteristics into intellectual (discriminative) and cognitive (directive) components. In a general sense, intelligence is an abstract quality of the mind and is common to all mental processes such as perception, memory, and reasoning. In human psychology, intelligence means the capacity to perceive and handle relationships, and the various intelligence tests are based on this definition of intelligence.

Psychologists attempt to measure intelligence by measuring a child's performance on a standardized test and comparing it with norms established with children of the same chronologic age for that particular test. The value obtained is expressed as the standard deviation (SD) from the

TABLE 8-1. CLASSIFICATION OF MENTAL RETARDATION

	Standard Deviation	Wechsler Score	Binet Score
Mildly retarded	3 SD below the mean	69–55	67–52
Moderately retarded	4 SD below the mean	54–40	51–36
Severely retarded	5 SD below the mean	39–25	35–20
Profoundly retarded	6 SD below the mean	below 25	below 20

(Based on the classification suggested by the American Association for Mental Deficiency.)

mean (which is arbitrarily set at 100). This is reported as intellectual quotient (IQ), though in reality the value represented is the mean developmental index or age for that child for that test. Based on this number, various levels of intelligence can be classified (Table 8-1). The reader is referred to other texts for details of the various tests of intellectual functions.

Behavior

Interpretation of behavior to the parents and anticipatory guidance are important functions of the pediatrician. Assessment of behavior requires an understanding of normal and abnormal behavior. Behavior is the response of an individual to internal and external stimuli.

There are no special techniques for assessing child behavior. It is essential to know the stages of normal emotional development, to know the basic personality traits of children, to take a detailed history, and to observe the children in various settings before one can interpret abnormal behavior. Some of the common problems that have behavioral-developmental components are listed in Table 8-2. These problems are listed according to the age groups in which they are seen most often.

The *severity* of a particular behavior problem or deviation depends on its *intensity, duration,* and *pervasiveness.* These characteristics help determine when the child should be referred to a psychiatrist.

MINOR NEUROLOGIC SIGNS

There are a number of children with a history of clumsiness, "hyperactivity," behavior problems, and true learning disabilities who have normal findings on classical neurologic examination but present "soft" neurologic signs suggestive of neurologic maturational deficit. These children have been variously classified as "minimal cerebral dysfunction," "hyperactive children," "children with learning disabilities," and "attention deficit disor-

TABLE 8-2. COMMON PROBLEMS WITH BEHAVIORAL-DEVELOPMENTAL CONTENT

Age-related	
Infancy	Failure to thrive Child abuse Child neglect Excess crying Sleep disturbances Infantile colic
Infancy to preschool	Failure to thrive Delayed development Child abuse Thumb sucking Breath holding Rhythmic body movements Sleep disturbances Hyperactivity
School age	Learning problems School phobia Bed-wetting Loss of control of bowel Sleep disorders Masturbation Abdominal pain Recurrent headache
Adolescence	Acting-out behavior Chronic fatigue Drug abuse Recurrent headache Swings in mood and behavior Suicidal attempts Teenage pregnancy Venereal diseases Juvenile delinquency
Situational	Hospitalized child Adopted child Child with chronic illness Child with terminal illness Institutionalized child

ders." There have been no demonstrated cause–effect relationships between the presence of "soft" neurologic signs and various developmental and behavioral problems, but their presence should suggest lack of maturation of the central nervous system.

Minor neurologic signs include abnormalities which are recognizable but not recorded during routine neurologic examinations (such as the presence of mirror movements when a child attempts to perform repetitive movements) or those elicited by special testing. Indications for examination of the CNS with emphasis on minor neurologic signs are: (1) detection of a neurologic disease early in the course—if there is a clinical suspicion by history; (2) an obvious disorder, such as cerebral palsy, to elicit abnormalities of movements which in time will help prepare for planning; (3) a child with behavior or learning problems without apparent neurologic disorder.

Touwen has described a set of well-standardized tests with precise instructions and a scoring system. Interested readers are referred to his monograph on this subject. Briefly, the examination includes assessment of the child in various positions and during various movements. With the child sitting, both the gross and fine motor movements are evaluated for quantity and quality, such as speed and smoothness (nonjerky). The child's posture, ability to retain balance when being pushed against the shoulder, and ability to follow an object by rotating the trunk are observed. Next the child is examined in a standing position. The posture, quality, and quantity of spontaneous movements and involuntary movements are noted.

A number of tests are mentioned to detect lack of coordination and the presence of associated movements. The following are some examples: (1) With the wrist held by the examiner and the hand allowed to relax, ask the child to open the mouth as wide as possible. Ask the patient to close the eyes lightly and stick the tongue out. Spreading and extension of the fingers during the above maneuver is abnormal after 4 years of age; (2) Perform rapid pronation-supination movements with the elbows flexed; normally these movements should be smooth and continuous without associated movements. Abnormalities in this test are significant after 7 or 8 years of age; (3) conduct a finger-nose test similar to the procedure described on page 236; (4) Ask the child to sequentially touch each of the fingers with the thumb of the same hand. Most children over the age of 6 years can do this smoothly; (5) Ask the child to use an index finger held 1 cm from the examiner's index finger, to follow the movement of the examiner closely, while the examiner's hand makes patterns in vertical and horizontal directions. Smoothness of movement is seen in children over 6 to 7 years of age.

The child is then examined during walking. Abnormalities such as asymmetric arm swing, circumduction, hyperextension of the knee are looked for. Ability to walk on tiptoes, to hop on one foot, and to walk a straight line are also tested.

In addition, examination of other systems such as the eyes (for acuity, strabismus) and ears (for acuity, localization), the involuntary movement of the tongue and asymmetric movement of the palate are also included in this assessment.

PSYCHIATRIC EXAMINATION

Detailed history taking is very essential in evaluation of children with psychiatric problems. It is hard to obtain an adequate history from most children. It is harder and even less reliable when dealing with children having psychiatric problems. A history obtained from parents may not be totally reliable either. One has to be aware not only of what the child and the parents say but how they say it. One should be alert to discrepancies between the histories given by the two parents, between the parents and child, between details of history given on different occasions, and between the history and what we actually see during observation.

During the period of history taking, information should be obtained on the following topics: the reason why the child was brought to see the physician; details on general health, previous consultations, and treatments; any medications the child is taking; daily history of activities; details of performance in school; recreational interests; peer relationships; family relationships; and the child's fears and anxieties. It is also important to know what the ethnic and cultural background of the family is, how intact the family is, whether there are other members of the family with mental illness, and what support structures (for emotional, physical, and spiritual sustenance) are available for the family.

During the period of observation and psychiatric examination, observations should be written down in simple terms and without interpretation. Dr. J. E. Simmons suggests organizing and recording the observations under the following headings:

1. Appearance: child's size, appearance, mannerisms, and speech
2. Mood (affect): is it appropriate? Does it fluctuate?
3. Orientation to people, places, objects, and time as appropriate to the child's age
4. Coping mechanisms: describe how the child handles anxiety and impulses—does the child deny, avoid, or project?
5. Neuromuscular integration
6. Thought-process and speech
7. Fantasy, as observed during play and when the child describes dreams and wishes
8. Superego—the child's ideals and value system
9. Concept of self—is the child's self-estimation that of being ugly or pretty? Good or bad?
10. Awareness of problems
11. Intelligence quotient

BIBLIOGRAPHY

Frankenburg WK, Thornton SM, Cohrs ME: Pediatric Developmental Diagnosis. New York, Thieme-Stratton, 1981.

Hodas GR, Sargent J: Psychiatric emergencies. In: Fleisher GR, Ludwig S (eds): Textbook of Pediatric Emergency Medicine. Baltimore, Williams & Wilkins, 1983, pp. 1074–1106.

Holt KS: Developmental Pediatrics. In Apley J (ed): Postgraduate Pediatric Series. London, Butterworth, 1977.

Knobloch H, Pasamanick B: Gesell and Amatruda's Developmental Diagnosis, 3rd ed. Hagerstown, Md., Harper & Row Pub., 1974.

Levine MD, Carey WB, Crocker AC, Gross RT: Developmental-Behavioral Pediatrics. Philadelphia, Saunders, 1983.

Simmons JE: Psychiatric Examination of Children, 1st ed. Philadelphia, Lea & Febiger, 1969.

Touwen BCL: Examination of the Child with Minor Neurological Dysfunction, 2nd ed. Clinics in Developmental Medicine, no. 71. London, Heinemann Medical Books, 1979.

CHAPTER 9

Physical Examination of the Newborn Infant

Alan R. Spitzer

The physical examination of the newborn infant represents one of the greatest joys in medical practice. Rarely does a physician have the opportunity to participate in an event so filled with unlimited hope for the future. Two questions are invariably asked of the pediatrician within moments of delivery: "Is it a boy or girl?"—usually very straightforward—and "Is everything normal?" The answer to this latter question is the primary concern of this chapter.

The emphasis of this section will be on the normal child, but the physician must have some appreciation of the variability of "normal" newborn findings to assess the young infant. At times, this borderline between normal and abnormal is difficult to distinguish.

Common abnormalities which the physician is likely to encounter will be discussed. In addition, the physical examination of the prematurely born and postmature infant have assumed increasing importance in recent years. Some attention will be given also to these classes of infant. Since the assessment of the neonate begins in the delivery room immediately after birth, it is appropriate that the discussion of neonatal physical examination begin at that point.

DELIVERY ROOM EVALUATION OF THE NEWBORN INFANT

The physiologic changes that occur during the birth process are extremely complex and beyond the scope of this book. The newborn infant, however, must accomplish these changes within a matter of moments. Failure to do so, regardless of the cause, potentially places the infant's life in danger. The primary responsibility of the physician in the delivery room is to determine whether the neonate has successfully accomplished the cardiopulmonary changes necessary to initiate life: closure of the ductus arteriosus, cessation of umbilical circulation, functional closure of the foramen ovale, and initiation of air breathing. The standard clinical evaluation that has been routinely used for the past 3 decades has been the screening system devised by Dr. Virginia Apgar (Table 9-1).

The Apgar score is primarily a reflection of cardiopulmonary and neuromuscular changes in the first minutes of life. The single most important feature of the scoring system is the heart rate. Depression of heart rate, especially below 100 beats per minute, is direct evidence of significant perinatal asphyxia. Failure of the physician to respond to such asphyxia can result in hypoxic encephalopathy or death. Other features of the scoring system cannot be overlooked, however, and are generally supportive in one's overall assessment of the infant. Thus, the baby with an Apgar score of 4 or less is clearly at risk. In general, Apgar scores of 7 or greater are considered to be normal, 4 to 6 are borderline, and 3 or less are abnormal.

While the Apgar score is a valuable part of the delivery room examination, it represents only a small part of the assessment. The primary purpose for the physician's presence in the delivery room is to be certain that the transition from intrauterine to extrauterine life has been successfully negotiated. Once the general well-being of the infant has been determined, the physician should routinely perform a quick screening examination of the baby, particularly looking for major malformations. Such findings should always be confirmed on subsequent, more careful examinations under less stressful conditions.

Routine procedures performed in the delivery room which may be diagnostic include passage of a nasogastric tube to assess patency of the nares and the esophagus and assessment of the volume of gastric fluid present at the time of birth. Excessive volume may indicate intestinal obstruction. In such infants, there may also be associated polyhydramnios prior to birth.

The final portion of the examination to be performed in the delivery room includes an evaluation for traumatic effects of delivery. These in-

TABLE 9-1. Apgar Scoring System

	Score		
Sign	***0***	***1***	***2***
Heart rate	Absent	Under 100 beats per minute	Over 100 beats per minute
Respiratory effort	Absent	Slow (irregular)	Good crying
Muscle tone	Limp	Some flexion of extremities	Active motion
Reflex irritability	No response	Grimace	Cough or sneeze
Color	Blue, pale	Pink body, blue extremities	All pink

clude findings such as caput succedaneum, cephalohematoma, brachial plexus palsy, clavicular fracture, femoral fracture, bruising of the skin, petechiae, or other similar findings of a stressful birth. Infants with these findings should be followed closely and appropriate therapy should be initiated.

GESTATIONAL AGE EXAMINATION (Fig. 9-1)

One of the most important parts of the physical examination of the neonate involves the determination of the gestational age of the infant. Frequently, the proper diagnosis cannot be made until the gestational age has been assessed. The diagnosis of hyaline membrane disease, for example, is one which is not appropriate for the term or postterm infant, but is common in the premature baby. Likewise, many diagnoses which might be acceptable for the term baby do not occur in the preterm infant. Thus, gestational age determination is often the first step toward specific diagnosis.

In general, infants are divided into the following categories based upon their gestational age examination:

1. Premature: 37 weeks or less gestational age
2. Full term: 38 to 42 weeks gestational age
3. Postmature: more than 42 weeks gestational age

The standard scoring system that is most commonly used to determine gestational age was described by Dubowitz, Dubowitz, and Goldberg in 1970. The test is divided into two separate sections, one of which evaluates external physical characteristics of the infant, and a second that assesses neuromuscular maturity. The examiner assigns a value to each of the tests and then sums the score to determine the gestational age. The test should be performed in the first 24 hours of life for the greatest reliability (Fig. 9-1). Although a great deal of statistical correlation has been used in devising this test, one should be aware that it is only an estimation of gestational age within the degree of accuracy of the individual performing the test. In addition, it is not uncommon to see infants in whom either the physical characteristics or the neuromuscular findings appear to be disproportionately mature.

Characteristically, the small-for-gestational age (SGA) infant born prematurely will appear to have neuromuscular findings that suggest greater maturity than the physical characteristics. In contrast, the infant of a diabetic mother who is large-for-gestational age will often demonstrate physical maturity advanced beyond neuromuscular maturity.

It is evident that the gestational age examination increases in value when one compares it to the infant's birthweight. An infant who has a birthweight below what would be expected for a determined gestational

External (superficial) Criteria

EXTERNAL SIGN	SCORE 0	1	2	3	4
OEDEMA	Obvious oedema hands and feet; pitting over tibia	No obvious oedema hands and feet; pitting over tibia	No oedema		
SKIN TEXTURE	Very thin, gelatinous	Thin and smooth	Smooth; medium thickness. Rash or superficial peeling	Slight thickening. Superficial cracking and peeling esp. hands and feet	Thick and parchment-like; superficial or deep cracking
SKIN COLOUR (Infant not crying)	Dark red	Uniformly pink	Pale pink: variable over body	Pale. Only pink over ears, lips, palms or soles	
SKIN OPACITY (trunk)	Numerous veins and venules clearly seen, especially over abdomen	Veins and tributaries seen	A few large vessels clearly seen over abdomen	A few large vessels seen indistinctly over abdomen	No blood vessels seen
LANUGO (over back)	No lanugo	Abundant; long and thick over whole back	Hair thinning especially over lower back	Small amount of lanugo and bald areas	At least half of back devoid of lanugo
PLANTAR CREASES	No skin creases	Faint red marks over anterior half of sole	Definite red marks over more than anterior half; indentations over less than anterior third	Indentations over more than anterior third	Definite deep indentations over more than anterior third
NIPPLE FORMATION	Nipple barely visible; no areola	Nipple well defined; areola smooth and flat diameter <0.75 cm.	Areola stippled, edge not raised; diameter <0.75 cm.	Areola stippled, edge raised diameter >0.75 cm.	
BREAST SIZE	No breast tissue palpable	Breast tissue on one or both sides < 0.5 cm. diameter	Breast tissue both sides; one or both 0.5–1.0 cm.	Breast tissue both sides; one or both > 1 cm.	
EAR FORM	Pinna flat and shapeless, little or no incurving of edge	Incurving of part of edge of pinna	Partial incurving whole of upper pinna	Well-defined incurving whole of upper pinna	
EAR FIRMNESS	Pinna soft, easily folded, no recoil	Pinna soft, easily folded, slow recoil	Cartilage to edge of pinna, but soft in places, ready recoil	Pinna firm, cartilage to edge, instant recoil	
GENITALIA MALE	Neither testis in scrotum	At least one testis high in scrotum	At least one testis right down		
FEMALES (With hips half abducted)	Labia majora widely separated, labia minora protruding	Labia majora almost cover labia minora	Labia majora completely cover labia minora		

Neurological Criteria

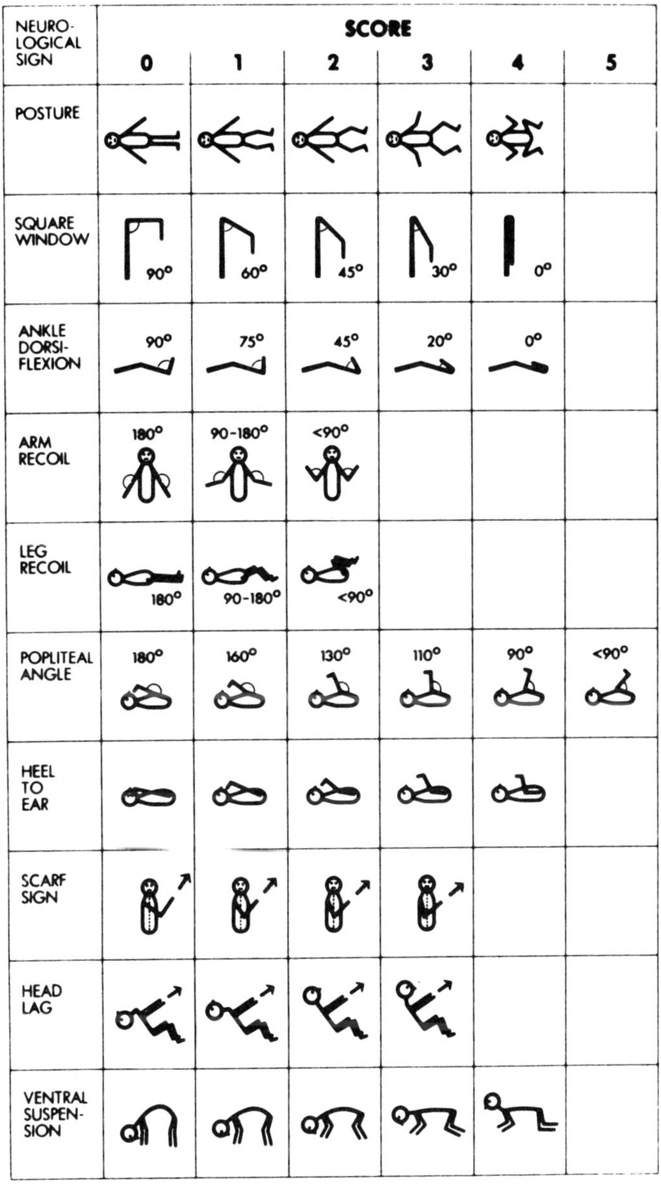

Figure 9-1. Gestational age examination. *(Reproduced with permission from Dubowitz LMS, Dubowitz V: Gestational Age of the Newborn: A Clinical Manual. Reading, Mass., Addison-Wesley, 1977.)*

age is regarded as a SGA infant. For the term infant, a birthweight of less than 2500 gm would place that baby in the category of small-for-gestational age. Figures 9-2 and 9-3 illustrate the expected percentile growth for infants of varying gestational ages. In contrast to the small-for-gestational age infant, the large-for-gestational age (LGA) baby has a birthweight above the expected norm for a given gestational age. Each of these categories of infants may have associated problems that the physician should

NEWBORN WEIGHT, BOYS

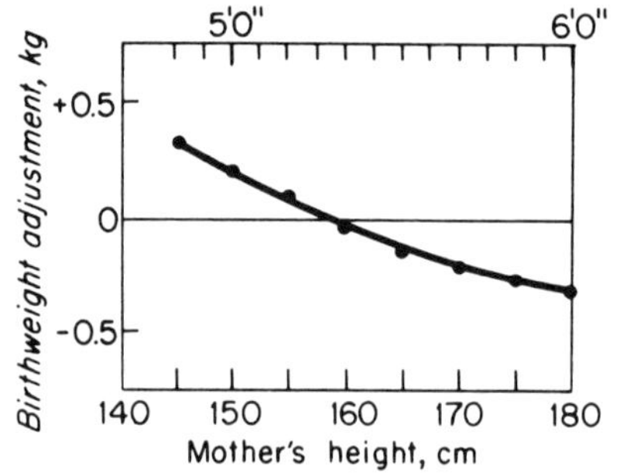

Adjustment for mother's height to be added or subtracted from birthweight when gestation is 37 weeks or more.

Figure 9-2. Newborn weights, boys. *(Reproduced with permission from Smith DW: Growth and Its Disorders. In Schaffer AJ, Markowitz M (eds): Major Problems in Clinical Pediatrics Series 15. Philadelphia, Saunders, 1977, p 30.)*

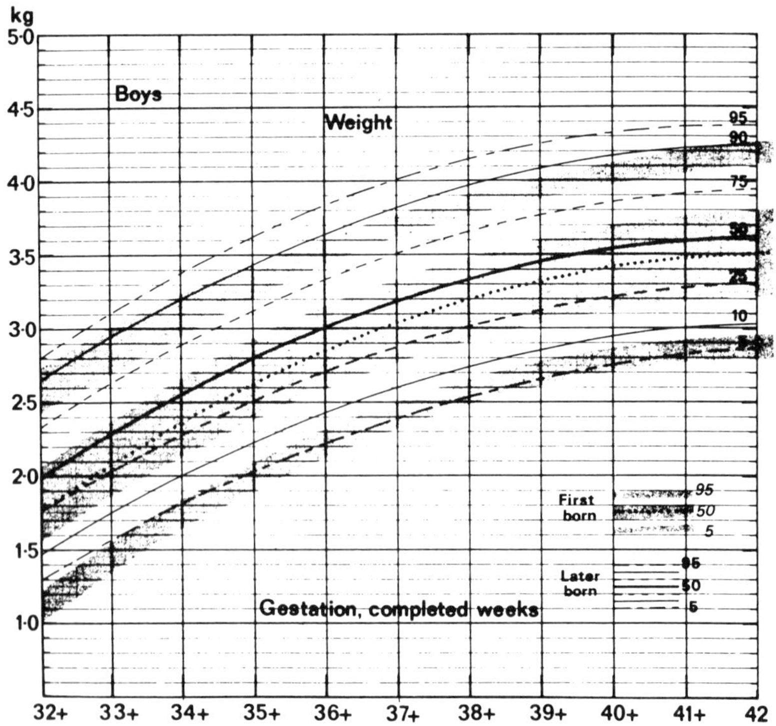

evaluate once these diagnoses have been made. Hypoglycemia, polycythemia, congenital infections, malformations, and long-term developmental problems may occur in the SGA infant. The LGA baby, most commonly born to a diabetic mother, may have hypoglycemia, hypocalcemia, respiratory distress, caudal regression syndrome, congenital heart disease, and other major physical anomalies.

NEWBORN WEIGHT, GIRLS

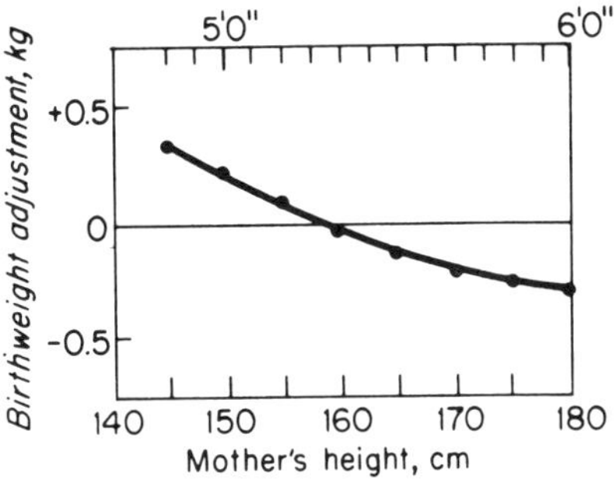

Adjustment for mother's height to be added or subtracted from birthweight when gestation is 37 weeks or more.

Figure 9-3. Newborn weight, girls. *(Reproduced with permission from Smith DW: Growth and Its Disorders. In Schaffer AJ, Markowitz M (eds): Major Problems in Clinical Pediatrics Series 15. Philadelphia, Saunders, 1977, p 31.)*

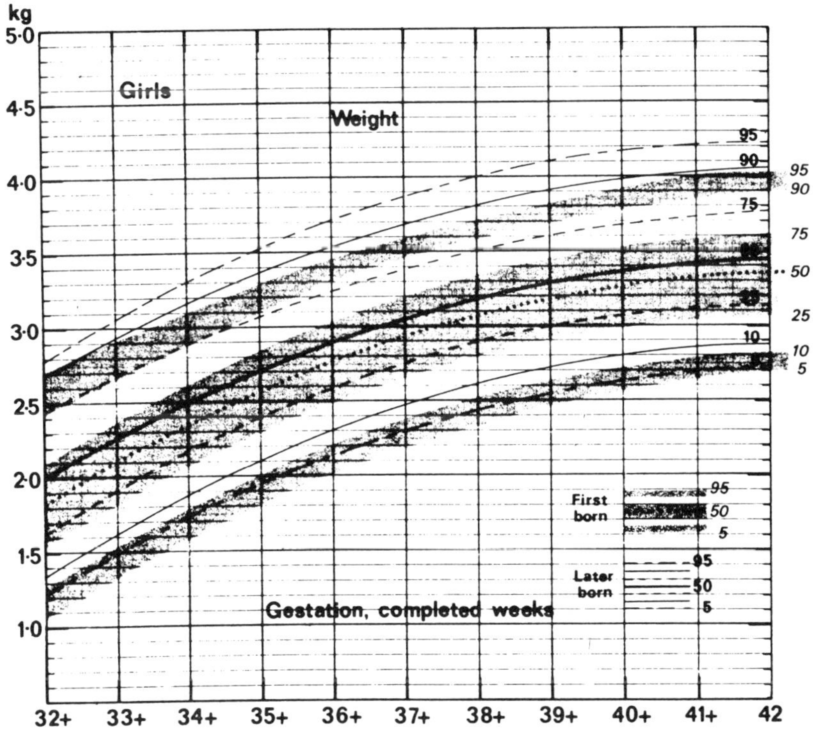

PHYSICAL EXAMINATION OF THE TERM INFANT

The first true systematic examination should be performed within 6 to 12 hours after birth, when the infant's temperature has stabilized and the infant has had an initial attempt at nursing. As with physical examination at any time of life, it is helpful if the examiner develops a specific routine that will avoid omission of any part of the examination. One must not force the examination, however. The baby who is screaming is not the ideal candidate for careful auscultation of the heart, and it would be better to allow the infant to quiet down in such cases before proceeding.

The following approach to the newborn examination is one that has worked well for the author. It is only one method, however, and is presented as a guide which can be followed or modified. The individual examiner has to develop a routine with which the examiner feels most comfortable.

General Appearance

In the case of the neonate, much can be learned by spending the initial moments of the examination simply observing the baby. Level of alertness of the baby is important. Most newborn babies sleep approximately 18 to 20 hours a day during the first week of life, waking mostly for feeding. The frequency of waking may vary significantly from infant to infant. Some babies may show little interest in feeding for the first 24 to 48 hours of life, waking very infrequently. Other children may wake on an hourly basis and appear hungry. This variation probably reflects the state of the infant in the uterus prior to birth as well as the relative degree of stress during delivery. By 3 to 4 days of life, however, most babies will have drawn sufficiently upon their nutritional reserves, so that hunger arousal should be a cyclic phenomenon. Excessive lethargy at this time should be cause for concern, with septicemia being the most significant diagnosis to be considered if there has been no history of perinatal asphyxia.

During periods of arousal, the infant should show spontaneous movement of all extremities. The general posture of the full-term infant is predominantly in flexor tone. Even during sleep, this tone is well maintained in the healthy baby. During arousal, the infant should seem aware of his or her environment. Eye movement should be searching and give indication that the child is sensitive to various stimuli in the immediate vicinity.

The color of the infant is important. While very transient cyanosis may occur in the delivery room until respiration is well established, it should have cleared entirely thereafter. Acrocyanosis, blue discoloration of the extremities, often occurs in any child exposed to cold stress and is commonly seen. Central cyanosis, particularly noticeable in the perioral region, may indicate cardiopulmonary disease and should be evaluated.

Infants who deliver with facial presentations or who have precipitous deliveries may have diffuse ecchymoses of the face and scalp that initially may cause a cyanotic appearance from extravasation of blood into the skin.

Examination of the tongue in these babies will reveal no cyanosis, and the rest of skin is the normal pink color. Polycythemic infants with hematocrits above 68 percent may also look cyanotic at times if there is enough desaturation of hemoglobin (>5 gm%). In addition, these infants may demonstrate respiratory distress from hyperviscosity of blood within the lungs, making diagnosis difficult. A rare cause of cyanosis is methemoglobinemia, which may be congenital or acquired. Blood specimens drawn from such infants will appear brown in color. Babies who have had significant perinatal asphyxia and central nervous system injury may demonstrate cyanosis on the basis of central alveolar hypoventilation. The history in such babies usually suggests this diagnosis, and other signs of difficult delivery, such as brachial plexus or facial nerve palsies, and bone fractures may be present.

Parents often are dismayed to find that the newborn infant loses a moderate amount of weight after birth, primarily through fluid loss. This process is thought to result from withdrawal of maternal hormones and changes in renal function in the neonate. Weight loss of up to 10 percent of birth weight is considered acceptable.

The Skin

The skin of the newborn infant often provides many clues to the general state of well-being of the baby. In particular, changes in skin color and texture, as well as the appearance of various rashes, should be carefully evaluated.

The implications of *cyanosis* in the infant have been previously described. Pallor is also a significant sign in the neonate. Pallor may be the result of anemia from a variety of causes. Perinatal asphyxia with profound circulatory disturbance, hypoglycemia, seizures, and thermal cold stress are other factors that may be associated with pallor. In contrast to pallor, the *plethoric* infant with a reddish coloration to the skin may have polycythemia, neonatal fever with early septicemia, or be an infant of a diabetic mother (with or without polycythemia).

Jaundice is the change in skin color that is probably most commonly observed in the newborn period. Infants with jaundice due to deposition of unconjugated bilirubin have a yellow-orange tint to the skin, while babies with conjugated hyperbilirubinemia often demonstrate a yellow-green coloration. Recently, the development of transcutaneous bilirubinometry has enabled the examiner to more accurately estimate the level of hyperbilirubinemia with a simple, noninvasive device. One may use the following schematic for clinical estimation of the degree of jaundice:

- Face only: 5–8 mg%
- Face and upper trunk: 8–12 mg%
- Lower trunk and extremities: > 12 mg%

At the nurseries of the Hospital of the University of Pennsylvania, approximately 25 percent of all term neonates will have sufficient jaundice to require testing during their 3 to 4 days of hospitalization after birth. Most commonly, the jaundice appears on the second to third day of life, peaks at day 3 to 4, and declines rapidly thereafter. Breast-fed infants may have persistence of their jaundice for an additional day or two, probably caused by increased enterohepatic circulation of bilirubin from the relative decrease in oral intake during the first days of life, when they receive only colostrum.

Jaundice that appears during the initial 24 hours of life should never be considered physiologic. Hyperbilirubinemia presenting this early is often due to hemolytic disease, either Rh or ABO incompatibility, or to sepsis, bacterial or viral. Further investigation in such infants is essential.

Minor abnormalities of the skin are common in newborn infants and rarely pose any threat. Capillary hemangiomas ("stork's bites") are found on the forehead, the eyelids, and the nape of the neck. Often very prominent at birth, they usually fade during the first months of life. The lesions are irregular, flat, erythematous lesions that blanch on pressure. Larger hemangiomas such as strawberry or cavernous lesions, which are irregular, raised, erythematous irregularities in the skin often begin as barely perceptible hemangiomas in the newborn period and then increase rapidly in size over the next 2 months. They may occur anywhere over the body surface and can cause marked disfiguration. Rarely do they need any therapy and virtually always involute spontaneously. Large ones, however, may consume large numbers of platelets (Kasselbach-Merritt syndrome). Cutaneous hemangiomas may be associated with arteriovenous malformations of underlying organs, especially the liver, gastrointestinal tract, and central nervous system. Very large arteriovenous malformations may increase cardiac output excessively and cause cardiac failure.

Papular and pustular lesions often arouse significant concern in the newborn period, yet, for the most part, are entirely benign. *Milia,* or small white papules, are usually found over the nose, the cheeks, and the forehead and represent retained sebaceous material. These disappear over the first weeks of life. *Miliaria* represents obstruction of eccrine sweat glands. These lesions therefore usually appear as a pinpoint vesiculopapular rash over the scalp, forehead, and skinfold regions. The rash may be superficial (miliaria crystallina) or more deep-seated with a reddish appearance (miliaria rubra). This rash usually will disappear within 1 to 2 weeks if the infant is not overheated to any substantial degree.

Erythema toxicum is the most common rash appearing during the newborn period. Eosinophilic inclusions can be found in the skin on biopsy, which is rarely indicated. It usually begins on the 2nd or 3rd day of life, but may not be seen until as late as 7 to 10 days. The rash consists of white papulovesicular lesions on an erythematous base that may be present over any skin surface except the palms and soles. Erythema toxicum is entirely benign and fades after several days.

Pustular melanosis may be confused with milia, miliaria, or erythema toxicum. These lesions are also papulovesicular and occur at any body surface, including the palms and soles. The lesions subsequently rupture, leaving a pigmented macule, surrounded by a scaly ring. These occur more commonly in the black infant. The pustular lesions that cause the most concern are true pustules produced by *Staphylococcus aureus* infection. Because of the enormous risk of septicemia in the newborn infant, lesions that appear to be pustular with significant surrounding erythema should be cultured for *Staphylococcus aureus.*

Vesicular lesions are most often associated with *Herpes simplex* acquired from the maternal birth canal during labor. Because of the life-threatening nature of this infection, vesicles should be investigated with skin scrapings and appropriate culture techniques.

Pigmented nevi may be seen in many infants. The most common type of nevus is the so-called Mongolian spot. This lesion is a large, flat, greyish-blue spot, most often seen over the lower trunk or buttocks, usually in black or oriental infants. They are benign and fade over periods of months to years. *Cafe-au-lait spots* are seen in many children and usually have no significance. They are light brown macules with irregular borders that may appear over any skin surface. If the lesions are large and numerous, however, they may reflect underlying neurofibromatosis (see page 174).

Eczema rarely occurs during the first days of life, but often is seen as the infant matures. Eczema represents a reaction of the skin to some allergen in the immediate environment of the infant. The skin in such lesions is red or reddish-yellow with weeping or scaling. Seborrheic eczema, when it involves the scalp, is termed *cradle cap.* An eczematoid rash appearing in the intertriginous areas of the skin, particularly if surrounded by smaller satellite lesions, is usually due to *Candida albicans* infection.

The hair of the infant may also be suggestive of a diagnosis. Unusual hair pattern, particularly denoted by odd-appearing whorls over the back of the scalp may indicate abnormal brain development and may be associated with certain neurologic syndromes. Brittle hair or kinky hair may also be associated with various genetic syndromes (see page 95).

Examination of the Head, Eyes, Ears, Nose, and Mouth

The newborn infant's skull provides protection for the underlying brain. Because of the lack of bony fusion, it is able to pass readily through the birth canal, often with substantial molding. This molding is observed as elongation of the skull in the anterioposterior diameter with overriding of the sutures. Although significant injury is uncommon during birth, one frequently finds some evidence of minor skull trauma. The most commonly observed phenomenon is a *caput succedaneum* which is the result of edema in the presenting area of the skull. The caput is differentiated from the *cephalohematoma,* which is a collection of blood in the periosteum and is usually localized to a single bone. Cephalohematomas have fractures associated with them in about 10 percent to 20 percent of cases. These rarely extend through the table of the skull and do not require intervention. The caput resolves over several days. In contrast, the cephalohematoma often liquifies in the center over the first few days, while the periphery begins to calcify, giving the impression of a depression in the skull. The cephalohematoma resolves over days to weeks. At times, a small nodular calcification may be left that can take months to resolve.

The configuration of the skull at birth is thus related to type of presentation. The infant born by normal vaginal delivery is more likely to have molding of the skull and an elongated, asymmetrical appearance. In contrast, the baby born by caesarean section or breech vaginal delivery usually has a well-rounded skull. Breech presentations of the baby may result in significant trauma because of the difficulty in delivering the head as the cervix begins to close. Molding disappears over 48 to 72 hours, although slight overriding of the sutures may persist in some babies.

Skull defects should be carefully checked. A defect in the skin overlying the skull, cutis aplasia, may be associated with other anomalies but is frequently an isolated benign finding. An encephalocele represents a failure of anterior neural tube closure with herniation of brain and meninges through the skull defect. Most occur in the occipital region and are associated with some degree of neurologic deficit. Anencephaly, which represents failure of hemispheric development of the brain, is fortunately rare. These infants may or may not have skin closure over the residual brain and may be stillborn. Prognosis is extremely poor in all cases.

The *fontanels* should be carefully examined. Infants have two major fontanels, an anterior fontanel, formed at the site of future fusion of the frontal and parietal bones, and a posterior fontanel at the potential site of fusion of parietal and occipital bones. Both fontanels may be difficult to appreciate in the hours immediately after birth because of the overriding sutures. By 48 hours of life, the anterior fontanel has a diameter of 2 to 3 cm, while the posterior fontanel is about 1 cm diameter. The fontanels should be slightly sunken and soft, with some tenseness only during crying. A persistently tense fontanel may indicate increased intracranial pressure, from infection (meningitis), fever, intracranial hemorrhage (subdural hematoma), or intracranial mass lesions. Arterial pulsations may be appreciated in the anterior fontanel in an otherwise well child and do not necessarily indicate increased intracranial pressure (see page 93).

In contrast, a depressed fontanel usually indicates dehydration, most often seen in somewhat older children with poor oral intake, vomiting, or diarrhea. Over the first several days of life, the overriding sutures separate so that suture lines can usually be palpated. These sutures are illustrated in Figure 7A-1. Craniosynostosis, the premature closure of suture lines, is usually not seen in the perinatal period. The examiner must therefore be rigorous in monitoring head circumference measurement. Inadequate growth, especially if accompanied by odd head shape, may indicate craniosynostosis. Excessive head growth may be the result of hydrocephalus, from either increased secretion or failure of flow and reabsorption of cerebrospinal fluid. Head circumference measurements should be carefully performed by taking the largest circumference when a measuring tape is placed around the skull. This circumference is most often obtained when the tape rests over the glabella and the occipital prominence. Normal head circumference for the term infant ranges from 32 to 37 cm. In addition to palpation, auscultation of the skull may reveal bruits from arteriovenous malformations. Transillumination remains a useful technique in the era of ultrasound and CT scanning (see page 94). It may be helpful in diagnosing a fluid collection such as hydrocephalus, hydranencephaly, subdural hematoma, or cephalohematoma.

Examination of the *eye* in the newborn infant frequently provides clues to diagnosis, yet is difficult to perform. In the otherwise healthy neonate, a rapid screening examination can be performed to diagnose serious difficulties of an urgent nature. If a more detailed examination needs to be carried out, this requires the help of an ophthalmologist capable of performing indirect ophthalmoscopy in young infants.

The newborn baby usually is crying or has the eyes shut at the time that the examination is to be carried out. Gentle rocking of the baby in a side-to-side manner, or holding the baby in a vertical upright fashion will often induce the child to open the eyes and look around. Forcible attempts to pry open the lids will invariably be met with resistance and crying. There clearly will be times, however, when examination must be performed on an uncooperative infant. In such cases, two people are required—the examiner and an aide to gently retract the infant's lids. Dilatation of the pupil with phenylephrine (2.5 percent) or tropicamide (1 percent) may also be required if careful fundoscopic examination is needed.

The shape of the eyes and their position should be noted (see page 102). A lateral upward slope of the eyes with an associated inner epicanthal fold is suggestive of Trisomy-21 in the non-Oriental child. In the absence of other findings of Down's syndrome, however, these may be regarded as a normal variant. A lateral downward slope is associated with some genetic syndromes, as well as with renal dysplasia or hypoplasia (Potter syndrome). Narrow palpebral fissures and a reduced intercanthal distance is found in fetal alcohol syndrome.

The conjunctiva should be inspected for abnormalities of development (coloboma of the lid) or discharge. Chemical irritation of the eyes from instillation of silver nitrate drops at birth may produce erythema and discharge during the first 24 to 48 hours. Gonococcal ophthalmia usually appears after the second day of life, as does other bacterial conjunctivitis acquired during the birth process. Inclusion blenorrhea caused by chlamydial infection and viral conjunctivitis are usually first noted after 4 to 5 days of life. It is not uncommon for chlamydial infection to appear after several weeks, at which time it may be associated with pneumonia and eosinophilia in the blood. One should not be falsely reassured by the degree of redness of the conjunctiva, the amount of discharge, or the age of presentation.

The sclera of term infants is usually white. Blue sclera are associated with osteogenesis imperfecta or cutis laxa but may be seen in some normal infants. Small hemorrhages in the sclera may be seen in the days immediately following birth. Subconjunctival hemorrhages occur from the increase in venous pressure that results during delivery. They are benign and resolve over several days, although they may leave some pigmentary changes for prolonged periods in some babies.

When one flashes an ophthalmoscope light through the newborn eye, a so-called red reflex should be observed. In actuality, the color seen is more orange than red. Clouding of the cornea may indicate cataracts or glaucoma. In this instance, the red reflex is not seen, and the eye has a hazy grey appearance. Lens opacification (cataracts) also prevents visualization of the retinal red reflex. A grey-white appearance of the lens can be observed in such cases. Cataracts may be associated with congenital infections, especially rubella, and disturbances of calcium metabolism. Rarely, a white reflex replacing the red may be a sign of retinoblastoma.

The iris should be briefly examined for congenital defects (coloboma) which may indicate defects in other organ systems. Small white spots (Brushfield spots) may surround the periphery of the iris. These may be a normal finding but are associated with Trisomy-21. Iris color tends to change as the infant matures, although the author's experience suggests that the change is not as dramatic as tradition suggests. The newborn pupil should constrict when exposed to bright light.

Ophthalmologic indirect observation is indicated in premature infants, infants who have had stressful deliveries, or infants suspected of congenital infection. The retina of the premature infant who has been exposed to oxygen may show neovascularization that progresses to retinal detachment. This entity is known as retrolental fibroplasia.

The infant who has had a difficult delivery may show numerous flame-shaped hemorrhages throughout the retina. Most newborns who are delivered vaginally will show some retinal hemorrhages that resolve within days. The small-for-gestational age infant may demonstrate a salt-and-pepper appearance of the retina that is the retinitis of congenital infection, particularly cytomegalic inclusion disease and toxoplasmosis.

Abnormalities of the *ear* may give clues to many genetic syndromes. For example, absence of the ear (anotica) is seen in Treacher-Collins syndrome whereas preauricular pits may be seen in normal infants. Ears that are low-set and posteriorly rotated are seen in other genetic syndromes.

It is difficult to see the tympanic membranes of the newborn infant because the external auditory canals are often filled with vernix caseosa and amniotic fluid debris. In certain circumstances, however, the membrane must be visualized, especially in the neonate with fever. In such instances, one should irrigate the canal with lukewarm saline to remove any debris. The ear should be dry before one approaches it with an otoscope. In the neonate, the tympanic membrane is angled somewhat more acutely than in the older child, so that visualization is more difficult. Retracting the pinna of the ear upward and anteriorly may be more effective than the usual posterior retraction normally used in the older child. Often the speculum of the otoscope must be used to gently probe the canal, while retracting the pinna in a number of directions until the tympanic membrane can be clearly seen. The tympanic membrane at this age is less translucent than in the older infant and the vascularity is slightly increased. Crying causes substantial injection. A red, bulging tympanic membrane supports the diagnosis of otitis media.

Hearing is difficult to assess in the immediate neonatal period. The infant should respond to loud sounds, however, with a typical startle response (Moro reflex). One must be careful in trying to assess hearing in this way. Be certain that the baby is exposed to sound alone and no other vibratory or tactile sensation. If there is any question about a child's hearing, careful audiologic evaluation can be performed at a very early age by trained audiologists.

The *nose* of the newborn infant is usually broad in appearance. In addition to inspecting for gross external developmental anomalies, a small catheter should be passed through both nares to be certain that choanal atresia or stenosis is not present. The infant with choanal atresia often presents in the delivery room with cyanosis at rest that disappears with crying. Nasal flaring refers to a widening of the alae nasae with inspiration and is a characteristic sign of respiratory insufficiency.

The *mouth* examination may reveal many localized or generalized conditions. Perioral cyanosis has been discussed previously. Cleft lip and cleft palate are readily visible and represent a failure of fusion of these midline structures during development. They may involve the nose and the nasal cavity and be associated with midline defects of the central nervous system. The lips should symmetrically retract with crying. Failure to do so may indicate a facial nerve palsy or underlying central nervous system disorder (asymmetric crying facies).

A large tongue relative to the size of the oral cavity is typical of the newborn infant. An excessively large tongue may be caused by or associated with a hemangioma or lymphangioma. Large tongues may also be seen with hypothyroidism, mucopolysaccharidoses and Beckwith syndrome. The frenulum of the tongue in the newborn often appears to attach to the very tip of the tongue, producing a significant indentation in the anterior portion. Parents are often concerned that their child may develop "tongue-tie." In actuality, the anterior portion of the tongue grows substantially so that rarely, if ever, is clipping of the frenulum indicated.

Teeth may occasionally be seen at birth. These may be fairly loose and attempts to remove them may result in the absence of a primary tooth in that area. Since there is a risk of aspiration of such teeth, however, some physicians recommend their removal. Retention cysts (ranula) may line the margin of the gums and are entirely benign, resolving with time. Small epithelial inclusion cysts of the palate are also benign and are referred to as "Epstein's Pearls."

A small jaw may be seen as a normal feature in some infants. If excessive and associated with glossoptosis and high-arched palate, one may diagnose Pierre-Robin syndrome. Feeding is often difficult for these infants and may require special treatment until the child grows sufficiently.

Salivation does not occur appreciably during the first 2 months of life. The infant who produces excessive secretions soon after birth should be suspected of esophageal atresia and an attempt should be made to pass a catheter. If esophageal atresia is present (often in accompaniment with tracheoesophageal fistula), the catheter will curl in the esophagus. Dye does not have to be injected in such babies and may result in aspiration. Other infants reported by parents to have excessive secretions most often have gastroesophageal reflux. This finding is seen in many infants during the first months of life and is usually benign. Some babies, however, will have apnea or esophagitis with reflux.

Examination of the Neck

The neck of the newborn infant is short and normally not readily visible for inspection during physical examination. To examine the neck, the physician should place a pad beneath the baby's shoulder blades to mildly hyperextend and bring the neck into view. The neck is examined by palpation, auscultation, and transillumination.

Masses are often readily visible in the neck. A very common mass seen in the young infant is a hematoma in the area of the sternocleidomastoid muscle due to birth injury. Cystic hygromas represent the most common masses seen in the neck in this age group. They are soft swellings that arise from lymphoid tissue and readily transilluminate. They most commonly arise in the anterior triangle of the neck. Firmer masses, seen along sternocleidomastoids, are branchial cleft cysts and do not readily transilluminate.

The most common midline mass is the thyroglossal duct cyst. Goiters may also be seen in hypothyroid infants, but are relatively rare except in countries where goiter is endemic.

Excess skin in the posteriolateral region of the neck is referred to as "webbing" and is seen in syndromes such as Turner syndrome, Noonan syndrome, and Klippel-Feil syndrome.

Flexing of the neck should always be performed as part of the examination. The neck should be supple and easily moved. An excessively resistant neck may indicate meningitis or subarachnoid hemorrhage with meningeal irritation.

Auscultation over the neck may reveal bruits in the area of the thyroid gland. Such findings are occasionally present in the infant born to a hypothyroid mother receiving thyroid replacement or in the hyperthyroid mother on suppressive medication. In either case, the infants may be transiently hyperthyroid.

Examination of the Thorax and Lungs

Because of the critical nature of the transition from intrauterine to extrauterine life, the examination of the lungs is of paramount importance. Again, the routine should proceed from inspection to palpation to auscultation. Percussion may occasionally be helpful, but because of the small size of the neonatal chest cage, its value is limited.

The shape of the newborn infant's thorax is normally rounder than that of the older infant or adult. This barreled appearance may be accentuated in the baby who has aspirated meconium. The circumference of the chest immediately after birth should be approximately 2 cm less than the head circumference and averages about 33 cm. Within a short time after birth, respiration normally should be easy and the chest should move minimally and symmetrically with each breath.

Breathing is predominantly abdominal during the newborn period with little help from accessory muscles unless respiratory distress is present. Retractions are the most important sign of lung disease in the neonate and are seen with respiratory distress, atelectasis, airway obstruction, aspiration syndromes, and other entities that either reduce lung volume or produce hypoxemia. Retractions may occur in the intercostal spaces, the supraclavicular spaces, and the suprasternal space. They are produced by forceful contraction of accessory respiratory muscles in these regions. Asymmetry of chest movement is associated with a paralyzed diaphragm from a traumatic delivery, pneumothorax, or cystic malformation of the lungs. If traumatic delivery is the etiology, one should carefully inspect for evidence of clavicular fractures, brachial plexus injury, and facial nerve palsy.

Examination of the lungs is extremely variable in the newborn infant. The timing of the examination, especially in the hours immediately after birth, strongly influences the range of normal physical findings.

The newborn respiratory rate is variable, altering substantially with sleep and wakefulness. In general, the respiratory rate ranges from 30 to 60 breaths per minute, with the mean for most infants being about 40 breaths per minute. Breathing is usually easy and primarily abdominal with little use of accessory muscles. It is not uncommon to see significant retractions and cyanosis during the first hours of life as the infant clears its lungs of fetal lung fluid. By 8 to 12 hours, however, respiration should essentially be normal.

Continued nasal flaring, tachypnea, and cyanosis after this time should be pursued with appropriate investigations. Other signs of abnormal lung status include grunting at the end of expiration, which is an attempt by the infant to increase functional residual capacity and improve gas exchange, and irregular or slow respirations in the face of cyanosis, usually a sign of brain injury. Cheyne-Stokes breathing patterns are rare in the newborn period.

Apnea (Fig. 9-4) which usually refers to a cessation of breathing greater than 15 seconds, or less than 15 seconds but with accompanying bradycardia, is occasionally seen in some infants after difficult deliveries. It should not persist for more than 24 hours, and one should always be aware that apnea may be one of the first manifestations of neonatal sepsis. The infant with apnea always deserves close observation and frequently needs thorough evaluation. Periodic breathing refers to periods of respiration for less than 20 seconds separated by periods of apnea for less than 10 seconds duration occurring at least three times in succession. This finding has implications similar to those regarding apnea.

The breasts of both male and female newborn infants should be inspected. They may appear full and engorged as a result of maternal hormonal secretion that has transferred across the placenta. This phenomenon becomes apparent on days 2 and 3 of life and persists for days to weeks. Milky white secretions (witches' milk) may be expressed in some babies. Redness and induration should be watched for in infants with breast engorgement (neonatal mastitis).

Palpation should be performed to feel for masses or fractures. Fractures are often appreciated by the sensation of crepitus over the affected bone. Palpation and percussion of the chest are generally not as helpful in the newborn chest examination as in the older child. Because the neonatal

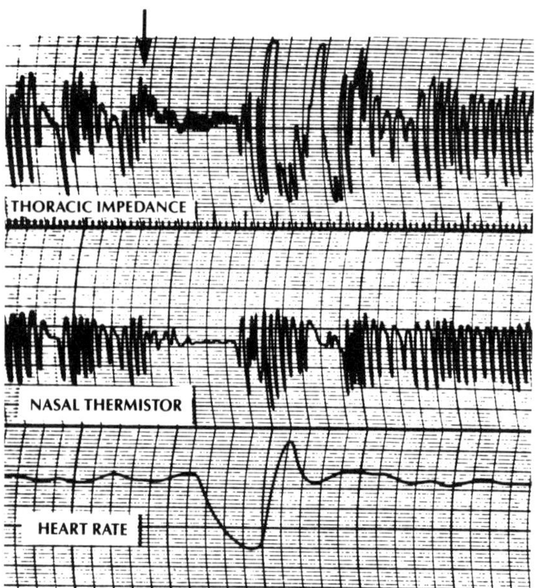

Figure 9-4. Nasal thermistor-pneumocardiogram recording demonstrating central apnea (*arrow*). Nasal air flow and thoracic impedance cease for approximately 15 seconds with a subsequent decline in heart rate from 150 to 78 beats per minute. Stimulation was required to terminate the episode of apnea. Note: Small cardiogenic artifact is noted in the thoracic impedance channel during apnea. *(Reproduced with permission from Dr. AR Spitzer, from Spitzer AR and Fox WW: Clinical Management of Infantile Apnea. Monograph Series. Port Washington, N.Y., D A S Communications, 1984.)*

chest is so compact and resonant, sound and percussion notes are readily transmitted throughout the thorax. It is thus more difficult to localize findings to a specific part of the lung on the basis of these examinations. A dull percussion note, however, can be helpful in determining pleural effusion or lobar atelectasis. A hyperresonant percussion note may be found in pneumothorax, lung cysts, or lobar emphysema.

Certain features of the chest in the newborn make the procedure of auscultation somewhat different than in the older child. The neonatal chest is relatively small and the chest wall is comparatively thin. As a result, breath sounds are readily transmitted, making it difficult to localize the findings to an individual segment or lobe of the lung. Ideally, auscultation should be approached with the infant awake and resting quietly. The head of the stethoscope should be warmed (as well as the hands!), so that the infant does not startle and cry. Ocassionally, if one wants deep inspirations, crying may produce the desired type of breath. The examiner then must be prepared to listen as the baby inspires following a loud cry. Breath sounds in the newborn infant can be ideally heard in the midaxillary line in the midthorax. Again, because of the chest dimensions, all lobes of the lungs on that side of the chest can be auscultated in that area. The stethoscope should be moved over the entire chest, however, to be sure that all regions are carefully heard. In general, a small diaphragm is most useful for auscultation, although in some infants (especially premature or SGA) firm application of the bell side may produce better results.

Breath sounds in the newborn and young infant tend to be more broncho-vesicular in character. Because the larger airways lie closer to the examiner's ear, the sounds generated in these structures are louder and more tubular sounding than those which are heard in adults.

Unilateral absence of breath sounds may be associated with atelectasis, pleural effusion, pneumothorax, and cystic malformations of the lung. The presence of bowel sounds in the chest should alert one to the possibility of congenital diaphragmatic hernia, especially if accompanied by respiratory distress, a shift in heart position, and a scaphoid abdomen.

Stridor on inspiration is most often associated with laryngomalacia in this age group and is usually benign. Other possible diagnoses, however, include tracheomalacia, laryngeal web, vocal cord paralysis (from birth trauma), vascular ring, or other internal masses causing tracheal compression. A rhonchus or wheeze is a continuous musical note (see page 135) and one may hear inspiratory rhonchi due to excessive mucus in the upper airway which clears when the infant coughs or cries.

Crackles or rales are discontinuous musical auscultatory noises (see page 135) and are associated with pneumonia, delayed reabsorption of fetal lung fluid, meconium aspiration, syndrome, and pulmonary edema.

Because of the relative lack of the development of the bronchial smooth musculature in the newborn infant, ausculatory findings of wheezing are rare. Some infants in the first months of life will wheeze with certain viral infections, such as respiratory syncytial virus or parainfluenza virus, typically during an episode of infantile bronchiolitis.

Examination of the Cardiovascular System

Several features of the newborn heart require some modification of the usual approach to examination. The normal resting heart rate of the term infant is 90 to 160 beats per minute. Auscultation, as a result, requires the development of a finely tuned appreciation of irregularities at a rate much higher than one is used to. The infant is rarely cooperative, and auscultation during crying is extremely difficult. Differentiation between functional, or benign, extraneous sounds and true organic heart disease is important, yet often problematic.

Examination begins, as always, with inspection. The cardinal signs of heart disease in the neonate are cyanosis or respiratory distress. The issue of cyanosis has been discussed previously. It is sufficient to reiterate that central cyanosis is the sign of greatest significance. Peripheral cyanosis alone rarely indicates heart disease of any consequence. Respiratory distress is a reflection of an inability of the cardiovascular system to meet the needs of the peripheral circulation. While it is most commonly associated with lung disease, it is frequently seen in infants with cardiac disease. In many heart lesions encountered in the newborn period, cyanosis and respiratory distress occur simultaneously. Other important signs of congenital heart disease include: pallor, mottling of the skin, diaphoresis, lethargy, irritability, poor weight gain, and slow feeding. Parents of infants with heart disease often report that feeding takes hours to complete. The energy expended by a baby in taking a four-ounce feeding has been compared to an adult walking up three flights of stairs.

Edema, the most common sign of adult heart disease, is less commonly observed in the newborn. Some infants with congestive heart failure may show edema in dependent areas of the body. Since sick infants often lie on their backs, the presacral area, the back, and the posterior scalp may show collections of fluid. Isolated edema (lymphedema) of the feet as seen in Turner syndrome (XO chromosomal syndrome) is very rare in the newborn with cardiac disease.

Following inspection, palpation often provides a number of clues to the etiology of an infant's heart disease. The point of maximum impulse (PMI) should always be determined. In infants, the heart is more centrally located within the thoracic cavity and the PMI usually is found at the fourth left interspace just medial to the midclavicular line. Although there can be some degree of variability in location of the PMI, significant movement of the PMI from the usual location should make one think of malposition of the heart (situs inversus, dextrocardia, pneumothorax, or mass lesions) that may have caused the heart to shift. Additional palpatory sensations such as thrills and heaves should also be noted at this time. Occasionally, thrills may be noted in otherwise well infants during the first hours of life and disappear by several days of age. The examiner should palpate the entire precordium during examination.

Examination of the peripheral pulses can be performed at this time as part of the cardiovascular examination. It is helpful in appreciating the pulses to have the infant in a relaxed, warm environment. It is extremely difficult to appreciate pulsations if the infant is crying or if the extremities are so cool that the peripheral pulses are diminished. Palpation of the pulses is very subjective and variable from one examiner to the other. It is important, however, that the individual examiner develop consistency in examination in order to appreciate the different pulses in one infant when compared to another. The pulses that one should examine are the carotid, brachial, radial, femoral, dorsalis pedis, and posterior tibial. In some infants, the latter two may not be palpable. This does not necessarily indicate cardiac disease. The quality of the pulse is important. A sharp, bounding type pulsation may be associated with a patent ductus arteriosus. Weak, thready pulsations are seen in shock and congenital malformations of the heart associated with decreased systemic circulation. Stronger pulses in the upper compared to the lower extremities should raise the question of coarctation of the aorta.

Palpation of the skin is also useful in assessing cardiac function. Determination of capillary filling time is helpful when one is attempting to assess the degree of skin perfusion. This test is performed by lightly pressing the skin to produce slight blanching and then assessing the time it takes for the capillary bed in that area to refill. In a healthy baby, capillary refilling should occur within 1 or 2 seconds. Infants with impaired peripheral circulation will take significantly longer. Refilling taking longer than 3 seconds is clearly abnormal. The examiner should establish skin sites upon which this test is usually performed. It is often helpful to use one central site (forehead, sternum) and one peripheral site (toes).

The next step in cardiovascular examination requires the use of tools. Blood pressure, often neglected in the infant, should always be checked. Selection of the appropriate size cuff is essential. The cuff should cover two thirds to three fourths of the length of the extremity for an accurate determination. The cuff should be inflated well above the systolic pressure and then gradually released. The point at which one first auscultates or palpates a pulse is a reasonable approximation of systole. Muffling of sounds may be hard to appreciate so that a diastolic pressure in the newborn is less accurate and one may have to indicate the diastolic as the point at which sounds disappear. An alternative technique is to use the point at which an extremity flushes as the systolic, as one releases the cuff pressure. The use of a Doppler technique in the newborn may help simplify the procedure. Upper and lower extremities should be checked.

Normal blood pressure in the newborn infant is extremely variable in the first hours of life, but tends to stabilize by around 12 hours of age. Blood pressure is also a function of weight and gestational age. The range of blood pressures one can expect is:

- Systolic 40–80 mm Hg
- Diastolic 20–55 mm Hg
- Mean 25–60 mm Hg

Hypertension in this age group is never benign and always has some pathologic etiology.

For ausculation of the heart, ideally the infant should be quiet. Even the most skilled examiner cannot appreciate the subtleties of cardiac sounds in an irritable infant. Sometimes, therefore, the examiner may have to repeat an examination several times to be certain that nothing has been missed. A helpful trick to quiet a crying baby is to offer a pacifier. Alternatively, one may have to wait to perform the examination at a time when the baby has been recently fed.

Auscultation begins with evaluation of heart rate. Normal resting heart rate in this age group ranges from 90 to 160 beats per minute with most full term infants having a rate of approximately 120 to 140 beats per minute. Evaluation of cardiac rhythm is difficult because of the rapidity of the heart rate.

One attempts to determine if there are occasional decelerations and accelerations of heart rate with respiration as normally occur in the newborn infant (sinus arrhythmia), or if there are true arrhythmias as manifested by occasional "skipped beats." If any question exists, an EKG should be obtained or continuous monitoring should be performed with a Holter monitor.

Heart sounds in this age group tend to be loud because of the thin chest wall, but difficult to analyze for clinical characteristics because of the fast heart rate. It is impossible to time heart sounds using carotid pulsations as is done in adults. In general, the first heart sound is heard best at the apex of the heart and the second heart sound is most prominent at the base of the heart in the second left interspace (pulmonic area). Splitting of the second heart sound may not be immediately appreciated because of the relatively high initial pulmonary vascular resistance. As resistance decreases over the first 24 to 48 hours, however, splitting becomes readily apparent. Third and fourth heart sounds are uncommon in newborns initially, but may be present in young infants in the absence of cardiac disease. Because of these characteristics, one should begin auscultation at the apex with a small diaphragm and gradually move the stethoscope upward to the base along the left side of the sternum, then across and down the right side of the sternum. In this way, the heart sounds can be appreciated and accurately characterized.

Heart murmurs often cause much consternation. It is often stated that every infant has a heart murmur at some time, but these are rarely pathologic in origin. Murmurs are produced by turbulence in the flow of blood through the chambers of the heart. When this turbulence is excessive, additional heart sounds are generated. These sounds are termed murmurs. Innocent (functional) murmurs are often heard during the first few days of life. These most commonly appear in the second left interspace, have a soft vibratory quality, and are intermittent. They are probably produced by rapid flow of high hematocrit blood through the pulmonic valve, changes in pulmonary vascular resistance, or closing of the ductus arteriosus. Another common innocent murmur heard throughout the entire thorax, but most prominently over the anterior chest and in the axillary regions, is thought to be produced by peripheral pulmonary stenosis and disappears with time.

Pathologic murmurs are more intense (usually grade 2 to 3 or louder) and persist beyond the first days of life. The degree of urgency in obtaining chest radiograph, electrocardiogram, echocardiogram, and cardiac consultation is determined by the general status of the newborn. Procrastination during the first few days is acceptable and occasionally desirable, in the noncyanotic newborn with a murmur who has no respiratory distress, hypertension, arrhythmia, or signs of congestive failure. The murmurs in many such babies will disappear and unnecessary anxiety for the parents can be averted.

Examination of the Abdomen in the Neonate

The abdomen of the newborn infant is normally rounded in appearance, soft, and moves synchronously with the respiratory movements of the chest wall. Often in the hours immediately after birth, the abdomen may have a full appearance until the first meconium stool is passed.

Meconium is the tarry black material consisting of desquamated intestinal cells, intestinal secretions, and swallowed amniotic material present in the intestine prior to birth. Normally, the infant should not pass meconium until shortly after birth. In stressed situations, however, the baby may defecate prior to birth, introducing meconium into the amniotic cavity. This may lead to the meconium aspiration syndrome, one of the leading causes of neonatal respiratory distress.

Inspection of the newborn abdomen will reveal slightly prominent veins over the surface of the abdomen. Very prominent venous engorgement, however, suggests venous obstruction above the level of the portal system or peritonitis. The umbilical cord initially has a jellylike consistency (Wharton jelly) and consists of two umbilical arteries and a single umbilical vein. The cord should always be inspected for the number of arteries, as a single umbilical vessel may be associated with genitourinary anomalies. The umbilical cord normally begins to dry to a hard consistency within hours following delivery and separates from the skin within 20 days. Occasionally, a small glistening pearllike structure (umbilical granuloma) may be seen after the cord separates and cauterization of the granuloma with silver nitrate may be necessary. Continued secretion from the umbilical stump after treatment may be evidence of a patent urachus or a patent omphalomesenteric sinus.

Abdominal auscultation, if indicated as part of the examination, should usually be performed prior to palpation, since palpation will often alter the findings. Most commonly, one performs auscultation only when bowel obstruction is a concern. In the newborn, the cardinal signs of intestinal obstruction are abdominal distension, failure to pass meconium, and bilious vomiting. In auscultating for possible obstruction, one may hear other high-pitched bowel sounds occurring frequently, most often present with mechanical obstruction, or one may not hear any significant bowel sounds, commonly observed with an ileus, often related to septicemia. Bruits heard in the abdomen may be due to renal artery stenosis.

Palpation of the infant's abdomen should be done gently with the infant as relaxed as possible. Although possible while the baby is crying, the examination in such circumstances is usually less than optimal. Firm pressure is rarely necessary to palpate the most common abdominal lesions. In particular, the examiner should be concerned with the detection of any masses and, therefore, should examine all abdominal quadrants systematically. The most common intraabdominal masses in the newborn are related to the genitourinary tract, typically involving some form of obstructive uropathy, such as posterior urethral valves, cystic malformations of the renal system, or solid masses.

The liver is palpated at the right costal margin and in the neonate is usually found to be 1 to 2 cm below the costal margin. When one is palpating for liver enlargement, it is helpful to gently begin palpation of the right lower quadrant and gradually ascend until the liver margin is noted. It is never necessary to push deeply into the abdomen to find the liver edge unless massive ascites is also present. The consistency of the liver is noted at this time. A hard or nodular liver is distinctly abnormal and suggests intrinsic liver pathology. A firm or rubbery consistency usually indicates extrinsic pathology, such as congestive heart failure.

Palpation of the spleen is performed in a similar fashion, but on the left side of the abdomen. Splenic enlargement beyond 1 cm below the left costal margin is usually abnormal. In circumstances in which one might expect an enlarged spleen, caution should be exerted to avoid vigorous or frequent palpation which may result in splenic rupture or subcapsular hematoma.

One may often note during palpation that there is a separation of the musculature of the abdomen in the neonate in the midline. This is referred to as diastasis recti and may be associated with a circular umbilical hernia. A large umbilical hernia may be associated with congenital hypothyroidism.

In palpating the abdomen, one should always observe the reactions of the infant. Unlike the older child who can express pain, the neonate shows discomfort by resisting palpation, crying, or grimacing in response to touch.

When examining the abdomen, it is easy to turn the infant over to examine the back. One should inspect and then palpate for masses and unusual prominences. Tufts of hair, pilonidal sinus, soft lumps may indicate spina bifida occulta. Clinically evident spina bifida includes a meningocele, in which there is failure of fusion of the dorsum of the spine with protrusion of the meninges, or a myelomeningocele, in which neural elements are found as well.

Examination of the Genitourinary System

Examination of the genitourinary system begins with inspection. Male infants should have a phallus of at least 1-cm length and the urethra should open at the tip of the phallus. A urethral opening proximal to the end of the phallus is referred to as hypospadias. Hypospadias may occur in degrees: In first-degree hypospadias, the urethral opening is on the glans of the penis but proximal to the tip. Often, the foreskin is not completely developed and the penis has a curvature caudally, referred to as a chordee. In second-degree hypospadias, the urethral opening is along the shaft of the penis. In third-degree hypospadias, the urethral opening lies anywhere from the perineum to the base of the penis. Ultrasound or radiographic evaluation should always be performed in the child with second- or third-degree hypospadias to look for other genitourinary anomalies.

The scrotum should be pigmented, and rugae and median raphe should be readily visible. Testes should be easily palpable in the scrotum. Commonly in the older infant, the testes are retracted into the inguinal canal because of a brisk cremasteric reflex. One should be able to gently push the testes into the scrotum. Inability to find the testes or get them into the scrotum suggests undescended testicles. Scrotal enlargement, especially if it transilluminates, indicates a hydrocele and associated hernia. The hydrocele may be communicating or noncommunicating. A unilaterally cyanotic scrotum appearing shortly after birth is seen with intrauterine testicular torsion. Usually, it is painless for the neonate, but the testes can rarely be saved.

Inspection of the female genitalia is equally important in the newborn physical examination. In the full term female infant, the labia majora are large and completely enclose the labia minora. The labia are pigmented and often appear somewhat red and edematous, especially in the hours immediately following birth. The labia majora should be gently separated and the genitalia inspected. Often a white discharge is noted. In addition, some infants will have a blood-tinged discharge beginning on the second or third day of life that may persist for several days. This discharge occurs because of the withdrawal of hormones passed across the placenta during gestation.

The urethral and vaginal openings should be inspected. The vagina should not have any membrane covering its opening. Presence of a membrane may lead to hydrometrocolpos at a later time requiring minor surgical intervention.

The inguinal canals should be palpated in female infants as well as in male infants. The presence of a silk sign (see page 160) produced by gently rubbing the inguinal canal may be indicative of an indirect hernia. Hydrocele in the male and a prominence of the labia majora in the female are the usual signs of indirect hernia seen in affected infants.

Ambiguous genitalia may occur for many reasons in the newborn, and the appearance of the genitalia in such babies may vary significantly. Most commonly, congenital adrenal hyperplasia is the diagnosis for this anomaly of development. If the sex of the newborn is not readily determinable, the infant should be referred for an endocrinologic workup. This should include chromosomal analysis (karyotype). Presence of a labial mass in the phenotypically female infant may indicate a testis and maldevelopment of the genitalia.

The kidneys may be readily palpated in most infants by gentle deep palpation of the abdomen. Because of the presence of the liver on the right side of the abdomen, the right kidney is usually more easily felt. The kidney should be approximately 4 cm in the longest axis, with a rubbery consistency and a lobulated margin. Kidney enlargement is most often the result of lower urinary tract obstruction.

The female ovaries and uterus are accessible to palpation through the rectum. The rectal examination should be performed gently with the smallest finger. Ovarian enlargement may be due to a cyst or torsion, while uterine enlargement occurs with hydrometrocolpos.

The perianal area should be inspected as part of the genital examination. One should be sure of the patency of the anus and rectum. Often, a small fistula may be present that is confused with the anus in some forms of anal and rectal atresias. This fistula, through which feces may pass, is never found in the appropriate position, and in severe cases may connect to some organ of the genitourinary system.

Examination of the Musculoskeletal System

Examination of the newborn musculoskeletal system, together with the neurologic examination, provides the examiner with a great deal of information regarding the success or failure of intrauterine development. Certain features of the musculoskeletal system are readily apparent with even cursory examination. The limbs should be symmetrical and move spontaneously and equally in the appropriate directions. Unequal limb size is associated with congenital malformations, hemangiomas and lymphangiomas, and intrauterine positional anomalies. There should be the usual complement of the fingers and toes with no extra digits or fusion of digits (syndactly). Occasionally, one encounters familial inheritance of extra digits. These should be distinguished from skin tags that usually occur on the lateral aspect of the hands or feet and which contain no bones.

The nails should be examined. Ingrown-appearing toenails are commonly seen in newborns and appear imbedded deep within the skin. These simply grow out in time and require no therapy. Hypoplastic nails may be seen in many genetic syndromes.

One examination that is essential in the newborn examination is the examination of the hip joint. Although all joints should demonstrate proper degrees of flexion and mobility, dislocation of the hip, if not detected early, can lead to gait problems. The hip should be tested by the Barlow and Ortolani maneuvers (see page 72 and Fig. 6-14). The infant is placed in a supine position and the knees and hips are flexed at 90° angles. The examiner grasps the infant's thigh with the thumb over the femoral triangle and the forefinger positioned along the lateral shaft of the femur and greater trochanter. The hips are then abducted, internally rotated with a forward pressure with the forefinger on the greater trochanter. If there is difficulty with abduction or if the femoral head moves anteriorly during this maneuver one should suspect congenital dislocation of the hip. Asymmetry of the gluteal folds may also be seen in the congenital hip dislocation.

Infants delivered by breech extraction may often demonstrate positional abnormalities of an extreme degree that appear worrisome in the period immediately after birth. These usually resolve over the course of time with no therapy. Of more concern, however, is the child born with fixed contractures of the joints (arthrogryposis multiplex congenita). The etiology of this phenomenon is debated, but many of these infants will have significant associated neurologic problems.

Neurologic Evaluation of the Newborn

The neurologic evaluation of the newborn infant is one of the most critical parts of the neonatal examination. For most parents, once the sex of the infant has been learned and the baby has been found to have no major malformations, the next question relates to neurologic status. While the neurologic examination cannot predict the future, it can help to determine if development to that point has proceeded appropriately and if one may anticipate problems.

Certain aspects of the neurologic examination have already been described. Infant posture, sleep state, feeding, breathing, and cardiac status may all reflect the neurologic status of the baby. As a result, much has already been determined about the state of the central and autonomic nervous systems earlier in the examination. Performance of the neurologic examination may vary significantly over a relatively short period of time depending upon factors such as the sleep state or time since the last feeding. The optimal time to perform an examination is usually immediately prior to feeding. The infant is awake at that time and very responsive to environmental stimulation. Assessment is thus most accurate.

Level of consciousness should be assessed first. This may vary from a hyperalert state, often encountered in the first 24 hours of life to lethargy, stupor, or coma, which may accompany serious illness. Coma, with no response to stimuli whatsoever, fortunately is exceedingly rare and is usually indicative of profound neurologic injury.

Posture of the baby should be observed next. For full-term infants, the normal posture should be predominantly flexor, with arms and legs partially flexed while at rest. There should be symmetry between sides. Abnormalities of posture include frog-leg position (seen in hypotonic infants and in normal premature babies), opisthotonic posturing, and asymmetry of posture. More extensive neurologic evaluation is indicated with such findings. Muscle tone may be assessed at the same time, usually by performing maneuvers included in the Dubowitz assessment of gestational age (Fig 9-1).

Newborn infants should demonstrate spontaneous movement of all extremities. It is often difficult to determine whether movements are entirely normal. Jittery or tremulous movements may be seen in some entirely normal infants. These can, at times, be indistinguishable from seizures. Neonatal seizures may occur in many forms, ranging from classical tonic-clonic activity to lip-smacking, bicycling-like movement of the lower extremities, or apnea. Unusual movement patterns should be studied by electroencephalography.

The sensory system of the baby is difficult to assess since the neonate is entirely uncooperative. When one assesses for sensory loss, the primary sensation tested is superficial pain. The test is performed by pinprick evaluation at various dermatome levels. If the infant feels the stimuli, crying or grimacing is usually elicited. Withdrawal from pain stimulus is a local reflex phenomenon and does not necessarily indicate pain perception.

Cranial nerve evaluation (see also page 215*ff*) is difficult in evaluation of the neonate, but the major sensory and motor functions of these nerves can usually be assessed. Olfaction (cranial nerve I) is rarely tested because disturbances in olfaction are not easy to elicit in the infant.

Vision (cranial nerve II) can be tested by response to both bright light and the ability of the baby to follow a face or brightly colored object over an arc of approximately 60°. In addition, the second cranial nerve should be studied by ophthalmoscopic examination, with special attention to abnormalities of the optic disc. The remainder of the fundoscopic examination has been discussed previously.

Extraocular movement is controlled by cranial nerves III, IV, and VI, and can be assessed by observation of the infant in an upright position (see also page 220). Conjugate gaze and doll's- eye movements should be readily elicited. It is not uncommon, however, for some degree of disconjugate gaze to persist for as long as 6 months of life, especially immediately after sleep.

Cranial nerve V can be tested by pinprick over the area of the distribution of the trigeminal nerve, as well as by observing the ability of the infant to securely close the mouth during sucking. The facial nerve (VII) controls expression and its effects are readily seen during crying. Asymmetric crying facies may indicate a facial nerve injury.

The auditory component of the VIII cranial nerve can be tested only grossly by exposing the baby to loud sounds and observing the reaction, usually a startle response. If there is a question of the baby's ability to perceive sound, auditory-evoked potentials should be performed. The vestibular function confirmed by VIII nerve has already been tested with elicitation of the doll's-eye movements when the baby is held at arm's length and rotated from side to side.

Effective coordination of swallowing assesses nerves IX and X. Cranial nerve XII must function during effective sucking and milk expression as the tongue is necessary for this process. Cranial nerve XI can be observed by turning the infant's head to one side while restraining it at the opposite shoulder. One observes for muscle contraction of the sternocleidomastoid.

Testing of basic reflexes can usually be readily performed in the neonate with the use of a reflex hammer. If possible, this procedure should be carried out when the infant is at quiet rest. During crying, the reflexes tend to be dampened, as the child fights the examiner. Since most infants tend to have slightly increased tone, the reflexes tend to be somewhat brisk, especially at the antecubital fossa, the knee, and the Achilles tendon. Often, the plantar response appears to be extensor when elicited, but the large toe often can be noted to move in a flexor posture initially, then extend as the leg undergoes more of a withdrawal response to the stimulus.

"Primitive" reflexes (see page 248) are thought to represent adaptive behavior related in some way to man's evolution from more primitive ancestors. These reflexes include the Moro response, elicited by a startle or by a sudden movement of the infant by the examiner. The most common method is to elevate the head off the bed, cradling the occiput in the palm of the examiner. The head is then suddenly lowered several centimeters. The infant's hand should open and extend with subsequent abduction of the upper extremities. The lower extremities may also extend and a cry is often elicited. The Moro begins to appear at about 28-week gestation and should be complete at 37 weeks. It disappears by 4 months of age in most babies.

The palmar grasp is elicited by inserting a finger into the infant's palm and observing the contraction of the fingers around the digit. This reflex appears at 28 weeks, is well developed by 32-weeks gestation, and disappears at 2 to 3 months of age.

The asymmetric tonic neck response is seen when one rotates the baby's head to one side. This movement is accompanied by extension of the upper extremity on the side toward which the face is turned and flexion of the contralateral extremity and similar movements of the lower extremities. The term "fencing posture" is often used to describe this position. This reflex appears at 35-weeks gestational age, is greatest at about 1-month postnatal age, and disappears by 6 months of age.

The placing and stepping responses (involuntary walking) appear at about 35 to 36 weeks of gestation. The former is produced by touching the dorsum of the foot to the examining table and observing the movement of the foot as the infant places it on the surface. These disappear by 2 months of age (other neurodevelopmental reflexes are described in Chapter 7F, page 248).

A highly integrated central nervous system is necessary for these reflexes to be present. In testing for them, the examiner is ascertaining a basically intact neurologic development.

PHYSICAL EXAMINATION OF THE PREMATURELY BORN INFANT

The introduction of newborn intensive care units throughout the world during the past 2 decades has dramatically changed the approach to the preterm infant. Mechanical ventilation, intravenous alimentation techniques, improvement of thermal environment, and other advances in therapy have enabled the premature infant to survive conditions that used to be rapidly fatal until recently. At the same time, previously unknown diseases such as bronchopulmonary dysplasia, necrotizing enterocolitis, and retrolental fibroplasia have appeared. It is therefore essential that the practicing physician be familiar with the physical examination of the premature baby.

As described previously, the examination of the baby begins with the gestational age examination. In the case of the preterm infant, this practice is essential. Based upon weight and gestational age, premature infants can be divided into several groups:

- *Severe prematurity:* babies less than 1000 gm birthweight and 24 to 28 weeks gestational age.
- *Moderate prematurity:* 1000 to 2000 gm birthweight and 29 to 35 weeks gestational age.
- *Mild prematurity:* 2000 to 2500 gm birthweight and 35 to 37 weeks gestational age.

The separation of babies into these categories is valuable for several reasons. First, it enables the physician to deal with the critical questions of likelihood of survival and chances for intact survival. Secondly, the problems which each group of babies faces are somewhat different, and it thus prepares the examiner for the possibility of encountering those problems. For example, hyaline membrane disease will occur in approximately 50 percent of babies in the moderately premature group, but only 5 to 10 percent of mildly premature babies will have this syndrome. In contrast, the severely premature baby will not initially demonstrate hyaline membrane disease because the infant has minimal alveolar development. These infants instead will show pulmonary insufficiency of prematurity, a distinctly different clinical entity. One should note, however, that even these classifications of babies may not be completely adequate, since the moderately premature 1100-gm infant may be very different from the 1900-gm baby in that category. The premature examination will therefore be described in terms of progressive maturity and changes that can be expected from postconception.

General Appearance

The appearance of premature infants ("premies") is strikingly different from that of the term infant. Premies are scrawny with little fat deposition. Muscular tone is diminished. In many infants, severe respiratory distress is most prominent as the baby struggles to breathe with immature lungs. Activity is minimal if the baby has respiratory problems, and, even in the baby without respiratory disease, activity may consist of little more than myoclonic jerks. Cyanosis may be prominent; without immediate medical intervention, many babies cannot survive.

Skin

The skin of the very premature baby is shiny and translucent. Blood vessels may be readily apparent in the skin. As gestation proceeds, fat is deposited subcutaneously and skin keratinization increases so that the normal skin appearance is gradually developed. In the stages of early viability (24 to 26 weeks gestation) the skin is densely covered with lanugo, most prominent over the scalp, forehead, shoulders, and extremities. The lanugo recedes as the infant approaches term. Creases in the plantar surface of the feet are absent initially, again increasing with increase in the gestation period.

Premature babies often have ecchymoses and petechiae from blood extravasation into the skin during delivery. These findings are the result of sudden stresses on very fragile superficial skin vessels. Forceps marks may also be readily visible in the form of ecchymoses.

Head, Eyes, Ears, Nose, Mouth

The very immature infant has a fragile calvarium. With any period of nutritional deficiency, the calcification of the skull may be reduced to the point of easy indentation of the skull with very little pressure. Bruising soon after delivery is often prominent, as previously mentioned; molding is usually not substantial, since the head is relatively small compared to the size of the birth canal. Sutures should not be prominently split, although as the very premature infant grows, there may be some widening of sutures. Significant splitting, especially of the squamosal sutures, may indicate hydrocephalus.

The eyes of the premature infant are immature and difficult to examine. There is usually fusion of the lids until approximately 24 weeks gestational age, and the presence of fused lids is often used as a criterion for assessing approximate gestational age in the marginally viable baby. The examination of the anterior capsule of the lens is also used as a technique for assessing gestational age. The uveal tract may have membranous remnants present and the red reflex may be diminished by these findings (as well as the red blood cell concentration being lower than of the term infant). In addition, there may be some degree of lens opacification that usually clears by 32 weeks gestation. Examination for retrolental fibroplasia, which produces an aberrant vascularization of the retina that can lead to retinal detachment in the most severe forms, can only be seen by indirect ophthalmoscopy.

The ears of the preterm baby have varying degrees of cartilage present, increasing as the baby approaches maturity. Hearing is probably present even in the most immature infant.

The nose and mouth are examined as described in the section on the term infant.

Chest and Lungs

The chest wall is very compliant in the very premature infant and does not serve its normal function of acting as a fixed strut against which the muscles of respiration can act. As a result, breathing is much less effective in the premature baby, with the result that atelectasis often occurs over the course of time, often accompanied by apnea. This entity is referred to as pulmonary insufficiency of prematurity. On physical examination these babies will be noted to have marked respiratory effort (assuming that they are not apneic), dramatic sternal retractions and intercostal retractions, and, often, cyanosis. Breath sounds will be greatly diminished and barely audible at times, since little of the tidal volume enters the lungs. Often intubation and mechanical ventilation is necessary. This problem usually affects babies who are less than 1000 gm birthweight.

The slightly more mature infant, usually of a birthweight ranging from 1000 to 2500 gm, also is often beset by respiratory difficulties. These babies commonly have hyaline membrane disease. This syndrome, due to surfactant deficiency, results in several characteristic physical findings: tachypnea, nasal flaring, marked sternal and intercostal retraction, and cyanosis. Of interest is the audible grunting sound made at end-expiration by these babies in an attempt to maintain lung volume.

Heart

The cardiac examination is essentially identical to the examination of the more mature infant. One must be careful not to forget that heart disease can occur in the premature baby, an error of omission that occurs occasionally when faced with apparent pulmonary disease. At times, especially in the mildly immature infant, the distinction between cardiac and pulmonary disease is not made readily. A test which is helpful in such instances is the hyperoxia test. The infant is placed in 100 percent oxygen for a 5 minute period of time and an arterial blood gas is obtained. If the PaO_2 is greater than 100 torr, the likelihood of cardiac disease involving a right-to-left shunt is small, since significant bypassing of the lungs would be incompatible with blood oxygenation to that degree. Thus, a PaO_2 above 100 torr when the baby is in 100 percent oxygen most commonly indicates lung disease.

The entity most commonly associated with premature infants is a patent ductus arteriosus. Clinically, this problem appears on the 3rd or 4th day of life, when the premature infant with respiratory distress syndrome has begun to improve. Suddenly, the child may deteriorate and become cyanotic, develop apnea, and show decreased skin perfusion. Peripheral pulses become prominent and bounding in quality. A loud systolic murmur that begins after the first heart sound and ends prior to the second heart sound may be noted. The murmur occasionally extends into diastole, but is not usually "machinery-like" as in adults. The liver may rapidly enlarge and the heart rate may increase substantially to 180 to 200 beats per minute. Medical or surgical treatment may be required quickly.

Abdomen

The abdominal examination proceeds as in the term infant. Because of diminished musculature, the organs are often easily palpable. Physical findings, which often cause much concern in this age group include abdominal distension, prominent loops of bowel, decreased bowel sounds, feeding intolerance and residuals of the previous feeding being present in the stomach, vomiting, and bloody diarrhea. This constellation of signs is associated with necrotizing enterocolitis, a severe and devastating disease of the immature baby.

Genitalia

The genitalia of premature infants undergo dramatic changes with gestation, and, as a result, are used in the gestational age examination to help quantitate maturity. Otherwise, examination is the same as for the older neonate.

Neuromuscular

The neuromuscular examination of the preterm infant comprises a major portion of the gestational age examination. As a result, it need not be recounted here. In general, there is a rapid progressive increase in neuromuscular tone throughout gestation that is clearly reflected in the previously detailed section (see page 275).

Certain types of behavior in the preterm infant often raise unnecessary concern and should be noted. Sudden twitching movements involving all extremities (myoclonic jerks) or tremulousness of single extremities are often thought of as seizures. In fact, most often these are normal types of activity that simply reflect an immature, poorly myelinated central nervous system. True seizure activity in this age group is often extremely subtle and may range from no clinically apparent signs to cyclic flexing of a digit or extremity, lip-smacking or repetitive mouthing movements, yawning, apnea, or autonomic instability. If any questions exist about the nature of any such behavior, an electroencephalogram should be performed.

The single most devastating problem for the premature baby, however, is intraventricular hemorrhage. These infants may suddenly deteriorate with apnea, cyanosis, and autonomic instability. The anterior fontanel may become firm and prominent, and the sutures may split widely. An ultrasound or CT examination will confirm the diagnosis. Hydrocephalus may ensue either acutely or weeks later. The hydrocephalus may first manifest itself by splitting of suture lines and rapidly increasing head circumference.

BIBLIOGRAPHY

Apgar VA: A proposal for a new method of evaluation of the newborn infant. Anesth Analg 32:260, 1953.

Avery GB: Neonatology. Philadelphia, Lippincott, 1981.

Dubowitz LM, Dubowitz V, Goldberg C: Clinical assessment of gestational age in the newborn infant. J Pediatr 77:1, 1970.

Fanaroff AA, Martin RJ: Behrman's Neonatal-Perinatal Medicine. St. Louis, Mo., C. V. Mosby, 1983.

Harrison H: The Premature Baby Book. New York, St. Martin's Press, 1983.

Oski FA, Naiman JL: Anemia in the Neonatal Period. In: Hematologic Problems in the Newborn. Philadelphia, Saunders, 1982, pp 56–86.

Phibbs RH: Evaluation of the Newborn. In: Rudolph AM (ed.): Pediatrics. Norwalk, Conn., Appleton-Century-Crofts, 1982, p. 123.

Ziai M, Clarke TA, Merritt TA: Assessment of the Newborn. Boston, Little, Brown, 1984.

CHAPTER 10

Examination of the Adolescent

Youth Is a Disease that Time Cures:
Goethe

Insanity Is Inherited—You Get It from Your Teenagers:
Bumper Sticker

Adolescence is the metamorphic period from which the callow child emerges as a mature adult. It would seem logical that pediatricians, whose careers are tethered to monitoring the progressive changes of childhood, continue patient care through those maturational stages; but, prior to the pioneer studies of Dr. Roswell Gallagher, pediatricians treated only those adolescents whose physical maturation occurred in the preteen years. In contemporary pediatrics, however, care of the adolescent has become a recognized subspecialty. The concerns are unique and the relationships different than with children, but the need to recognize orderly progression of developmental processes is analogous.

Much of the published work during the 35 years since the first appearance of Gallagher's work relates to social, behavioral, psychologic, and physiologic problems. This chapter will emphasize the distinctive features of the adolescent physical examination, the changes associated with growth and maturation. We will describe the body in its transition. Most of the descriptions earlier in this book also are applicable to the adolescent, so the "systems" sections of this chapter should be read in conjunction with the similar "system" section in the appropriate earlier chapter.

APPROACHING THE EXAMINATION

The adolescent, weaning from attachments to childhood, may feel ambivalence about the examination, and the parents also may have doubts as to whether their teenager should continue with the pediatrician or move on to an "older doctor" (pediatricians never seem to get "older"). The need for roots, however, and the confidence engendered in a long-standing, nonjudgmental relationship can establish a foundation for most satisfactory interaction. The pediatrician needs fine-tuned sensitivity to make patient and parents comfortable—with each other, with the doctor, and with their presence in the office.

A "teenage" waiting area, partially partitioned from the toys and games of the section used by younger children and with appropriate reading material, can be helpful. Examining tables of adequate size and availability of stirrups for pelvic examination are also important.

The decision as to whether a parent should be present in the examining room should be determined by the patient and parent. The physician should broach the question of the parent's presence but not resolve it, unless asked to do so.

The examination is an anxiously anticipated occasion for the teenager, so it is essential that the doctor maintain conversation directed to the mechanics and nature of what is being done, the normal physiologic findings, and complete discussion of any abnormality. After the patient has dressed, time should be allotted for discussion, preferably in a relaxed consultation room. Conference should be held first with the teenager alone for review of the examination and an opportunity for a private, confidential exchange. The parent can then be invited to join in a three-way talk.

HISTORY TAKING

The taking of a history should be directed toward the patient. The parent, if present, may feel free to interject or remind. Insight can be gained into the relationship between the two by observing how frequent and how appropriate is the parent's contribution.

History taking can be informal but should be meticulous. It can be introduced casually and continued during the course of the examination, with questioning related to the area of the body or the organ system being examined.

History to be explored that is particularly appropriate for the adolescent includes: rate of growth, development of secondary sexual characteristics, onset and regularity of menstruation, weight gain or loss, appetite, sleep patterns, energy levels, peer and family relationships, school and work activities, academic satisfaction, skin blemishes, recurrent sore throat, recurrent chest or abdominal or head pain, awareness of skipped or rapid heart beat, extremity pain or swelling, genital discomfort or discharge, and presence of tumors or growths or "swollen glands."

Much can be learned about the patient's personality, self-image, and relationships during the history-taking process. Do they seem self-confident? Depressed? Hostile? Articulate? Do they look at the examiner or avoid eye contact? Can they speak frankly and openly? Do they have unexpressed fears regarding health? For themselves? Their families? Their friends? Why? Careful communication with the patient can provide clues as to the possible origin of such symptoms as chest or abdominal pain or headache. All complaints should be listened to seriously and evaluated carefully.

A common complaint is that of being "tired," of just not having much energy. Careful history taking may reveal that the patient is in tenth grade, growing rapidly, taking a full academic load, worried about college entrance exams, playing in the school band, on the basketball team, working at a part-time job some evenings and weekends: trying to do more than the body is capable of doing.

There should be an opportunity to discuss sexuality, smoking, alcohol, and drug use, best done during private, confidential time with the patient. The parent can be included, without breaching confidentiality, if the patient so requests or if the parent wants a "referee" for an ongoing dispute.

GROWTH

Adolescence is a time of very rapid growth. The average female grows about 9 inches (22 cm) between the ages of 10 and 14 years; the average male, about 13 inches (33 cm) between 11 and 17 years. At each percentile, from 5 through 95, the absolute height increments are about the same during those ages. Height measurements should be taken with the patient standing erect, feet together, barefoot, stomach held in, chest out, and spine straightened.

The average female gains about 38 pounds (18 kg) and the average male 60 pounds (27 kg) during those same time frames (see stature and weight charts, Figs. 6-18, 6-19, 6-22, and 6-23, pages 76, 77, 80, and 81). Weight should be measured on an accurately calibrated scale, preferably of the balance type. For consistency and comparability, the patient should always be weighed while wearing only underclothing. Skin fat can be documented with calipers designed for that purpose (see page 80).

The most rapid periods of growth occur in the year or two prior to menarche in the female (at about Tanner Stage III) and between Tanner Stages III and IV in the male (see below). Most females grow only an additional 2 to 5 cm after menarche and have completed their growth by the time they have been menstruating 2 years. For the male, markers for the end point of growth are not as well-defined, though the transition from Tanner Stage IV to Stage V (below) is a good physical diagnostic end point. Physiologically, growth ends with the closure of the skeletal epiphyses.

Girls begin and end their growth spurt at an earlier chronologic age than boys. As a result, at about eighth grade (or about age 13), the average female is taller than the average male, a predicament which may be embarrassing to the tall girl or the short boy. By tenth grade (age 15), this is remedied; most females have just about achieved their final height, while most males are heavily into their growth spurt and have outgrown their female counterparts.

A normal child may shoot up to a higher percentile or lag back to a lower one during the growth spurt. The patient who achieves sexual maturation early may seem quite tall as a 14-year-old boy or as an 11-year-girl. They may stop growing, however, at these early ages and be passed in physical stature by most of their peers. Any attempt at making a prediction of ultimate height during adolescence must take into consideration the stage of sexual maturation and the skeletal epiphyseal development.

Many adolescent concerns are related to height and weight. A physician who is a careful listener and observer can work with the patient to understand realistic height potential and to establish weight objectives compatible with the patient's concerns and health.

DEVELOPMENT OF PRIMARY SEXUAL CHARACTERISTICS

The unique features of adolescence and, indeed, a definition for the period are the striking changes of sexual maturation which mark the transition from the prepubertal state to adulthood. The primary characteristics are best described with relation to growth of the breasts in females, the genitals in males, and the development of pubic hair in both. The secondary characteristics relate to body shape, hair, and growth velocity and are discussed in other sections of this chapter. The hormonal changes that govern sexual maturation are discussed beautifully in a number of the listed references. We will describe only the observable physical features.

The work by Marshall and Tanner in England, first published in the late 1960s, has become the standard with which all discussion of the sexual maturation of adolescence begins. They established criteria, which have been modified only slightly over the years, for staging the phases of primary sexual development (Tables 10-1, 10-2, and 10-3). The tables include means and ranges for the first appearance of each of the stages. Failure to attain Stage II by the upper age of the second standard deviation may be defined as pubertal delay. Figure 10-1 allows for understanding of normal stages of breast development. Testicular development in the male or breast enlargement in the female almost always precede the appearance of pubic hair.

Marked disparities in the sequences of staging, particularly if accompanied by disturbances in stature or weight, awaken suspicion for unusual endocrinologic abnormalities. As examples, the presence of significant amounts of pubic hair for a length of time in the male, without the ex-

TABLE 10-1. MALE GENITAL DEVELOPMENT

Stage		Age at Onset Mean	Age at Onset Range (± 2SD)
I	Preadolescent. Testes, scrotum and penis are of about the same size and proportion as in early childhood.	—	—
II	Early enlargement of scrotum and testes. Skin of scrotum reddens and changes in texture. Little or no enlargement of penis.	11.64	9.50–13.78
III	Enlargement of penis, at first mainly in length. Further growth of testes and scrotum.	12.85	10.77–14.93
IV	Increasing length and breadth of penis and glans size. Pigmentation of scrotal skin. Enlarging testes and scrotum.	13.77	11.73–15.81
V	Adult size and shape of genitalia.	14.92	12.72–17.12

(Reproduced with permission and modified, after Rosenfeld RG: Pediatrics in Review, 4:176, 1982. Copyright American Academy of Pediatrics, 1982.)

pected changes in the genitalia, may be associated with Klinefelter syndrome or with an excessive degree of adrenal androgen secretion. Although breast development usually begins before the appearance of pubic hair in the female, a patient with stage V breasts and no pubic hair should be evaluated for the possibility of testicular feminization syndrome. On the other hand, a female who has had pubic hair for a considerable length of time and no breast development may have a failure of gonadal hormone

TABLE 10-2. FEMALE BREAST DEVELOPMENT

Stage		Age at Onset Mean	Age at Onset Range (± 2SD)
I	Preadolescent. Elevation of papillae only.	—	—
II	Breast bud stage; elevation of breast as a small mound. Widening and elevation of areola, with pigmentation of areola.	11.15	8.95–13.25
III	Further enlargement and elevation of breast and areola, with no separation of their contours.	12.15	9.97–14.33
IV	Projection of areola and papilla to form a secondary mound above the level of the breast.	13.11	10.81–15.31
V	Mature stage; projection of papilla only, due to recession of the areola to the general contour of the breast.	15.33	11.85–18.81

(Reproduced with permission and modified after Rosenfeld RG: Pediatrics in Review, 4:177, 1982. Copyright, American Academy of Pediatrics, 1982.)

TABLE 10-3. MALE AND FEMALE PUBIC HAIR

Stage		Age at Onset			
		Male		*Female*	
		Mean	Range (± 2SD)	Mean	Range (± 2SD)
I	Preadolescent. No pubic hair.	—	—	—	—
II	Sparse growth of long, slightly pigmented downy hair, straight or slightly curled, at base of penis, or along labia or mons.	13.4	11.2–15.6	11.7	9.3–14.1
III	Darker, coarser, more curled. Spread sparsely over the pubis or mons.	13.9	11.9–16.0	12.4	10.2–14.6
IV	Adult-type hair, more abundant. Still limited to pubis or mons. No spread to thighs.	14.4	12.2–16.5	13.0	10.8–15.1
V	Adult in quality, quantity, and distribution with spread to medial aspect of thighs. Spread up linea alba occurs later (?Stage VI).	15.2	13.0–17.3	14.4	12.2–16.7

(Reproduced with permission and modified after Rosenfeld RG: Pediatrics in Review, 4:177, 1982. Copyright, American Academy of Pediatrics, 1982.)

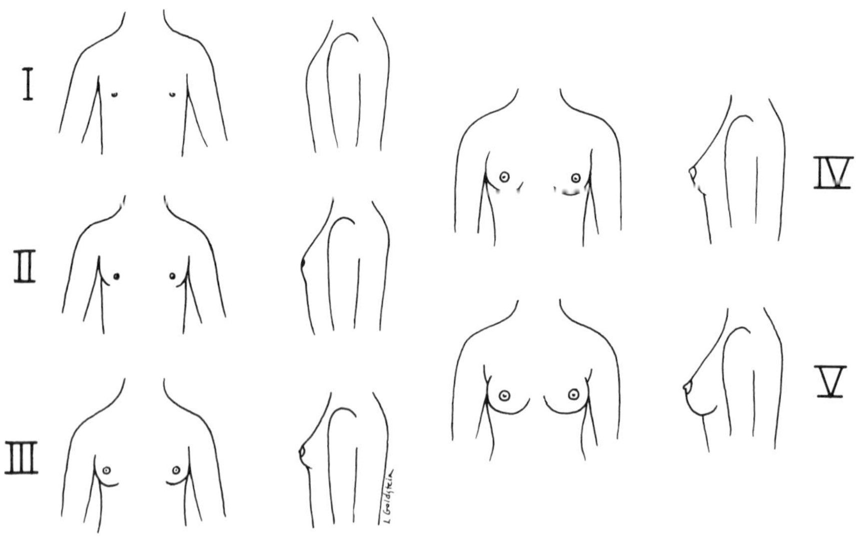

Figure 10-1. Stages of breast development. *(After Marshall and Tanner.)*

TABLE 10-4. PERCENTAGE OF PATIENTS IN STAGES I THROUGH V AT MENARCHE

Stage	Breast (%)	Pubic Hair (%)
I	0	1
II	1	4
III	26	19
IV	62	63
V	11	14

(Reproduced with permission from Marshall WA, Tanner JM: Variations in Patterns of Pubertal Changes in Girls. Arch Dis Child 44:291, 1969.)

secretion. Normal development usually proceeds in an orderly fashion, following the approximate sequences suggested in the tables.

The average age for menarche for the American female is about 12.6 years, slightly earlier for black, slightly later for white. Menarche usually occurs at Tanner Stage III or later (Table 10-4). Rarely, however, it can occur before the appearance of any significant development of primary characteristics. Primary amennorhea may be defined as failure of menarche by the 17th birthday. There are regional and geographic variations, and local norms should be used where available and applicable.

SKIN AND HAIR (see also Chapter 7D)

Acne vulgaris is the physiologic price adolescents pay for transition through the stages of sexual development. Androgenically induced, it is generally more common and more severe in the male, but it does appear to a greater or lesser extent in close to 100 percent of teenagers. The lesions involve the sebaceous follicles and can be referred to, in order of increasing severity, as comedones (whiteheads and blackheads), papules, pustules, nodules, and cysts. Resolution is accompanied by transient redness and hyperpigmentation. Scarring may ensue from the more severe pustular, nodular, and cystic lesions. The most common and disturbing site is the face, where it is estimated there are 15,000 to 20,000 sebaceous glands. Other affected areas are the chest, back, and shoulders.

Impetigo is characterized by clusters of lesions, about 0.5 to 3.0 cm in diameter, varying in appearance from bullous to abraded purulence to crusted. These are caused by skin infection and are most commonly found in intertriginous areas—axillae, intergluteal, groin—but may occur on any skin surface.

Red to purplish plaquelike, *discoid* lesions, with scaling, prominent capillaries, and areas of atrophy may be signs of lupus erythematosus. These can be found on any skin area, most commonly the face and upper extremities, and are usually asymmetrical.

Nevi increase in number during adolescence. Compound nevi are flesh-colored to brown, smooth to warty in contour. Intradermal nevi are nonpigmented through brown to black, dome-shaped to pedunculated, usually less than 1 cm in diameter, and may occur anywhere on the skin surface. Malignant melanomas are thick, irregular, nodular, and deeply pigmented. They are extremely rare in adolesence, but rapid changes in growth, pigmentation, or ulceration of a dark nevus should be regarded suspiciously.

Striae are shallow, linear, parallel-oriented, slightly depressed lesions, which are pink initially and later become white. They occur where the skin has been "stretched" because of rapid growth, particularly the lower abdomen, upper thighs, and female breasts.

A number of circular-to-ovoid, macular-to-slightly raised lesions, localized on the trunk and extremities, occur with increased frequency in late childhood and adolescence. *Pityriasis rosea* (Fig. 7D-3) presents as oval lesions, flat to slightly raised, pink to brown, peripherally scaled, distributed mostly on the trunk with the long axis parallel to the lines of cleavage, giving a "Christmas tree" appearance. Rarely, the distribution is reversed, with predominance on the extremities and face. The "herald patch" that precedes the major outbreak of pityriasis can be confused with *Tinea Corporis.* The latter consists of one or more well-defined ovoid scaly patches with clear centers, but a spreading border which may be papular or vesicular. *Tinea Versicolor* consists of oval, macular lesions with superficial scaling, distributed mostly over the upper trunk, arms, and neck and frequently confluent. The lesions tend to be hypopigmented and, as a result, more prominent by contrast in the summer when the surrounding skin is tanned; in winter; the lesions are darker and colored tan to brown.

Body hair becomes widely distributed during adolescence. Facial, extremity, chest, axillary, and perianal hair appear under androgenic stimulation, and therefore more profusely in the male. Excessive growth of body hair in the female is hirsutism and may be physiologic or suggestive of excessive androgen-producing or insufficient estrogen endocrinologic abnormalities (Cushing, polycystic ovary syndrome). Children who have blond-colored hair in early childhood tend to darken somewhat. Look for premature greying or whitening of the hair, particularly of the scalp (early sign of thyroid disease; associated with pernicious anemia, vitiligo, neurofibromatosis, Waardenburg syndrome). Early hair loss may be physiologic as in premature balding, or associated with fungal skin infection or alopecia areata.

The *Nails* should be inspected carefully for clubbing (see p. 71) and for loosening (onycholysis—tetracycline reaction; trauma).

EENT (see also Chapter 7A)

Eyes (see p. 100)

Visual acuity should be checked with an eye chart or electric projector; myopia and astigmatism may manifest during this period. Prominent, bulging eyeballs (exophthalmos) should be noted as unilateral (retroorbital tumor or cellulitis) or bilateral (thyrotoxicosis). Eye muscle patterns should be examined and nystagmus evaluated. When indicated, fields should also be checked. A painful, photophobic, tearing, red eye with a small pupil and no purulent discharge should arouse suspicion of uveitis (juvenile rheumatoid arthritis, sarcoidosis, trauma). The optic nerve should always be examined through the ophthalmoscope for cupping and elevation (tumor, pseudotumor cerebri, drusen).

Ears (see p. 108)

The ear canal becomes angulated, so the drums are best visualized by pulling the lobe out from the skull and upwards, thereby straightening the canal. The canal is wider and, if not occluded by cerumen or increased growth of hair, the drum should be easily visualized. The malleus is readily visible through the translucent drum; the incus and stapes, less so. The continuity of the pars flaccida (superior to the short process of the malleus) should be checked for a cystlike accumulation (cholesteatoma). A particularly shiny normal short process may be mistaken for cholesteatoma, as may areas of scarring from old infections or from previously removed ventilatory tubes (tympanosclerosis).

Hearing should be evaluated, either crudely with a ticking watch, or preferably with audiometric screening.

Nose (see p. 107)

The external surface of the nostril becomes more prominent, somewhat broader. Frequently, a protuberance develops at the junction of the cartilaginous and bony parts.

The mucous membranes overlying the turbinates should be examined for continuity, discoloration, and congestion. Persistent watery congestion and grayish discoloration, particularly if accompanied by edema and venous congestion of the skin below the orbits, suggests allergy; pedunculated protrusions of edematous hyperplastic mucosa are polyps, almost always allergic in origin. Congestion with ulceration should arouse suspicion of drug snorting. Unilateral congestion, particularly if purulent, suggests foreign body.

Teeth

In normal occlusion, the upper teeth slightly overlap the lower, with upper and lower incisors, cuspids, and molars in appropriate contact. The teeth interdigitate to allow satisfactory closure.

The second permanent molars erupt in early adolescence; the third begin erupting in the late teens.

NECK (see p. 96)

Enlargement and protrusion of the thyroid cartilage, along with the hyoid bone and cricoid cartilage, occur on either side of the midline of the anterior neck and are associated with the deepening voice of adolescence. The thyroid gland, overlying the cartilage, may become visible. It is best seen from in front and can be better visualized by having the patient swallow. Palpation for swelling, tenderness, and consistency should be performed carefully from the front and the back. Feel for enlargement of a single lobe or of the entire gland and for discrete nodules (Hashimoto thyroiditis, thryrotoxicosis, adenocarcinoma, benign goiter).

LYMPHATICS

Lymph nodes of less than 1 cm commonly are palpable in the neck, axillae, and groin areas. They are moderately firm, round to slightly ovoid, and usually nontender.

Tender nodes larger than 1 cm should be investigated for an infectious origin. Nodes of 2 to 4 cm in the anterior and posterior cervical area, but also occurring in other lymph node groups, and accompanied by shaggy gray exudative tonsillitis and splenomegaly, may be due to Epstein-Barr virus (infectious mononucleosis). Tender nodes mostly confined to the anterior cervical or submental chains are related to pharyngitis or stomatitis (*Streptococcus,* mycoplasma, coxsackie) or to dental disease. Tender or fluctuant nodes occurring in other areas also drain local sources of infection or inflammation. Matted nodes with doughy consistency suggest tuberculous infection.

Though infection or inflammation is by far the most common cause of lymph node enlargement, nontender nodes, particularly in the neck, persisting at a size greater than 1.5 cm for longer than a few weeks or enlarging rapidly before that time, should be considered suspiciously as possible malignant lymphoma (Hodgkin, non-Hodgkin). The incidence of the former increases strikingly during adolescence, the latter just prior to adolescence.

BREASTS

The areola of the male breast develops in a manner similar to the female up to Tanner Stage II. Small (1 to 3 cm), round, cystlike lesions, tender to pressure, directly underlying the nipple are breast buds. They are physiologic and disappear later in puberty. An excess of tissue (gynecomastia) is usually physiologic and can be a source of embarrassment.

After having evaluated the female breast for Tanner staging (Fig. 10-1 and Table 10-2), palpate for masses by compressing breast tissue between the examining fingers. Start centrally and proceed circumferentially to the periphery. Unilateral, small cystlike lesions under the nipple are breast buds, as in the male, and should not be confused with tumor. Multiple masses or bilateral masses in the breast tissue are likely to represent hypertrophy. A unilateral, firm, rubbery mass in an outer quadrant may be tumor, almost always a benign fibroadenoma or cyst. Malignancy is extremely rare under the age of 20.

Marked asymmetry in breast size may be related to chest deformity secondary to scoliosis or to distortion caused by previous chest or cardiac surgery. It may occur rarely without an explanation.

Compression of the female nipple and subareolar tissue ("milking") may elicit excretion of a white discharge (galactorrhea), the presence of which may be normal, but may be a sign of hypothyroidism, prolactin-secreting tumor, or drug administration (diazepam, tricyclic antidepressants).

CARDIOPULMONARY (see also Chapter 7B)

Chest

The chest wall in the adolescent has a transverse configuration, with the lateral diameter greater than the anterior-posterior. A rounded chest wall may be secondary to chronic respiratory obstruction (asthma, emphysema, pulmonary hypertension).

Unilateral bulging of the wall may be related to scoliosis. Localized anterior bulging may be a result of long-standing ventricular enlargement (left parasternal bulge, right ventricle; left midclavicular to midaxillary, more likely left ventricle). Visible rocking pulsations of the anterior chest are associated with intracardiac shunting or aortic regurgitation.

Palpable pulsations of the intercostal arteries at the lower rib margins, best felt over the back with the patient leaning forward, are due to collateral circulation (coarctation of aorta). These may also be heard, as to-and-fro murmurs.

The degree of chest expansion can be derived by measuring chest circumference during both peak expiration and peak inspiration, using a conventional tape and measuring at the fourth intercostal space, and subtracting the difference between the two measurements. Normal values for adolescent boys is 7.0 cm (range 3 to 11 cm) and for girls 5.5 cm (range 2.5 to 9.0 cm). Markedly diminished expansion occurs in chronic pulmonary disease and neuromuscular diseases.

A history of pain in the chest should be studied with careful cardiopulmonary evaluation but, in the adolescent, usually proves to be of tension or stress origin (psychosomatic).

Pulmonary (see p. 133)

Respirations normally are regular, shallow, and not accompanied by rib retraction. The rate is about 12 to 20 respirations per minute.

Expiratory wheeze, bronchospasm, and retraction may appear during or following exercise (exercise-induced asthma).

"Attacks" or "spells" of rapid or intermittent deep breathing, may be associated with chest pain, palpitations, numbing, tingling, air hunger, and occasionally loss of consciousness (psychogenic hyperventilation syndrome, salicylism, organic CNS disease).

Cardiovascular (see p. 136)

Blood pressure (Chapter 6, p. 86) needs to be measured as part of every physical examination. For most adolescents, a 12-cm cuff is appropriate. In obese patients and for measurements in the lower extremities, an 18-cm cuff may be necessary. A mercury manometer is more accurate than an aneroid and is adequate for most purposes. For extreme accuracy, electronic devices based on the Doppler principle are available.

Every patient should have blood pressure taken in both arms at least one time, in a search for marked differences between the two upper extremities (aortic root, subclavian, or innominate anomalies). Lower extremity pressures should also be taken at least once; systolic pressure should be 10 to 40 mm higher than the upper extremity (otherwise, think of coarctation of the aorta).

Normal values for both male and female are graphed in Figures 6-26 and 6-27. Systolic pressure over the 90th percentile associated with normal diastolic pressure in an otherwise well patient may be related to the anxiety and stress of the examination process and should be rechecked on several occasions under relaxed conditions. Diastolic pressure over the 90th percentile, confirmed on several readings, should be studied (cardiac, renal, endocrinologic, metabolic). Pressures below the 5th percentile may be physiologic (familial, highly conditioned athletes) or abnormal (Addison, shock).

The *pulse* (Chapter 6, p. 85) is best palpable just medial to the distal radius proximal to the base of the first metacarpal (radial artery). It should also be palpated at other sites: the groin (femoral), foot (dorsalis pedis), neck (carotid).

Pulse volume is the difference in force between the maximal and minimal expansion of the pulsation and correlates with the pulse pressure, which is the difference between systolic and diastolic blood pressure (bounding in aortic regurgitation; weak in shock).

The rate during adolescence should be between 65 and 110. Slower rates may be quite normal in highly conditioned athletes (sinus bradycardia), but careful simultaneous palpation and auscultation of the heart should be performed to determine dropped beats. The pulse rate may be extremely rapid and regular (over 190) with the patient at rest (supraventricular tachycardia; atrial flutter with regular A-V block) or in shock (ventricular tachycardia).

A regularly irregular pulse that slows during expiration and picks up during inspiration is sinus arrhythmia, a normal variant common in early adolescence. A regularly irregular pulse with normal rate may be ventricular contractions at regular intervals (bigeminy, trigeminy). An irregularly irregular pulse with good volume and normal rate may represent inconsistent premature ventricular contractions. An irregularly irregular pulse with weakened pulse volume is found in fibrillation or in atrial flutter with inconsistent A-V block.

Heart Auscultation (Chapter 7B, p. 139) may be more difficult because of the thickened chest wall. Nevertheless, Hoffmann, in Rudolph's *Pediatrics,* describes five innocent murmurs, one or more of which may be detected easily in 15 to 20 percent of adolescents. The three systolic innocent murmurs are: (1) *Still,* midsystolic and vibratory, best heard at the apex and lower left sternal border; (2) *basal ejection,* midsystolic and high pitched, best heard at the upper right or left sternal border; and (3) *carotid bruit,* early systolic and high pitched, best heard above the clavicles. In addition, there are two continuous murmurs: (1) *venous hum,* low pitched and unrelated in timing to the cardiac cycle, heard under the clavicle and in the neck; and (2) *mammary souffle,* heard over the breasts of pregnant or lactating females.

ABDOMEN AND GENITALIA (see also Chapter 7C)

Abdomen (see p. 151)

The musculature enclosing the abdominal cavity in the teenager is thicker and the adjacent bones heavier. Examination of the abdominal and retroperitoneal contents is therefore more difficult.

The liver and spleen normally are not palpable, except that in an asthenic individual it may be possible to feel the edge of a normal liver. A normal-sized kidney is not palpable. A suprapubic mass, palpated on both sides of the midline, is likely to be distended bladder, but the possibility of it being a pregnant uterus should be considered in postpubertal females.

Hernia (see p. 159) is found more commonly in males. It presents usually as a soft scrotal mass, possibly containing intestine with an inclusive fluid and gas mixture. The mass usually is easily reducible by gently squeezing the sac and its contents back into the abdominal cavity with the patient in either an erect or, preferably, supine position. In the female, the mass may present intralabially. Incarceration is uncommon in adolescence.

A femoral presentation, below the inguinal ligament, is uncommon. Hydroceles, with their clear transillumination, first appearing in adolescence, are usually traumatic or secondary to inflammation.

Rectal examination (see p. 165) should be performed in any patient with a history of passage of bright red blood per rectum or in whom there is suspicion of undefined abdominal or retroperitoneal pathology. With the patient either in a left lateral or a supine position, use a rubber or disposable glove or finger cot properly lubricated. On external inspection of the anus, look for dilated vessels containing clots and covered with mucous membranes (hemorrhoids), linear cuts at the mucous membrane–cutaneous junction (fissures), mucous-membrane-covered pedunculated masses (polyps), skin tags, pinworms, and skin eruptions (impetigo, herpes, verrucae, fungus). Multiple fissuring, herpetic vesicles, purulent discharge, or condylomata may be related to sodomization. After inspection, insert a finger gently and slowly. Get a sense of the perianal muscle tone. Feel within the rectum for internal hemorrhoids and polyps. Use the finger to explore the perirectal area for masses—retroperitoneal sarcoma, enlarged nodes. The appendix can be palpated on the right at the distal cecum; tender, of course, in appendicitis. Bimanual palpation, with the fingers of the opposite hand on the external surface of the abdomen, can be helpful in better defining organs, masses, and areas of inflammation. In the male, palpate the prostate anteriorly for tenderness and to help elicit urethral discharge for culture; prostatic tumor is rare in adolescence. In the female, palpate the cervix for tenderness and feel the body of the uterus bimanually for enlargement or tenderness; palpate the adnexal area for ovarian masses and for tubal tenderness or enlargement (ectopic pregnancy).

Genitalia (see p. 160)

Male: The penis grows during adolescence from the average prepubertal length of about 5 to 6 cm to the average adult range of about 8 to 16 cm. Testicular volume can be measured, and direct readings obtained in milliliters, by use of the Prader orchiometer. The average adult volume is about 20 ml. The diameter of the prepubertal testes, measured including the scrotal skin, is about 2.0 × 1.5 cm; at Tanner Stage IV, the average testis has enlarged to about 3.5 × 2.5 cm, with the longer axis vertical. The left testis is usually slightly lower than the right. Malignant tumors of the testes are firm, almost rock hard, and are incorporated within the testicular mass. A small slightly firm mass, adherent to but not attached to, the upper pole of the testes is the epididymis. The spermatic cord may be palpated between the upper lateral pole and the external inguinal ring; in torsion of the cord, the testicle becomes swollen and tender, and the cord more so. Doppler effect may be used to differentiate between epididymitis and testicular torsion if clinical diagnosis is uncertain. A narrow cylindrical-shaped mass, long axis vertical, very soft to the feel, lying adjacent to the testicle and extending along the spermatic cord, is a varicocele: more common on the left, present in about 20 percent of adolescent males. Urethral discharge should always be cultured (gonorrhea, chlamydia, nonspecific). Lesions on the shaft of the penis include inclusion cysts (about 1 to 2 mm and yellowish), abrasions, herpes progenitalis (vesicles which become ulcerated), syphilitic chancre (asymptomatic: round, about 1 cm, usually ulcerated). Two to 3 mm sized, crablike, crawling creatures within the pubic hair are pediculi.

Female: Changes in the female external genitalia are characterized by lengthening of the clitoral glans to an average of about 1 cm and by its widening to about 3 to 4 mm. The labiae, particularly the minora, become significantly more prominent. With estrogenization, the vaginal mucosa becomes thicker, more moist, and a dull pink in color. External examination should also include a search of the pubic hair (lice), and of the tissues for condylomata, pinworms, ulcerations (herpes), and visible discharge.

Internal *pelvic examination* is indicated if the patient is sexually active or contraceptives are to be prescribed, has vaginal discharge, abnormal bleeding or amenorrhea, has otherwise undiagnosable abdominal or pelvic pain, has been exposed *in utero* to diethylstilbesterol, or needs reassurance regarding the health of the pelvic organs. The patient should be properly informed about the nature and mechanics of the examination, if necessary over a series of visits. She should be in lithotomy position, with the feet in stirrups, and the bladder empty. Hymenotomy may be necessary prior to internal examination. Bimanual palpation, with the fingers of one hand in the vagina and the other on the lower anterior abdominal wall, can be used to find an enlarged or retroverted uterus, adnexal masses (ovarian tumors or cysts, ectopic pregnancy), tenderness of the adnexal organs (pelvic inflammatory disease, endometriosis), and retroperitoneal masses (sarcoma). Visual examination should be performed with a Huffman, Pederson, or Graves speculum (in order of increasing breadth). The pink vaginal mucosa is slightly less moist on the external surface of the cervix. Look for a redder erythematous area at the cervical os, which is endocervical columnar epithelium extending to the external surface of the cervix (ectropion). It is normal if localized; if extensive, think of *in utero* DES exposure or cervicitis. Evaluate the nature of any discharge seen—whitish to yellow, mucoid, with little itching (leucorrhea); frothy, malodorous, yellow, and itchy (trichomonas); thick, cheesy, itchy (monilia); purulent and painful (gonorrhea); sanguinous and malodorant (think of a foreign body). Look for painful vesicles and small ulcers (herpes). Complete the examination with a Papanicolaou smear, appropriate cultures, and wet preparations.

MUSCULOSKELETAL (see also Chapter 7E)

The composition of body mass—lean (muscle) versus fat—undergoes change in adolescence. Traditionally, "baby fat" is known to lessen early in puberty in both boys and girls. In girls, it does so until menarche, after which fat, as a percentage of body mass, again increases. In boys, fat mass continues to decrease and lean mass increases so that, at maturation, fat is a far greater percentage of body composition in girls than in boys.

Upper/lower body-span ratio is determined with the patient standing. The distance from the top of the head to the symphysis pubis is the upper (U), and the distance from the symphysis to the floor is the lower (L). U/L is about 1.0 immediately prepubertal, diminishes to 0.9 in early puberty as the extremities grow more rapidly, and returns to 1.0 in later puberty. Arm span is measured as the distance between the fingertips of outstretched arms and is usually equal to or only minimally greater than total height. Marked variations in the U/L or arm-span ratio may suggest endocrine-mediated growth disturbance.

Of the musculoskeletal problems not immediately precipitated by acute trauma, probably the most common in adolescence are scoliosis, Osgood-Schlatter disease, and slipped capital femoral epiphysis.

Scoliosis (see p. 197) is a lateral curvature of the spine, with convexity to the left or to the right, and may not be detectable until the rapid growth period of adolescence. Severe, undetected scoliosis is accompanied by marked deformities in the shape of the chest wall, with a posterior muscular hump on the convex side of the curve and an anterior depression on that side.

Osgood-Schlatter disease. Pain over the lower edge of the anterior aspect of the knee, aggravated by activity, particularly flexion of the joint, suggests Osgood-Schlatter disease. The pain is not over the joint, but below the knee. Look for a prominent tibial tubercle. Pressure on the tubercle elicits tenderness. The knee area is otherwise normal. There may be unilateral or bilateral involvement. Osgood-Schlatter was an almost exclusively male disease, but with the increasing participation of females in strenous physical activity, it is seen almost equally commonly in both sexes. It occurs in early adolescence and usually subsides with the closure of the proximal tibial epiphysis at ages 14 to 16.

Slipped Capital Femoral Epiphysis. The disease is much more common in boys than girls, and is elicited as explained in the following paragraph. Vague, continuing complaints of pain in the hip, anterior thigh, or knee in an adolescent with a limp, should arouse suspicion of slipped capital femoral epiphysis. Usually, these patients are obese. On examination, there may be some tenderness over the involved hip and adjacent groin, but this will be minimal. With the patient supine, medial rotation of the hip is found to be restricted, and passive flexion results in even more lateral rotation. The involved extremity tends to be slightly shorter in length than the normal one; this has to be evaluated carefully because bilateral involvement is not uncommon. Trendelenburg sign is positive.

Trendelenburg test. This test is designed to evaluate the strength of the gluteus medius muscle. Normally, when a person stands on one leg, the gluteus medius on the supported side should contract and maintain the level of the pelvis on the unsupported side. But if the gluteus medius is weak (either due to neuromuscular disease or mechanical reasons, such as in dislocated hip) when a person stands on the side with the weak gluteus medius, the pelvis on the opposite side drops or descends. This is called positive Trendelenburg sign.

BIBLIOGRAPHY

Barnes HV: Physical growth and development during puberty. Med Clin North Am 59:1305, 1975.

Dahlquist LM, Gil KM, Kalfus GR, Boyd MS: Enhancing an autistic girl's cooperation with gynecological examinations. Clin Pediatr 23:193, 1984.

Emans SJH, Goldstein DP: Pediatric and Adolescent Gynecology, 2nd ed. Boston, Little, Brown, 1982.

Fleisher G, Ludwig S: Pediatric Emergency Medicine. Baltimore, Williams & Wilkins, 1982.

Gallagher JR, Heald FP, Garell DC: Medical Care of the Adolescent, 3rd ed. New York, Appleton-Century-Crofts, 1976.

Goldstein, DP, Miler V: Breast masses in adolescent females. Clin Pediatr 21:17, 1982.

Hofmann A: Adolescent Medicine. Menlo Park, Calif., Addison-Wesley, 1983.

Liss IF, Cohen MI: Adolescent sexuality. Adv Pediatr 26:119, 1979.

Marshall WA, Tanner JM: Variations in patterns of pubertal changes in boys. Arch Dis Child 45:13, 1970.

Marshall WA, Tanner JM: Variations in patterns of pubertal changes in girls. Arch Dis Child 44:291, 1969.

Nadas AS, Fyler DC: Pediatric Cardiology, 3rd ed. Philadelphia, Saunders, 1972.

Rapp, CE Jr: The adolescent patient. Ann Intern Med 99:52, 1983.

Recommendations of the diethylstilbestrol-adenosis (DESAD) project for the identification and management of exposed individuals. NIH pub. no. 81-2049. Bethesda, Md., National Cancer Institute, 1981.

Rosenfeld RG: Evaluation of growth and maturation in adolescence. Pediatrics in Review, 4:175, 1982.

Rudolph AM, Hoffman JIE: Pediatrics, 17th ed. Norwalk, Conn., Appleton-Century-Crofts, 1982.

Scoles PV: Pediatric Orthopedics in Clinical Practice. Chicago, Year Book Med., Pub., 1982.

Index